Case Studies from the Medical Records of Leading Chinese Acupuncture Experts

Companion volumes

Basic Theories of Traditional Chinese Medicine
Edited by Zhu Bing and Wang Hongcai
ISBN 978 1 84819 038 2
International Acupuncture Textbooks

Diagnostics of Traditional Chinese Medicine
Edited by Zhu Bing and Wang Hongcai
ISBN 978 1 84819 036 8
International Acupuncture Textbooks

Meridians and Acupoints
Edited by Zhu Bing and Wang Hongcai
ISBN 978 1 84819 037 5
International Acupuncture Textbooks

Acupuncture Therapeutics
Edited by Zhu Bing and Wang Hongcai
ISBN 978 1 84819 039 9
International Acupuncture Textbooks

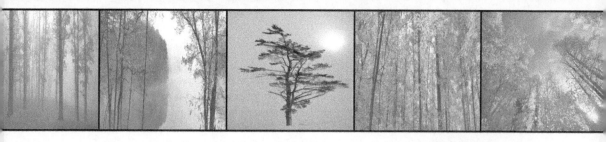

International
Acupuncture
Textbooks

Case Studies from the Medical Records of Leading Chinese Acupuncture Experts

Chief Editors: Zhu Bing and Wang Hongcai

Advisor: Cheng Xinnong

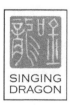

SINGING
DRAGON

LONDON AND PHILADELPHIA

China Beijing International Acupuncture Training Center
Institute of Acupuncture and Moxibustion
China Academy of Chinese Medical Sciences
Advisor: Cheng Xinnong
Chief Editors: Zhu Bing, Wang Hongcai
Deputy Editors: Liu Zhaohui, Zheng Zhenzhen, Wang Huizhu
Members of the Editorial Board: Han Bin, Hu Jinsheng, Ji Xiaoping, Liu Jiaying, Liu Taoxin, Liu Zhaohui, Meng Hong, Wei Lixin, Wu Zhongchao, Yang Jinhong, Zhou Yunxian, Wang Hongcai, Wang Huizhu, Yu Min, Zhu Bing

First published in 2011
by Singing Dragon (an imprint of Jessica Kingsley Publishers)
in co-operation with People's Military Medical Press
116 Pentonville Road
London N1 9JB, UK
and
400 Market Street, Suite 400
Philadelphia, PA 19106, USA

Library of Congress Cataloging in Publication Data
A CIP catalog record for this book is available from the Library of Congress

British Library Cataloguing in Publication Data
A CIP catalogue record for this book is available from the British Library

ISBN 978 1 84819 046 7

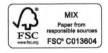

CHINA BEIJING INTERNATIONAL ACUPUNCTURE TRAINING CENTER

China Beijing International Acupuncture Training Center (CBIATC) was set up in 1975 at the request of the World Health Organization (WHO) and with the approval of the State Council of the People's Republic of China. Since its foundation, it has been supported and administered by WHO, the Chinese government, the State Administration of Traditional Chinese Medicine (SATCM) and the China Academy of Chinese Medical Sciences (CACMS). Now it has developed into a world-famous, authoritative training organization.

Since 1975, aiming to popularize acupuncture to the world, CBIATC has been working actively to accomplish the task, 'to perfect ways of acupuncture training and provide more opportunities for foreign doctors', assigned by WHO. More than 30 years' experience has created an excellent teaching team led by the academician, Professor Cheng Xinnong, and a group of professors. The multiple courses here are offered in different languages, including English, German, Spanish and Japanese. According to statistics, so far CBIATC has provided training in acupuncture, Tuina Massage, Traditional Chinese Medicine, Qigong, and so on for over 10,000 medical doctors and students from 106 countries and regions.

The teaching programmes of CBIATC include three-month and various short courses, are carefully and rationally worked out based on the individual needs of participants. Characterized by the organic combination of theory with practice, there are more than ten cooperating hospitals for the students to practice in. With professional teaching and advanced services, CBIATC will lead you to the profound and wonderful world of acupuncture.

Official website: www.cbiatc.com
Training support: www.tcmoo.com

ABOUT THE AUTHORS

ZHU BING

Zhu Bing, Ph.D. studied Life Science at Paris University in France and graduated in 1989. Now he is the member of China Society of Integrated Traditional Chinese and Western Medicine, China Association of Acupuncture–Moxibustion, and Chinese Association for Physiological Sciences, and the vice director of Beijing Physiology Specialized Committee.

In recent years, he has been engaged in scientific research on the mechanism of acupuncture analgesia and pain physiology and the specific relationship between the meridians and Zang Fu organs. He has published more than 90 academic papers and 26 of them have been quoted by SCI. He is a doctorial supervisor at the China Academy of Chinese Medical Sciences.

WANG HONGCAI

Wang Hongcai, Ph.D. is a professor and doctorial supervisor at the China Academy of Chinese Medical Sciences, and the assistant director of China Beijing International Acupuncture Training Centre.

Invited to more than 30 countries for academic exchanges and treatment, he has fulfilled many significant medical tasks that have been assigned by the Ministry of Foreign Affairs and State Administration of Traditional Chinese Medicine in the People's Republic of China, including treating the president of India and the leaders of Iraq and Indonesia.

PREFACE

More than 2000 years ago, a Chinese doctor named Bianque saved the life of a crown prince simply with an acupuncture needle. The story became one of the earliest acupuncture medical cases and went down in history. It is perhaps since then that people have been fascinated by the mystery of acupuncture and kept on studying it. In 1975, at the request of the World Health Organization, an acupuncture school was founded in Beijing, China, namely the China Beijing International Acupuncture Training Center. As one of the sponsor institutions, the Center compiled a textbook of Chinese Acupuncture and Moxibustion for foreign learners, published in 1980 and reprinted repeatedly afterwards, which has been of profound, far-reaching influence. It has been adopted as a 'model book' for acupuncture education and examination in many countries, and has played a significant role in the global dissemination of acupuncture.

Today, with the purpose of extending this 'authentic and professional' knowledge, we have compiled a series of books entitled *International Acupuncture Textbooks* to introduce incisively the basic theories of Traditional Chinese Medicine (TCM) and acupuncture–moxibustion techniques, by building on and developing the characteristics of the original textbook of Chinese Acupuncture and Moxibustion; and presenting authoritatively the systematic teaching materials with concise explanation based on a core syllabus for TCM professional education in China.

In addition, just as the same plant might have its unique properties when growing in different geographical environments, this set of books may reflect, in its particular style, our experience accumulated over 30 years of international acupuncture training.

Zhu Bing and Wang Hongcai

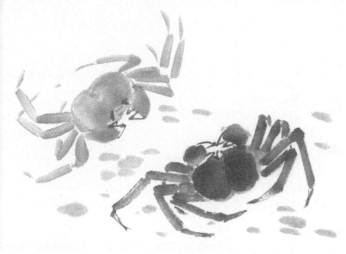

CONTENTS

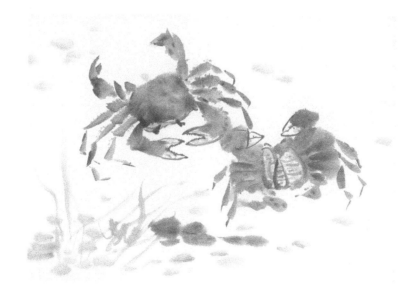

FOREWORD

The important aspect of acupuncture study is to absorb the abstract theory into clinical practice. In our 35 years' teaching, our experience is that the case study is the most difficult aspect for students in their study. *Case Studies from the Medical Records of Leading Chinese Acupuncture Experts* has been written to help them to learn how to understand and practise the differentiation of syndromes. Students often ask: 'Which point can I use for this disease?' Different from the ideas of Western medicine, the approach in Traditional Chinese Medicine (TCM) is that a disease does not point directly to a particular kind of drug or a certain kind of treatment. The same disease manifests differently in different patients. The treating principle is therefore different for each individual patient, and so are the acupuncture points used. After reading this book, students will get to know that we are treating patients through the art of differentiation, not just the disease using only this or that point. Acupuncture strengthens the patient to fight the disease to restore the balance of Yin and Yang, not to give him something to use to mend his diseased left foot with the Blood of his right foot.

Case Studies from the Medical Records of Leading Chinese Acupuncture Experts includes 176 cases, covering 76 kinds of diseases, and teaches the student how to apply the theory in practice. In particular, the 'Differentiation and analysis' and 'Essentials' in each case are the key links in telling the reader how TCM thinks for the treatment of individuals.

We will be greatly delighted if this book is of benefit to our readers. Your suggestions and comments are highly appreciated. We sincerely hope that more and more foreign friends will come to understand acupuncture and Chinese culture through the study of this book.

Finally, special thanks should be given to the Teaching and Translation Departments of China Beijing International Acupuncture Training Center and the Acupuncture Hospital of the Institute of Acupuncture and Moxibustion.

Liu Zhaohui

INTRODUCTION

Case Studies from the Medical Records of Leading Chinese Acupuncture Experts is a collection of cases for case study. Containing 176 cases, covering 76 types of disease, it is laid out in the following way for easy reading and clear understanding:

1. General data

2. Chief complaint

3. History of present illness

4. Present symptoms

5. Tongue and pulse

6. Differentiation and analysis

7. Diagnosis

8. Treating principle

9. Prescription

10. Effect

11. Essentials

The diseases are arranged as follows:

Chapter 1: Internal Diseases

Chapter 2: Gynaecological and Paediatric Diseases

Chapter 3: Diseases of the Eyes, Ears, Nose and Throat

Chapter 4: Skin Diseases, External Diseases

Chapter 5: Other conditions

An appendix with the name of the disease in Western medicine in alphabetical order is included for ease of reference.

Wang Huizhu

INTERNAL DISEASES

SECTION ONE • COMMON COLD

CASE I: YANG JIEBIN'S MEDICAL RECORD

1. General data

Yang, male, 35, paid his first visit on April 28, 1976.

2. Chief complaint

Headache and fever for 1 day.

3. History of present illness

He slept without covering himself warmly enough and on the following day began to have dizziness and headache.

4. Present symptoms

Dizziness, headache, aversion to Wind Cold, no sweating, then fever, running nose, itching throat, cough, lack of taste, normal urine and stools. Body temperature 40°C.

5. Tongue and pulse

White moistened tongue-coating, superficial tight pulse.

6. Differentiation and analysis

Invasion of Wind Cold to the body surface resulting in dizziness, headache, aversion to Wind Cold, and no sweating. Superficial pulse indicating an exterior syndrome and tight pulse indicating a Cold syndrome.

7. Diagnosis

TCM: Common cold (Wind Cold astringing the body surface).

Western medicine: Common cold.

8. Treating principle

Dispel Wind Cold, relieve the exterior syndrome by means of diaphoresis.

9. Prescription

Dazhui (GV 14), Fengmen (BL 12), Taiyang (EX-HN5), Hegu (LI 4).

Moxibustion was applied after needling Dazhui (GV 14). Cupping was applied after needling Fengmen (BL 12). Taiyang (EX-HN5) and Hegu (LI 4) were punctured with the reducing method.

10. Effect

After 1 treatment, he sweated and his fever was relieved. After 2 treatments, his symptoms were greatly reduced. After 3 treatments, he was cured.

11. Essentials

Taiyang (EX-HN5) and Hegu (LI 4) were reduced to relieve exterior syndrome by sweating and dispelling Wind. Fengmen (BL 12) was punctured and cupped to dispel Wind and promote the Lung in dispersing for relieving exterior syndrome. Dazhui (GV 14), a meeting point of all Yang channels, was punctured to strenghen superficies and treated with moxibustion to dispel Cold. Three treatments of acupuncture and moxibustion cured the patient.

CASE II: CHENG XINNONG'S MEDICAL RECORD

1. General data

Liu, male, 33, paid his first visit on September 6, 1986.

2. Chief complaint

Fever, cough, headache, neckache and backache for 10 days.

3. History of present illness

He was attacked by Cold during sleep at night 10 days ago. On the following day in the morning he had a fever and cough. He took Suxiao Ganmao Jiaonang (Quick Effect Capsule for common cold) and Banlangen Chongji (Radix Isatidis Granules) but without effect.

4. Present symptoms

He now felt cold in the back, with headache especially in the occipital region, soreness in the neck and back, and ache all over the body. He had a cough, sore throat, profuse thin yellow Phlegm, lack of taste, and poor sleep. His urine was dark yellow and stools normal.

5. Tongue and pulse

Tongue borders and tip red, coating thin white moistureless, pulse superficial rapid.

6. Differentiation and analysis

Invasion of Wind Cold to the body surface causes the failure of Lung Qi in dispersing, resulting in cough. The Cold is changing into Heat. Cold in the back, headache especially at the occipital region, soreness in neck and back, and ache all over the body, cough, and sore throat are the manifestations of exterior Cold, while the dark yellow urine, red tip and borders of tongue, thin white moistureless coating, superficial rapid pulse are signs of interior Heat.

7. Diagnosis

TCM: Common cold (exterior Cold and interior Heat).

Western medicine: Common cold.

8. Treating principle

Dispel Wind Cold, promote the Lungs in dispersing, reduce Heat.

9. Prescription

Dazhui (GV 14), Fengchi (GB 20), Feishu (BL 13), Yuzhen (BL 9), Tianding (LI 17), Taiyang (EX-HN5), Zanzhu (BL 2), Lieque (LU 7), Hegu (LI 4), Shaoshang (LU 11).

Shaoshang (LU 11) was pricked with a three-edged needle for bleeding. Other points were punctured with a filiform needle and the needles were retained for 30 minutes.

10. Effect

After 3 treatments the symptoms disappeared.

11. Essentials

Dazhui (GV 14) functions to disperse Yang Qi for relieving exterior syndrome. Fengchi (GB 20) functions to dispel Wind for relieving headache. Taiyang (EX-HN5), Zanzhu (BL 2), Yuzhen (BL 9), and Fengchi (GB 20) are used to treat headache. Hegu (LI 4), the Yuan-Source point, and Lieque (LU 7), the Luo-Connecting point, promote the Lungs in dispersing to relieve the exterior syndrome. Feishu (BL 13) promotes the Lungs in dispersing to stop the cough. Tianding (LI 17) and Shaoshang (LU 11) clear Heat to treat sore throat.

SORE THROAT

Pricking Shangyang (LI 1) and Shaoshang (LU 11) with three-edged needle plus puncturing Hegu (LI 4) with filiform needle and retaining the needle for 30 minutes is very effective for sore throat.

For carbon monoxide poisoning, in addition to routine treatment, puncturing Shaoshang (LU 11) and Renzhong (GV 26) with a filiform needle can speed resuscitation.

CASE III: XIAO SHAOQING'S MEDICAL RECORD

1. General data

Zhang, male, 39, paid his first visit on October 5, 1979.

2. Chief complaint

Headache and fever for 4 days.

3. History of present illness

Four days ago, he began to have a headache and fever due to not enough clothing.

4. Present symptoms

Headache, fever, cough, nasal obstruction and pain in the lower back. Throat congestion, body temperature 38.5°C.

5. Tongue and pulse

Flabby tongue, thin yellow and slightly sticky coating, rolling and rapid pulse.

6. Differentiation and analysis

The prevalent epidemic pathogen attacks the Lungs and blocks the exterior, causing fever and aching all over the body. The thin yellow and slightly sticky coating and rolling and rapid pulse are the signs of invasion of Wind Heat.

7. Diagnosis

TCM: Common cold (Wind Heat attacking the Lungs).

Western medicine: Common cold.

8. Treating principle

Dispel Wind, clear Heat, relieve exterior syndrome.

9. Prescription

Dazhui (GV 14), Fengmen (BL 12), Feishu (BL 13), Shenshu (BL 23), Hegu (LI 4).
   Acupuncture was given once a day with the needles retained for 20 minutes.

10. Effect

After one treatment, his headache and nasal obstruction disappeared, and his fever gradually lowered. After two treatments, he was cured.

11. Essentials

Dazhui (GV 14), the meeting point of all the Yang channels, relieves exterior syndrome by circulating Yang, calming the Mind and clearing Heat. Shenshu (BL 23) is to communicate between the child (Kidneys) and the mother (Metal), producing Water to reinforce the body resistance. Fengmen (BL 12), (the right Fengmen is known as Refu), a meeting point of Governor Vessel and Foot-Taiyang Channel, is to dispel Wind, promote the Lungs in dispersing, regulate Qi, and clear Heat. Used together with Fengchi (GB 20), Fengmen (BL 12) is stronger in dispelling Wind and relieving exterior syndrome. Feishu (BL 13), clearing the Lungs, in combination with Hegu (LI 4), is to promote sweating to relieve exterior syndrome.

CASE IV: MENG HONG'S MEDICAL RECORD

1. General data

Niu, female, 38 years old.

2. Chief complaint

Cough and headache for 3 days.

3. History of present illness

In the last 3 days she had a cough with Phlegm, headache, dizziness and discomfort all over the body.

4. Present symptoms

Red face, cough with yellow thick Phlegm, fever, sore throat, thirst with desire to drink water, yellow urine, dry stools.

5. Tongue and pulse

Red tongue, thin yellow coating; superficial rapid pulse.

6. Differentiation and analysis

Invasion of Wind Heat. The pathogenic Wind Heat invaded from mouth and nose, affecting the Lungs, the Qi of which failed to descend, so there is a cough with Phlegm. Wind, the Yang pathogenic factor, together with Heat, caused fever. The Lung Heat steamed and heated the throat, so thirst and preferring to drink water. Red tongue, thin yellow coating, and superficial rapid pulse are the manifestations of Wind Heat affecting the Lung defence.

7. Diagnosis

TCM: Common cold (Wind Heat type).

Western medicine: Common cold.

8. Treating principle

Eliminate Wind and clear Heat.

9. Prescription

Dazhui (GV 14), Feishu (BL 13), Fengchi (GB 20), Quchi (LI 11), Waiguan (TE 5), Hegu (LI 4), Lieque (LU 7).

Acupuncture. Dazhui (GV 14) and Feishu (BL 13) were pricked and cupped for bloodletting. In case the sore throat was serious, Yuji (LU 10) and Shaoshang (LU 11) were pricked for bloodletting, 5–15 drops of blood. Once a day, 3 times as 1 course.

10. Effect

One to 2 courses, successful result.

11. Essentials

The exogenous diseases are usually quick in onset and rapid in changes. The treatment should be flexible according to the changes of the symptoms. In the case of Lung Heat, pricking, bleeding, cupping and bloodletting through point pricking are applied to clear the Lung Heat. Moxibustion is not applicable.

SUMMARY

Common cold, known as Shangfeng (attacked by Wind), symptomized as nasal obstruction, running nose, cough, aversion to cold, fever, and aching all over the body, is a common disease seen all the year round, especially in winter and spring. It is caused by insufficiency of anti-pathogenic Qi, invasion of Wind Cold or Wind Heat, and disturbance of the Lungs in dispersing.

Main points: Dazhui (GV 14), Fengchi (GB 20), Hegu (LI 4) Taiyang (EX-HN5), Yintang (EX-HN3), and Zanzhu (BL 2) are added for headache. Yuji (LU 10) or Shaoshang (LU 11) is pricked to bleed for sore throat. Chize (LU 5) and Taiyuan (LU 9) or Feishu (BL 13) are added for cough. Yingxiang (LI 20) is added for nasal obstruction.

SECTION TWO • COUGH

CASE I: YANG JIEBIN'S MEDICAL RECORD

1. General data

Fu, female, 27, paid her first visit on July 29, 1998.

2. Chief complaint

Cough for 1 month.

3. History of present illness

One month ago, she was attacked by Cold and began to have a cough. Taking medicines and penicillin injection were not helpful.

4. Present symptoms

She coughed repeatedly with a heavy sound and white foamy Phlegm, which was difficult to spit. She felt fullness in the chest. She had dizziness, itching and sore throat, nasal obstruction, running nose, aversion to cold and Wind, aching and tiredness all over the body. The cough was aggravated especially at night. Her appetite was normal, and urine and stools normal.

5. Tongue and pulse

Light red tongue, thin white coating, deep and tight pulse.

6. Differentiation and analysis

The invasion of Wind Cold causes the failure of the Lungs in descending, thus cough. This is also the cause of itching and sore throat, nasal obstruction, running nose, aversion to cold and Wind, aching and tiredness all over the body, and the light red tongue, thin white coating, deep and tight pulse.

7. Diagnosis

TCM: Cough (Wind Cold invasion).

Western medicine: Acute bronchitis.

8. Treating principle

Promote the Lungs in dispersing, relieve exterior syndrome, dissolve Phlegm, stop the cough.

9. Prescription

- Dazhui (GV 14), Fengchi (GB 20), Hegu (LI 4), Fengmen (BL 12).
- Dazhu (BL 11), Zhongfu (LU 1), Feishu (BL 13), Zusanli (ST 36).

The above two groups of points were used by turns, once a day, one group each time. Strong stimulation was applied for reducing the pathogenic Wind Cold. The needles were retained after arrival of Qi and manipulated lifting-thrusting and rotating once every 5 minutes. Cupping was done at Dazhui (GV 14), Fengmen (BL 12), Dazhu (BL 11), Zhongfu (LU 1), and Feishu (BL 13) for 15 minutes after needling.

10. Effect

After 2 treatments, her cough was relieved and Phlegm reduced. After 4 treatments, her cough almost stopped. After 6 treatments, her cough with Phlegm and fullness in the chest disappeared. The follow-up after 1 month showed no recurrence.

11. Essentials

Dazhui (GV 14) is reduced to dispel Wind Cold. Dazhu (BL 11), Fengchi (GB 20), Hegu (LI 4) and Fengmen (BL 12) dispel Wind Cold, and promote the Lungs in dispersing to relieve exterior syndrome. Zhongfu (LU 1), Front-Mu, and Feishu (BL 13), Back-Shu, regulate Qi of the Lungs to dissolve Phlegm and stop the cough. Zusanli (ST 36), the Earth point, reinforces the Earth to produce the Metal, and eliminates Damp to dissolve Phlegm.

CASE II: RECORD IN *ACUPUNCTURE-MOXIBUSTION FOR DIFFICULT DISEASES*

1. General data

Liao, female, 62, paid her first visit on November 16, 1996.

2. Chief complaint

Cough with white Phlegm for more than 7 years.

3. History of present illness

She was constitutionally weak and likely to catch a cold. She had a cough often and she took antitussive often.

4. Present symptoms

Cough, aversion to cold, tiredness, fullness in the chest and epigastrium, loose stools.

5. Tongue and pulse

Pale tongue, white sticky coating, soft and rolling pulse.

6. Differentiation and analysis

The Spleen fails to do its task of transportation and transformation, thus the Phlegm is produced due to Damp retention, causing a cough with profuse Phlegm. The Spleen deficiency leads to Qi deficiency, thus the existence of tiredness and loose stools. Pale tongue, white sticky coating, soft and rolling pulse are the signs of Phlegm Damp.

7. Diagnosis

TCM: Cough (Phlegm Damp retention in the Lung).

Western medicine: Chronic bronchitis.

8. Treating principle

Strengthen the Spleen to dissolve Phlegm Damp and stop the cough.

9. Prescription

Pishu (BL 20), Taiyuan (LU 9), Taibai (SP 3), Zhangmen (LR 13), Fenglong (ST 40).

Moxibustion was applied to Pishu (BL 20). Other points were punctured with the reinforcing method.

10. Effect

Treated once every other day, she was cured after 30 treatments. Then medicinal vesiculation was applied once every 10 days for 6 months to consolidate the effect.

11. Essentials

The Yuan-Source point is the place at where the Zang Qi is confluent. For this reason, Taiyuan (LU 9) and Taibai (SP 3) are selected to reinforce the Lungs and Spleen. Pishu (BL 20) and Zhangmen (LR 13) are to strengthen the Spleen Qi and regulate the Lung Qi. Fenglong (ST 40), Luo-Connecting point, is to promote the Spleen Qi for dissolving Phlegm.

CASE III: ZHOU YUNXIAN'S MEDICAL RECORD

1. General data

Li, male, 62 years old, a worker.

2. Chief complaint

Cough and dyspnoea for 15 years, in the last month the attack was repeated.

3. History of present illness

Fifteen years ago, because of the rapid climate changes he got a cold, manifested as fever, cough, and asthmatic breathing. After taking Chinese and Western medicines, the symptoms got better, but were not cured. Every autumn and winter, a cough with asthmatic breathing would appear 3–4 times, each time lasting about 1 month. Only a large amount of antibiotics and anti-asthmatics could relieve it a little, but later it got worse. One month ago, the weather became cold suddenly, his common cold caused the attack of coughing and asthmatic breathing again, profuse sputum with Blood in it, and medication was useless. He came for acupuncture treatment.

4. Present symptoms

Paroxysmal cough with dyspnoea, worse in the morning and evening, profuse sputum with Blood in it, resting in half lying half sitting position because of difficult breathing. Usually he had shortness of breath, tiredness, and fullness in the chest, worse on exertion, sweating, no thirst, normal appetite, frequent urination (at night 3–4 times), loose stools, 1–2 times a day.

Now he has pale dark complexion, purplish lips, low speaking voice, sputum gurgling in the throat, and wheezing sound in auscultation.

5. Tongue and pulse

Pale tongue with toothmarks, white coating a little sticky; deep thready forceless pulse.

6. Differentiation and analysis

Initially, his Lung defence was not strong, so he caught cold often. A prolonged cough resulted in the deficiency of Lung Qi. The dysfunction of the Lungs in descending and dispersing made his cough and dyspnoea worse. The Kidneys were involved in the case of a long-term cough, the result of which would be failure of the Kidneys in receiving Qi, so cough and dyspnoea got worse on exertion and there was frequent urination as well. The Lung Qi deficiency caused Spleen Qi deficiency, manifested as profuse sputum in addition to shortness of breath, tiredness, and speaking in a low voice. Pale tongue with toothmarks, and thready and forceless pulse were also the signs of Qi deficiency.

7. Diagnosis

TCM: Cough with dyspnoea.

Western medicine: Chronic asthmatic bronchitis.

8. Treating principle

Reinforce the Lungs, Spleen and Kidneys, dissolve sputum to stop the cough. Select points mainly from the Lung, Kidney, Stomach and Ren meridians, and Back-Shu points.

9. Prescription

Dingchuan (EX-B1), Feishu (BL 13), Pishu (BL 20), Shenshu (BL 23), Zhongfu (LU 1), Lieque (LU 7), Hegu (LI 4), Shanzhong (CV 17), Qihai (CV 6), Zusanli (ST 36), Fenglong (ST 40), Taixi (KI 3).

The reducing method for Fenglong (ST 40), even method for Hegu (LI 4) and Lieque (LU 7), the reinforcing method for the others. Cupping on the upper back after needling.

10. Effect

After the first treatment, the patient breathed much better. Five treatments relieved his cough and dyspnoea greatly. He could lie flat in bed and walk from the bus stop to hospital without rest. In total he had 25 treatments.

11. Essentials

Lung and Spleen Qi deficiency, Lung and Kidney Qi deficiency.

Dingchuan (EX-B1) is a special point for relieving cough and asthma. Feishu (BL 13) and Zhongfu (LU 1), the combination of Back-Shu and Front-Mu points, are treating the Lung, together with Lieque (LU 7) and Hegu (LI 4), for stopping cough and asthma too. Shanzhong (CV 17), Qihai (CV 6), and Zusanli (ST 36) are for reinforcing the Lung, Spleen, and Kidney Qi. Shenshu (BL 23) and Taixi (KI 3) are for reinforcing the Kidneys in receiving Qi. Fenglong (ST 40) is for dissolving sputum.

TIANJIU

Tianjiu (medicinal vesiculation) is a therapy carried out by applying irritating medicines to certain acupoints so as to cause blisters. It is often used in the treatment of asthma, chronic bronchitis, allergic rhinitis, chronic cough, weak constitution, susceptibility to common cold, chronic gastroenteritis, insomnia, and pain of the lower back and legs, etc.

CASE IV: RECORD IN *ACUPUNCTURE-MOXIBUSTION FOR DIFFICULT DISEASES*

1. General data

Zhao, male, 42, paid his first visit on April 15, 1958.

2. Chief complaint

Cough for 1 year and haemoptysis for the most recent 3 days.

3. History of present illness

He had a history of pulmonary tuberculosis for 1 year with the treatment of streptomycin and isonicotinylhydrazide.

4. Present symptoms

He was emaciated, with a low voice, cough with bloody Phlegm, tidal fever, night sweating, and sometimes haemoptysis. The haemostatic injection was not effective for him.

5. Tongue and pulse

Pale tongue, white coating, thready pulse.

6. Differentiation and analysis

This is a case of Lung Yin deficiency, so the patient is emaciated with cough with bloody Phlegm, tidal fever, night sweating, and his pulse is thready.

7. Diagnosis

TCM: Pulmonary tuberculosis (Qi and Yin deficiency of the Lungs and Kidneys).

Western medicine: Pulmonary tuberculosis.

8. Treating principle

Warm the Kidneys, reinforce Yin of the Lungs and Kidneys, calm the Mind, stop the bleeding, stop the cough.

9. Prescription

In a prone position, he was treated with moxibustion at Yongquan (KI 1) for 20 minutes each time, twice a day.

10. Effect

After two treatments, the bloody Phlegm disappeared. With 3 days' treatment in succession, the symptoms were basically gone. He was asked to continue the treatment for his tuberculosis.

11. Essentials

This is Yin deficiency producing internal Heat, in the case of which, moxibustion can also be applied. Yongquan (KI 1), Jing-Well point, is good to open the orifices, tranquilize and calm the Mind, and is important for haemoptysis. It also follows the principle of using a lower point for an upper disease.

SUMMARY

Cough is *Kesou*. *Ke* is the cough with sound but no Phlegm and *Sou* is the cough with Phlegm but no sound. *Kesou* is cough with sound and Phlegm. It includes exogenous cough and endogenous cough.

The exogenous cough is caused by Wind, Cold, Heat and Dryness invading the Lungs. Invasion of Wind Cold causes a cough with thin Phlegm, nasal obstruction, running nose, aversion to cold, no sweating, thin white coating to the tongue, and superficial tight pulse. Invasion of Wind Heat causes a cough with yellow thick Phlegm, fever, headache, sweating, aversion to wind, and superficial rapid pulse. Invasion of Dryness and Heat causes dry cough or a cough with yellow Phlegm that is difficult to spit, dry and sore throat, and rapid pulse.

The endogenous cough is caused by dysfunctions of the Zang Fu organs, and mostly develops from acute cases. Spleen deficiency produces Phlegm Damp, fullness in the chest, poor appetite, white sticky coating to the tongue, and superficial soft pulse. Liver Fire attacking the Lungs produces a cough with hypochondriac pain, vomiting, scanty thick Phlegm, red face, dry throat, yellow tongue-coating, and wiry rapid pulse. Yin deficiency of the Lungs produces a dry cough, or a cough with bloody Phlegm, tidal fever, night sweating, irritability, hot sensation in palms and soles, red tongue, little coating, and thready rapid pulse.

Main points: Feishu (BL 13), Tiantu (CV 22). Fengmen (BL 12) and Hegu (LI 4) for exogenous cough; Dazhui (GV 14) for fever; pricking Shaoshang (LU 11) to bleed for sore throat; Chize (LU 5) and Kongzui (LU 6) for haemoptysis; Zusanli (ST 36) and Fenglong (ST 40) for profuse Phlegm and poor appetite; Yanglingquan (GB 34) for hypochondriac pain; and cupping after needling for aversion to cold and pain in the back.

SECTION THREE • ASTHMA

CASE 1: SHAO JINGMING'S MEDICAL RECORD

1. General data

Zhao, female, 13, came for the first time on July 20, 1963.

2. Chief complaint

Asthma for more than 7 years.

3. History of present illness

When she was 6 years old, she had a cough due to common cold. In winter her cough became worse and it developed into asthma gradually.

4. Present symptoms

She had asthma attacks whenever she was exposed to cold. During the attack, she had dyspnoea, purple lips, Phlegm wheezing in the throat. She was emaciated with cold limbs.

5. Tongue and pulse

Light red tongue, thin white moistened coating, deep thready weak pulse.

6. Differentiation and analysis

This patient had invasion of pathogenic Wind when she was young. The pathogenic factor hid in the Lungs for a long time and caused the weakness of defensive Qi. She gets asthma attacks when she is exposed to Wind Cold.

7. Diagnosis

TCM: Asthma (Cold Phlegm in the Lungs).

Western medicine: Asthma.

8. Treating principle

Promote the Lungs in dispersing, dissolve Phlegm, stop asthma.

9. Prescription

Dazhui (GV 14), Fengmen (BL 12), Feishu (BL 13).

The needles were retained for 15 minutes after the arrival of Qi. During the retaining, they were manipulated 2–3 times. After removing the needles, moxibustion was applied for 5–7 minutes. The treatment was given once a day.

10. Effect

Her asthma was quickly relieved with moxibustion. After 10 treatments, she could breathe normally. One week was then allowed for rest, then the treatment changed to once every other day. With 10 more treatments to consolidate the effect, she didn't have an attack in the winter that year. In the following year, she was treated with the same method for 20 treatments. In the third year, 10 treatments were given again. Since then, she has not had any attacks of asthma.

11. Essentials

Dazhui (GV 14) promotes the Lungs in dispersing and regulates Qi. Fengmen (BL 12) dispels Wind to stop asthma. Feishu (BL 13) regulates the Lung Qi and strengthens the resistance so as to stop cough and asthma.

CASE II: SHAO JINGMING'S MEDICAL RECORD

1. General data

Wu, male, 20, came for the first time on May 23, 1996.

2. Chief complaint

Asthma for 12 years and worse for the last 2 years.

3. History of present illness

Twelve years ago, a common cold induced fullness in her chest and asthmatic breathing. With treatment, this was relieved. But since then, she has had attacks from time to time and it became worse in the last 2 years. With aminophylline and prednisone, her bronchial asthma could be relieved but not cured. This time, it lasted for more than 1 month and the medicinal treatment was not effective.

4. Present symptoms

She was emaciated with dyspnoea, Phlegm wheezing, and yellow Phlegm that was difficult to spit. There was wheezing sound in both her Lungs.

5. Tongue and pulse

Her tongue was dark without moisture. Her pulse was rapid and slightly rolling.

6. Differentiation and analysis

Dyspnoea, Phlegm wheezing, yellow Phlegm, wheezing sound in the Lungs, rapid and rolling pulse are all the signs of Phlegm Heat.

7. Diagnosis

TCM: Asthma (Phlegm Heat retention).

Western medicine: Bronchial asthma.

8. Treating principle

Promote the Lungs in dispersing, regulate Qi, dissolve Phlegm, stop asthma.

9. Prescription

Feishu (BL 13), Dazhui (GV 14), Fengmen (BL 12). The needles were retained for 30 minutes.

10. Effect

She felt relieved immediately when the arrival of Qi was achieved in acupuncture. After removing the needles, her fullness in the chest was greatly improved but the wheezing sound in her Lungs didn't disappear. The same treatment was applied 5 times in succession and the asthmatic breathing and wheezing sound stopped. Two courses (20 times) of treatment made all her symptoms disappear. Her 5-year follow-up found no recurrence.

11. Essentials

Dazhui (GV 14) disperses Yang to relieve exterior syndrome to stop asthma. Fengmen (BL 12) dispels pathogenic factors to stop asthma. Feishu (BL 13) regulates the Qi of the Lungs to strengthen the superficies to stop asthma.

CASE III: XIAO SHAOQING'S MEDICAL RECORD

1. General data

Zheng, male, 50, came for the first time on September 21, 1994.

2. Chief complaint

Cough and asthmatic breathing for more than 30 years and worse for the last month.

3. History of present illness

He began to have a cough and asthmatic breathing after he had measles when he was a child. Thereafter, the attacks were induced often when he was exposed to cold or had seafood. One month ago, the attacks started again. With medicinal spraying, the asthmatic breathing could be relieved.

4. Present symptoms

He had a cough, asthmatic breathing, fullness and pain in the chest, especially worse at night, profuse white thick Phlegm that was difficult to spit, and thirst with desire to drink. His appetite was normal, urine and stools normal. Rough breathing, rales in the Lungs.

5. Tongue and pulse

Pale tongue, white sticky coating, thready wiry rolling pulse.

6. Differentiation and analysis

The patient suffered from asthma for 30 years and his Lungs, Spleen and Kidneys must be weak, based on which, invasion of Wind Cold disturbed the Lungs in dispersing. With Qi deficiency of the Lungs, Spleen and Kidneys, the water metabolism was disordered, producing Phlegm Damp which was the cause of the cough and asthma.

7. Diagnosis

TCM: Asthma (invasion of Wind Cold, Phlegm Damp in the Lungs).

Western medicine: Allergic asthma.

8. Treating principle

Dispel Wind Cold, promote the Lungs in dispersing, dissolve Phlegm, stop the cough and asthma.

9. Prescription

Shanzhong (CV 17), Tiantu (CV 22), Dingchuan (EX-B1), Fenglong (ST 40), Antiguan (PC 6), Hegu (LI 4), Lieque (LU 7).

   Tiantu (CV 22) was punctured with a 3 cun filiform needle, which was inserted perpendicularly and obliquely along the posterior border of manubrium of sternum to about 2.5 cun, rotated and withdrawn quickly. Shanzhong (CV 17) was also punctured with a 3 cun filiform needle, which was obliquely inserted to the depth about 2.5 cun and rotated while lifting-thrusting to produce a strong needling sensation. Other points were punctured with even method and the needles retained for 20 minutes. Manipulation of needles was done once every 10 minutes. Once every day.

10. Effect

On the second visit, he showed a great relief of the cough, asthmatic breathing, and chest pain. The same treatment was applied again.

On the sixth visit, his cough and asthmatic breathing stopped, the Phlegm became much less and thin, the rales in the Lungs became less. It was thought that the exogenous pathogenic factors had been expelled, but the anti-pathogenic Qi was weak. Feishu (BL 13) and Shenshu (BL 23) were used instead of Hegu (LI 4) and Lieque (LU 7). Acupuncture with the reinforcing method and cupping were adopted and moxibustion was done at Guanyuan (CV 4) and Qihai (CV 6). One more course of treatment cured him completely.

11. Essentials

In acute cases, the asthmatic breathing should be controlled immediately, for the purpose of which, Shanzhong (CV 17), Tiantu (CV 22) and Dingchuan (EX-B1) were selected to descend Qi to stop the cough and asthma. Neiguan (PC 6) was to regulate Qi to relieve fullness and pain in the chest. Fenglong (ST 40) was to dissolve Phlegm. Lieque (LU 7) and Hegu (LI 4), the combination of Yuan and Luo, dispelled Wind Cold. After the acute symptoms were relieved, the fundamental cause was treated by using Feishu (BL 13) and Shenshu (BL 23) to reinforce the Lungs and Kidneys, and using Guanyuan (CV 4) and Qihai (CV 6) to build up the resistance. Moxibustion and cupping for this patient were important in the treatment.

SUMMARY

Asthma is an allergic disease of the respiratory tract. Characterized by repeated attacks of paroxysmal dyspnoea with wheezing, it is difficult to treat. Professor Shao Jingming is experienced in treating such a disease. According to him, asthma is of Benxu (resistance deficiency) and Biaoshi (pathogen excess). The former refers to hypofunction of the Lungs, Spleen and Kidneys and the latter to Phlegm Damp, Blood stasis and exogenous invasion. Promoting the Lungs in dispersing, regulating Qi, and dissolving Phlegm are the principles to follow for its treatment.

Main points: Dazhui (GV 14), Fengmen (BL 12), Feishu (BL 13).

Proven by clinical practice, Feishu (BL 13) is good for regulating Qi and strengthening resistance to stop coughs and asthma. Dazhui (GV 14) is good for dispersing Yang Qi to dispel Wind Cold and descending Qi to stop asthma. Fengmen (BL 12) is good for dispelling Wind Cold, reducing Heat, and regulating the Qi of the Lungs to stop the cough and asthma; especially when moxibustion is applied, it can activate body resistance to prevent common cold.

During an attack of asthma, these three points used together can lower the resistance in the respiratory tact. If used in the relieved stage, they can improve the functions of the Lungs for the long-term effect. They are especially effective for bronchial asthma.

Symptomatic points: Hegu (LI 4) is added for exogenous asthma; Chize (LU 5) and Taiyuan (LU 9) for cough; Zhongwan (CV 12) and Zusanli (ST 36) for profuse Phlegm; Tiantu (CV 22) and Shanzhong (CV 17) for Phlegm blocked in windpipe; Shenshu (BL 23), Guanyuan (CV 4) and Taixi (KI 3) for asthma of deficiency type; Jueyinshu (BL 14), Xinshu (BL 15) and Neiguan (PC 6) for palpitations; Yuji (LU 10) for dry throat; Yuji (LU 10), Kongzui (LU 6) and Chize (LU 5) for haemoptysis; Zhongwan (CV 12), Zusanli (ST 36), Tianshu (ST 25) and Qihai (CV 6) for epigastric fullness; Yinlingquan (SP 9), Shuidao (ST 28) and Zusanli (ST 36) for oedema of the lower limbs.

Treat once a day during the attack and every other day in the relieved stage. Ten times is 1 course of treatment. For adults, a 1 cun needle is used to insert 0.5–0.8 cun in depth. For children, a 0.5 cun needle is used to insert 0.2–0.3 cun. Retain the needles for half an hour. Manipulate the needles 2–3 times during retaining. Apply reinforcing or reducing according to the individual condition of the patient. For children less than 1 year old, don't retain the needles.

Moxibustion and cupping are adopted accordingly.

Statistically, the rate of effectiveness is up to 92%.

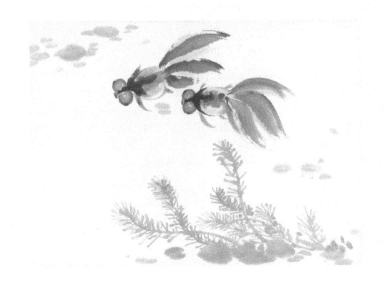

SECTION FOUR • HYPOCHONDRIAC PAIN

CASE I: CHENG XINNONG'S MEDICAL RECORD

1. General data

Xu, male, 47, came on July 25, 1987.

2. Chief complaint

Precordial discomfort for more than 2 years.

3. History of present illness

He had fullness and pain in the precardium when tired. Only nitroglycerin could relieve him when it was serious.

4. Present symptoms

Recently, the precordial pain became aggravated and radiated to the back and arm. Bed rest and glonoin could relieve his symptoms. He said he felt tired, short of breath, cold in the lower back, and distended in the abdomen after eating. His sleep was not good and urine yellow. Dark lips with petechiae, BP 120/80mmHg.

5. Tongue and pulse

Dark tongue, slightly thick coating, wiry thready hesitant pulse with missed beats.

6. Differentiation and analysis

The patient is constitutionally weak in Yang Qi, feeling cold in the lower back and distended in the abdomen after eating. Yang Qi in the chest is not energetic enough to circulate the Blood, causing Blood stasis, and therefore, precordial pain.

7. Diagnosis

TCM: Chest Bi (Qi deficiency and Blood stasis).

Western medicine: Precordial pain.

8. Treating principle

Reinforce Qi and dredge the channels and collaterals.

9. Prescription

Dazhui (GV 14), Shanzhong (CV 17), Zhongwan (CV 12), Qihai (CV 6), Neiguan (PC 6), Taiyuan (LU 9), Zusanli (ST 36), Sanyinjiao (SP 6), Jianyu (LI 15) (left).
They were punctured with even method.

10. Effect

11. Essentials

Dazhui (GV 14), a meeting point of all Yang channels, disperses Yang Qi effectively. Shanzhong (CV 17), the Influential point of Qi and Front-Mu of Pericardium, regulates Qi of the Heart to stop pain. Zhongwan (CV 12), the Influential point of the Fu organs and Front-Mu of Stomach, strengthens the Spleen and Stomach, activates Qi and Blood, reinforces Qi of the Middle Burner, and calms the Mind. Qihai (CV 6) enhances the Kidneys, the congenital Qi. Zusanli (ST 36) enhances the Spleen and Stomach, the acquired condition. Neiguan (PC 6) tonifies the Heart and removes obstruction of the channels to stop pain. Taiyuan (LU 9), the Influential point of the vessels, used together with Neiguan (PC 6) and Sanyinjiao (SP 6), reinforces Qi to circulate Yang to remove Blood stasis. Jianyu (LI 15) dredges the channels to circulate Qi and Blood to stop pain.

CASE II: CHENG XINNONG'S MEDICAL RECORD

1. General data

Zheng, male, 58, came on November 4, 1985.

2. Chief complaint

Left hypochondriac pain for 3 days.

3. History of present illness

The patient was habitually bad-tempered and had a quarrel with somebody a few days ago. Thereafter, he began to have a pain in the left hypochondrium, worse on coughing.

4. Present symptoms

Pain in the left hypochondrium, worse on coughing, no obvious swelling but a tenderness, limitation in movement, accompanied by poor appetite, abdominal distention, and acid regurgitation.

5. Tongue and pulse

Pale tongue, yellow thick sticky coating, wiry pulse.

6. Differentiation and analysis

This patient is habitually bad-tempered, anger damaging his Liver and causing Qi stagnation in channels running in the hypochondrium, thus he has pain. *Miraculous Pivot* says: 'If the pathogen is in the Liver, there will be pain in the hypochondrium'. His poor appetite, abdominal distention, acid regurgitation, and wiry pulse imply Liver Qi stagnation.

7. Diagnosis

TCM: Hypochondriac pain (Liver Qi stagnation).

Western medicine: Hypochondriac pain requiring further examination.

8. Treating principle

Soothe the Liver, regulate Qi, dredge the channels, stop pain.

9. Prescription

Yanglingquan (GB 34), Taichong (LR 3), Zusanli (ST 36), Zhigou (TE 6), Qimen (LR 14) (left).

They were punctured with the reducing method.

10. Effect

After the treatment, he felt greatly relieved immediately and his appetite improved and abdominal distension reduced. The tenderness became less. He was cured with four applications of the above treatment.

11. Essentials

Qimen (LR 14), Front-Mu of the Liver, Taichong (LR 3), the Yuan-Source of the Liver, together with Yanglingquan (GB 34), the He-Sea of the Gallbladder, are to regulate the Liver Qi, and together with Zhigou (TE 6), are to smooth Qi activities for removing Blood stasis. Zusanli (ST 36) is to strengthen the Spleen and Stomach, based on the good functions of which, his appetite is improved and abdominal distention reduced, thus all the symptoms are relieved.

CASE III: YANG JIEBIN'S MEDICAL RECORD

1. General data

Chen, female, 63.

2. Chief complaint

Right hypochondriac pain for 20 days.

3. History of present illness

Twenty days ago, at night, she suddenly had a serious pain in the right hypochondriac region. She hurried to the emergency room and the X-ray examination showed everything was normal in her Heart and Lungs. Administered painkiller, sleeping potion, analgesic injection, gentamycin, and herbal medicines, but she was not relieved.

Anamnesis: Hypertension.

4. Present symptoms

Serious pain in the right hypochondriac region, radiating to the back and especially worse on coughing and breathing. Accompanied by dizziness, tinnitus, and dry throat. Rosy-red complexion, fat body figure, suffering expression with groans, restlessness, tenderness in the right hypochondrium in the region of the 3rd to 7th rib.

5. Tongue and pulse

Slightly red tongue, little coating, wiry tight pulse.

6. Differentiation and analysis

The right hypochondrium is the attribution area of the Liver Meridian. Qi and Blood stagnation causes the obstruction of the Liver Meridian, resulting in pain. Wiry pulse indicates Liver Qi stagnation and pain. Tight pulse implies spasm of tendons and muscles.

7. Diagnosis

TCM: Hypochondriac pain.

Western medicine: Hypochondriac pain requiring further examination.

8. Treating principle

Dredge the channels and collaterals, regulate Qi circulation, stop pain.

9. Prescription

Right side: Zhigou (TE 6), Yanglingquan (GB 34), Rugen (ST 18), Tianchi (PC 1).

Zhigou (TE 6) was punctured penetrating to Jianshi (PC 5) with #28 2 cun filiform needle and strong stimulation for reducing, and Yanglingquan (GB 34) to Yinlingquan (SP 9). The needles were retained for half an hour, and in the duration, manipulated with lifting-thrusting and rotating once every 3 minutes. Cupping was done to Rugen (ST 18) and Tianchi (PC 1) for 15 minutes.

10. Effect

The pain stopped within 20 minutes and the patient was cured with half an hour's retention of the needles. The follow-up showed no recurrence of hypochondriac pain.

11. Essentials

Zhigou (TE 6) regulates the Shaoyang Channel and reduces the Ministerial Fire. Yanglingquan (GB 34), the He-Sea point, treats the Fu organs to regulate Fu Qi to stop pain. Cupping to Rugen (ST 18) and Tianchi (PC 1) removes the local Blood stasis to stop pain. The pain stops when obstruction of meridians and Qi stagnation are removed.

SUMMARY

Chest and hypochondriac pain is due to Qi stagnation and Blood stasis. The Heart Yang is inactive, the Lung Qi becomes stagnant, or overeating cold food causes Cold to accumulate in the Middle Burner and go upward to the chest, resulting in the obstruction of the channels in the chest region; therefore, there is pain in chest and hypochondrium.

Main points: Shanzhong (CV 17), Daling (PC 7), Taiyuan (LU 9), Neiguan (PC 6).

Add Dazhui (GV 14) and Xinshu (BL 15) to activate the Heart Yang. Add Feishu (BL 13), Zhongfu (LU 1) and Lieque (LU 7) to disperse the Lung Qi. Add Tiantu (CV 22) and Fenglong (ST 40) to dissolve Phlegm. Do moxibustion at Feishu (BL 13), Xinshu (BL 15) and Shanzhong (CV 17) after needling to relieve the radiating pain to the back to dispel Cold due to excessive Yin. Add Xingjian (LR 2), Xuehai (SP 10), Hegu (LI 4), Sanyinjiao (SP 6) to activate Qi and Blood circulation for those prolonged cases with Qi stagnation and Blood stasis.

Hypochondriac pain is related to the Liver and Gallbladder diseases because of the distribution of running course of the Shaoyang channels. *Miraculous Pivot* (*Five Pathogenic Factors*) says: 'The pathogenic factor is in the Liver, causing the pain in the hypochondrium.' *Miraculous Pivot* (*Channels*) says: 'Patients with Gallbladder diseases have a bitter taste, sigh frequently, and suffer from pain in the Heart and hypochondriac regions with difficulties in turning the body.'

The intercostal neuralgia and pleurisy and the hypochondriac pain caused by traumatic injury can be treated with the principle mentioned here.

Main points: Yanglingquan (GB 34), Zhigou (TE 6), Qimen (LR 14).

The hypochondriac pain due to Liver Qi stagnation is symptomized as distending pain, chest fullness, bitter taste and wiry pulse. Ganshu (BL 18), Danshu (BL 19) and Qiuxu (GB 40) should be added.

The hypochondriac pain due to Blood stasis caused by trauma is symptomized as stabbing pain, especially at night, dark tongue with Blood spots and wiry hesitant pulse. Geshu (BL 17) and Taichong (LR 3) should be added.

Hypochondriac pain due to Phlegm retention caused by prolonged cough and Damp retained in chest and hypochondrium is symptomized as dyspnoea, white moistened coating and thready soft pulse. Zhongwan (CV 12), Zusanli (ST 36) and Pishu (BL 20) should be added.

SECTION FIVE • EPIGASTRIC PAIN

CASE I: CHENG XINNONG'S MEDICAL RECORD

1. General data

Yan, male, 29, came on December 2, 1985.

2. Chief complaint

Pain in the epigastric region for 7 years.

3. History of present illness

He began to have pain fixed in the epigastric region 7 years ago. The diagnosis was duodenal bulbar ulcer and medicinal treatment not effective.

4. Present symptoms

The dull pain usually started 1–2 hours after a meal and was relieved by pressure. His complexion was sallow. He preferred warm drinks. His appetite was normal, with no nausea or vomiting. His urine and stools were normal.

5. Tongue and pulse

Tip of tongue red, slightly yellow coating, weak wiry pulse.

6. Differentiation and analysis

The Spleen and Stomach are both diseased. The Spleen Yang is not sufficient, and the Stomach Qi not harmonized, thus there is a dull pain in the epigastric region. The pain getting better by pressure, sallow complexion, preference for warm drinks are all the signs of Cold stagnation in the Stomach.

7. Diagnosis

TCM: Epigastric pain (Cold stagnated in Stomach).

Western medicine: Duodenal bulbar ulcer.

8. Treating principle

Warm the Middle Burner, dispel Cold, circulate Qi, stop pain.

9. Prescription

Zhongwan (CV 12), Qihai (CV 6), Neiguan (PC 6), Gongsun (SP 4), Zusanli (ST 36), Sanyinjiao (SP 6).

The reinforcing method and even method were applied. Moxibustion was applied to Zhongwan (CV 12).

10. Effect

After 1 treatment, he felt relieved. He was treated once daily for 10 consecutive treatments and the pain disappeared.

11. Essentials

Zhongwan (CV 12), Front-Mu of Stomach, is used to warm Yang and dispel Cold to harmonize the Stomach. Zusanli (ST 36), the Lower He-Sea of Foot-Yangming Channel, with Sanyinjiao (SP 6), are to strengthen the Stomach and promote the Spleen. Gongsun (SP 4), Luo-Connecting of Foot-Taiyin Channel, connecting with Neiguan (PC 6) of Pericardium Channel through Yinwei Channel, relaxes the chest, regulates Qi and harmonizes the Stomach.

With the treatment of these points in combination, the Stomach Qi is harmonized, transportation and transformation of the Middle Burner promoted, thereafter the pain is stopped.

CASE II: CHENG XINNONG'S MEDICAL RECORD

1. General data

Run, female, 60, came on April 6, 1992.

2. Chief complaint

Pain in the epigastrium for 10 years.

3. History of present illness

Because of the distending pain in the epigastrium she had had B-ultrasonic examination and the diagnosis was cholecystitis.

4. Present symptoms

The stone in the Gallbladder was 0.6 × 1.5cm and the cyst 1.4cm in the right lobe of the Liver. The pain involved the hypochondrium and was accompanied with hiccups which could be relieved by warmth. She had hiccups and sometimes palpitations. Her complexion is lustreless and her stools loose.

5. Tongue and pulse

Purple tongue, thin yellow coating, right pulse deep thready, left pulse deep wiry.

6. Differentiation and analysis

Emotional depression makes the Liver Qi stagnated, attacking the Stomach, the Qi of which fails to descend, thus there is distending pain, hiccups and loose stools.

The stagnation transforms into Fire, which then involves the Blood, thus there is purple tongue and yellow coating.

7. Diagnosis

TCM: Epigastric pain (Liver Qi attacking Stomach).

Western medicine: Chronic cholecystitis.

8. Treating principle

Soothe the Liver, regulate Qi, harmonize the Stomach, stop pain.

9. Prescription

Shanzhong (CV 17), Zhongwan (CV 12), Qihai (CV 6), Riyue (GB 24), Neiguan (PC 6), Weishu (BL 21), Danshu (BL 19), Yanglingquan (GB 34), Zusanli (ST 36), Taichong (LR 3), Qiuxu (GB 40).

   The reducing method and even method were applied.

10. Effect

The distending pain in the epigastrium was gradually relieved and 40 treatments totally cured her.

11. Essentials

Zhongwan (CV 12), Riyue (GB 24) and Danshu (BL 19), Front-Mu and Back-Shu in combination, harmonize the Stomach, soothe the Liver, and regulate Qi to stop pain. Danshu (BL 19), Yanglingquan (GB 34), Taichong (LR 3), and Qiuxu (GB 40) descend the upward rushing of Liver Qi to harmonize the Stomach. Neiguan (PC 6) and Shanzhong (CV 17) relax the chest and circulate Qi. Zhongwan (CV 12) and Neiguan (PC 6) harmonize the Stomach to stop pain. Qihai (CV 6) consolidates Yuan Qi and harmonizes Qi and Blood.

CASE III: TIAN CONGHE'S MEDICAL RECORD

1. General data

Anonymous female, 34, came on November 23, 2005.

2. Chief complaint

Repeated distending pain in the upper abdomen for 2 years, worse for 1 month.

3. History of present illness

Two years ago, she had a distending pain in the upper abdomen without clear reasons and it was diagnosed duodenal ulcer. Medicinal treatment was not effective. Over the last 1 month it became worse.

4. Present symptoms

She came with a distending pain after meals, acid regurgitation, belching, and being afraid of cold. Her bowel movement was 1–2 times a day with loose stools. Her urine was yellow.

Examination: The gastroscopy showed a chronic superficial antral gastritis and gastric peristalsis deficiency. The pathological findings were moderate chronic atrophic gastritis at the antral region, interstitial congestion, and glandular hyperplasia.

5. Tongue and pulse

Slightly red tongue, yellow sticky coating, wiry thready pulse.

6. Differentiation and analysis

The stagnated Liver Qi attacking the Stomach is the cause of distending pain in the upper abdomen, acid regurgitation, belching. Yellow sticky coating indicates the Damp transforming into Heat. Wiry pulse implies the pain syndrome and thready pulse indicates the Stomach Yin deficiency in the prolonged disease.

7. Diagnosis

TCM: Epigastric pain (Damp Heat retention in the Middle Burner, Liver Qi stagnation).

Western medicine: Duodenal ulcer.

8. Treating principle

Circulate Qi, dredge Triple Burner.

9. Prescription

The elongated needle (Mangzhen) 380mm in length was used to penetrate from Dazhui (GV 14) to Jizhong (GV 6) to clear the Governor Vessel of obstructions. Zhongwan (CV 12), Liangmen (ST 21), Zusanli (ST 36), Neiguan (PC 6), Qimen (LR 14), and Huangshu (KI 16) were punctured. Cupping was done at Pishu (BL 20) and Weishu (BL 21).

Three treatments a week, the long Mangzhen was used once a week only and changed to short (Mangzhen) and with less frequency when the symptoms relieved. Other necessary points were selected accordingly.

10. Effect

With nearly 2 months' treatment, the symptoms disappeared and the gastroscopy showed a cure of her chronic superficial antral gastritis.

11. Essentials

The Governor Vessel meets the Yang channels at Dazhui (GV 14). The Dai-Belt Channel originates from the second lumbar vertebra. The Yangwei-Link Vessel meets the Governor Vessel at Fengfu (GV 16) and Yamen (GV 15). The Yangqiao-Heel Vessel connects with Fengfu (GV 16) through the Foot-Taiyang Meridian. The Governor Vessel, connecting with the Kidneys which stores Yuan-Original Yang, and with all the Yang channels, externally protects from invasion of exogenous pathogenic factors, internally warms the Zang Fu organs, participating in the formation process of Essence and Blood. According to Professor Tian Conghe, the Governor Vessel is responsible for diseases of Yang of the entire body or any one of the Yang channels. Regulating the Governor Vessel with elongated needle penetrating points produces quick effects, but because it is a strong stimulation, it can be used only once a week or less. For this patient, the elongated needle penetrating method functioned well in circulating Qi and dredging Triple Burner. The symptoms ceased when the stagnant Qi of Liver was regulated and Damp Heat eliminated.

ELONGATED NEEDLE (MANGZHEN) REGULATING THE GOVERNOR VESSEL

The patient's position is very strictly requested according to whether it should be prone, lateral recumbent, or sitting erect with the back towards the doctor. Professor Tian uses Mangzhen penetrating downward with the thumb, index and middle finger of the puncturing hand holding the lower portion of the body of the needle, the ring finger supporting the body of the needle, and the pressing hand holding the handle of the needle. Press to insert the needle quickly with the force of the fingers and wrist of the puncturing hand and with the cooperation of the pressing hand. Then the puncturing hand manipulates the needle penetrated down along the posterior border of the spine and the pressing hand is used to control the direction of the needle. Reinforce or reduce when the tip of the needle arrives at the wanted depth. For safety, it is suggested to carry out the reinforcing-reducing by means of respiration, rotating or rapid and slow insertion and withdrawal, not lifting-thrusting. Ask the patient to inhale and manipulate the needle with the thumb turning forward, withdraw the needle quickly and press the hole means reinforcing, otherwise, reducing. The rotating should be gentle and agile with an amplitude of 180°-360°. The 125-175mm elongated needle may be retained for 20 minutes. The longer needles, 380mm, 500mm, 1200mm, are not retained. The needle should be kept straight when withdrawing it in order to prevent difficulties in removing, and violent withdrawing should be avoided.

CASE IV: SHAO JINGMING'S MEDICAL RECORD

1. General data

Liu, female, 29, came on June 25, 1999.

2. Chief complaint

Gastric pain and abdominal distention for 5 months.

3. History of present illness

One year ago she began to have discomfort in the upper abdomen and sometimes a bearing-down distention. In the last 5 months the gastric pain started because she was so busy that she could not have meals regularly. Metoclopramide relieved the pain but did not control it. The provincial hospital diagnosed her with gastroptosis (II) as a result of a barium meal examination. She was treated but the treatment was not effective.

4. Present symptoms

Gastric pain and abdominal distention, poor appetite, tiredness, poor sleep. Emaciation, pale complexion, spirit normal, boat-shaped abdomen with tenderness.

5. Tongue and pulse

Pale tongue, thin coating, deep but a slightly slow pulse.

6. Differentiation and analysis

This is due to the improper food intake, overworking and stress, prolonged disease, and weak constitution damaging the Spleen Yang, causing the sinking of Qi of the Middle Burner, which fails to keep the organs in the right position.

7. Diagnosis

TCM: Gastroptosis (sinking due to Yang deficiency).

Western medicine: Gastroptosis.

8. Treating principle

Strengthen the Spleen, harmonize the Stomach, lift and reinforce Yang Qi.

9. Prescription

Zhongwan (CV 12), Zusanli (ST 36), Weishang (Extra), Neiguan (PC 6), Shenmen (HT 7), Sanyinjiao (SP 6).

    Treated once a day.

10. Effect

After 6 treatments, her appetite and sleep were improved and her tiredness was gone. Then only the main points Zhongwan (CV 12), Zusanli (ST 36), and Weishang (Extra) were used every other day. After a total of 2 courses, her symptoms disappeared. X-ray examination showed that the Stomach had returned to the normal position. One year follow-up didn't find any recurrence.

11. Essentials

Gastroptosis is commonly seen in clinic. Professor Shao holds that it is mostly caused by irregular food intake, tiredness due to overwork, prolonged disease, and parturitions making the constitution weak and Spleen Yang exhausted, so that the Qi of the Middle Burner is too weak to hold the organs in the right position. The main points: Zhongwan (CV 12), Zusanli (ST 36), Weishang (Extra). The symptomized points: Neiguan (PC 6) for poor appetite, nausea and acid regurgitation. Pishu (BL 20) and Weishu (BL 21) for abdominal distension. Baihui (GV 20) for a bearing-down sensation in abdomen and diarrhoea. Shenmen (HT 7) and Sanyinjiao (SP 6) for insomnia. Moxibustion for Yang deficiency.

WEISHANG
Weishang (Extra), located 2 cun above the umbilicus and 4 cun lateral to anterior midline, functions quickly to reinforce Qi, strengthen the Spleen, and lift the Stomach, good for treating gastroptosis. A 3-4 cun filiform needle is used, after insertion, obliquely towards Shenque (CV 8) to a depth of 2.5-3.5 cun into the muscle. A medium strong stimulation is applied to produce a lifting and contracting sensation in the gastric region. The direction and depth are important. Give treatment when the Stomach is empty. A rest should be taken when the patient feels pain and discomfort during acupuncture.

SUMMARY

Gastric pain is common in gastroduodenal ulcer, acute and chronic gastritis, and neuroses. It is usually caused by irregular food intake, invasion of Cold and emotional depression. The pain is accompanied by nausea, vomiting, abdominal distension, and belching. It may be worse on pressure or better on warmth and pressure. A deep and rolling pulse indicates an excess and a deep thready wiry pulse suggests a deficiency syndrome. The treating principle is to harmonize the Stomach to stop pain.

Main points: Zhongwan (CV 12), Zusanli (ST 36), Neiguan (PC 6).

For distending pain due to food retention: Liangmen (ST 21), Neiting (ST 44), Gongsun (SP 4); for Cold stagnation in the Stomach causing clear fluid vomit, the pain relieved by warmth, and slow pulse: Pishu (BL 20), Weishu (BL 21), Qihai (CV 6), moxibustion; Liver Qi attacking the Stomach leading to hypochondriac pain: Yanglingquan (GB 34), Taichong (LR 3).

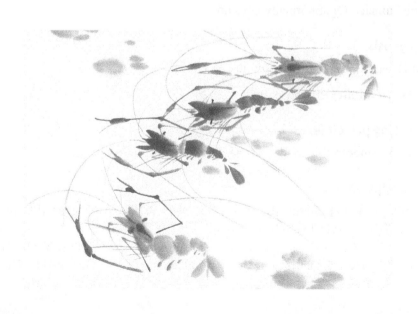

SECTION SIX • HICCUPS

CASE I: YANG JIEBIN'S MEDICAL RECORD

1. General data

Yang, male, 30.

2. Chief complaint

Sonorous hiccups for more than 10 days.

3. History of present illness

Eleven days ago, he began to have sonorous non-stop hiccups after lunch. Medicinal treatment was useless.

4. Present symptoms

Difficult breathing and speaking because of sonorous non-stop hiccups, accompanied by fullness of abdomen, acid regurgitation, feeling of heartburn, contracting pain in the head, chest and hypochondrium, and tiredness. Sturdy body figure, suffering complexion.

5. Tongue and pulse

Thin white coating, wiry rolling pulse.

6. Differentiation and analysis

In ancient times, this disease was called 'E'. Now it is called 'hiccups'. The cause is that the Stomach Qi abnormally goes up.

7. Diagnosis

TCM: Hiccups (Stomach Qi going up).

Western medicine: Phrenospasm.

8. Treating principle

Relax chest, smooth Qi circulation, harmonize the Middle Burner.

9. Prescription

Shanzhong (CV 17), Geshu (BL 17), Zhongwan (CV 12), Neiguan (PC 6), Jiaji (EX-B2) of 3–4 cervical vertebrae, Zusanli (ST 36).

Shanzhong (CV 17) was punctured penetrating to Zhongting (CV 16), Geshu (BL 17) obliquely 1.5 cun towards the spine, Neiguan (PC 6) penetrated to Waiguan

(TE 5), Jiaji (EX-B2) obliquely 1.5 cun towards the spine, Zhongwan (CV 12) and Zusanli (ST 36) punctured routinely.

Both needling and cupping were applied.

10. Effect

Ten minutes later, the hiccups decreased and half an hour later, they stopped. He slept for 10 hours that day. One more treatment was given to consolidate the good result on the following day. Observation for 1 week noticed no recurrence and he was discharged from the hospital.

11. Essentials

Hiccups are due to Qi going upward abnormally. Shanzhong (CV 17) and Geshu (BL 17) relax the chest to smooth the Qi circulation. Zhongwan (CV 12), the Influential point of the Fu organs and Front-Mu of Stomach, harmonizes the Stomach to send Qi downward. Neiguan (PC 6) penetrating to Waiguan (TE 5), the needling sensation goes to the chest directly to regulate the Qi activities of the Triple Burner. Zusanli (ST 36), the He-Sea point, regulates Qi of Stomach. Jiaji (EX-B2) comforts the chest to stop hiccups.

SUMMARY

Hiccups are usually caused by improper food disturbing the Stomach, the Qi of which fails to go downward. Professor Yang Jiebin treats it with the principle of harmonizing the Stomach to send the reversed Qi downward.

Main points: Shanzhong (CV 17), Geshu (BL 17), Zhongwan (CV 12), Neiguan (PC 6).

Assisting points: Jiaji (EX-B2) of 3–4 cervical vertebrae, Zusanli (ST 36).

These are nearby and distal points in combination. Use the #28 filiform needle to give strong stimulation for reducing, retaining for half an hour, lifting-thrusting and rotating once every 3 minutes. Arrival of Qi is essential. After needling, do cupping. Generally, a quick effect can be achieved. For mild cases, Neiguan (PC 6) or Jiaji (EX-B2) alone may stop the hiccups immediately. When the routine points are not very effective, pressing or puncturing Yifeng (TE 17) will be remarkably helpful.

SECTION SEVEN • ABDOMINAL PAIN

CASE I: FENG RUNSHEN'S MEDICAL RECORD

1. General data

Fan, male, 37 years old.

2. Chief complaint

Abdominal pain with a feeling of gas rushing upward from below the umbilicus.

3. History of present illness

He ate something cold and had gastric distention. When he went to bed, the pain started with a feeling of gas rushing upward from below the umbilicus, once every 3–5 minutes. It became worse at midnight.

4. Present symptoms

Greenish yellow complexion, purplish lips, cold extremities, tension in the abdominal muscles and the pain aggravated by pressure, vomiting, profuse sweating because of the pain, thirst with preference for warm drinks, scanty urine, with no bowel movement for the previous 2 days.

5. Tongue and pulse

Thin dry tongue-coating, thready wiry rapid pulse but weak on deep palpation.

6. Differentiation and analysis

This is a case of constitutional Kidney Yang deficiency. The cold food arouses and forces the Cold Qi of the Lower Burner to run upward, thus the pain is due to Cold Qi running upward.

7. Diagnosis

TCM: Bentun (due to Cold Qi running upward) abdominal pain (Cold Qi forcing upward).

Western medicine: Abdominal pain requiring further examination.

8. Treating principle

Warm and reinforce Spleen and Kidneys, dispel Cold, send reversed Qi downward.

9. Prescription

Guanyuan (CV 4), Zusanli (ST 36), Sanyinjiao (SP 6), Zhaohai (KI 6), Taichong (LR 3).

10. Effect

The reinforcing method was applied and warming-needle moxibustion led the warmth deeply to the points. The pain relieved at once. About 10 minutes later, the pain stopped.

11. Essentials

Guanyuan (CV 4) is to warm the Lower Burner, Zusanli (ST 36) to strengthen the Spleen and Stomach, Sanyinjiao (SP 6) to warm the Spleen Yang to restore the Kidney Yang, Taichong (LR 3) and Zhaohai (KI 6) to subdue the Liver Qi ascending. The pain is stopped because the Spleen Yang is warmed, Kidney Qi reinforced, Cold dispelled and reversed Qi regulated.

CASE II: CHENG XINNONG'S MEDICAL RECORD

1. General data

Jin, male, 25, first visited on January 21, 1984.

2. Chief complaint

Paroxysmal pain in the umbilical region for 1 year.

3. History of present illness

One year ago, a paroxysmal periumbilical colic suddenly started, each time lasting about 10 hours, and accompanied by nausea and vomiting, with a frequency of once a month. He had ascariasis.

4. Present symptoms

Paroxysmal periumbilical colic, accompanied with nausea, vomiting, poor appetite, sleep not good, stools dry but once a day, and urine normal.

5. Tongue and pulse

White coating, tip of tongue red, deep thready wiry pulse.

6. Differentiation and analysis

This is the abdominal pain related to ascariasis which over a long time creates disorders of Qi circulation. Nausea and vomiting result from ascarides blocking the Stomach and intestines, causing obstruction of the Qi of the Fu organs.

7. Diagnosis

TCM: Abdominal pain (deficiency Cold of the Middle Burner, ascarides blocking).

Western medicine: Ascariasis of biliary tract.

8. Treating principle

Warm the Middle Burner, reinforce the Spleen and Stomach, regulate Qi, stop pain.

9. Prescription

Neiguan (PC 6), Gongsun (SP 4), Zusanli (ST 36), Sanyinjiao (SP 6), Xiawan (CV 10), Qihai (CV 6), Tianshu (ST 25).

Moxibustion was applied to Tianshu (ST 25) and the even method applied to the other points.

10. Effect

11. Essentials

The abdominal pain is related to ascariasis which over a long time creates disorder of the Qi circulation. The principle of warming the Middle Burner, reinforcing the Spleen and Stomach, and regulating Qi should be followed to stop the pain.

SUMMARY

Abdominal pain refers to pain in the area below the xiphoid process and above the pubis. The divergent channels of Foot-Taiyin and Foot-Yangming enter into the abdomen, Liver Channel enters the lower abdomen, and the Conception Vessel runs in the interior of the abdomen. Abdominal pain is closely related with these four channels.

Main points: Zhongwan (CV 12), Tianshu (ST 25), Zusanli (ST 36), Sanyinjiao (SP 6), Taichong (LR 3).

Shenque (CV 8) and Gongsun (SP 4) are added for Cold retention in interior, Yinlingquan (SP 9) and Neiting (ST 44) added for Damp Heat stagnation, and Guanyuan (CV 4), Pishu (BL 20), Weishu (BL 21), and Zhangmen (LR 13) added for Spleen deficiency and Cold in Middle Burner.

SECTION EIGHT • DIARRHOEA

CASE I: RECORD IN *ACUPUNCTURE-MOXIBUSTION FOR DIFFICULT DISEASES*

1. General data

Sun, female, 58, first visited on June 8, 1988.

2. Chief complaint

Abdominal pain and diarrhoea in the morning for more than 2 years.

3. History of present illness

Every day in the morning, she began to have abdominal pain and diarrhoea, and medication was not effective.

4. Present symptoms

Every day in the morning from 6 o'clock, she began to have chills and abdominal pain, and diarrhoea 5–6 times. After 8 o'clock, the symptoms disappeared.

5. Tongue and pulse

Pale tongue, thin white coating, thready weak pulse.

6. Differentiation and analysis

Six o'clock in the morning is known as Mao (the fourth of the 12 Earthly Branches). During this period, Yang Qi arises. Yang Qi of this patient is deficient, failing to arise, so she has chills. Mao is also the period for the channel Qi of Yangming Large Intestine to flow. The deficiency Cold of this patient causes her diarrhoea. After Mao, her Yang Qi slowly arises, so her pain and diarrhoea stop.

7. Diagnosis

TCM: Diarrhoea (Yang deficiency with interior Cold).

Western medicine: Diarrhoea.

8. Treating principle

Warm Yang to stop diarrhoea.

9. Prescription

Zusanli (ST 36), Shangjuxu (ST 37), Dazhui (GV 14).

Zusanli (ST 36) and Shangjuxu (ST 37) were reinforced. Dazhui (GV 14) was applied with moxibustion for 30 minutes. Once a day, 6 treatments as 1 course.

10. Effect

After 2 courses, the chills, abdominal pain and diarrhoea were relieved. Another 2 courses cured her.

11. Essentials

Zusanli (ST 36) and Shangjuxu (ST 37) are Lower He-Sea points, good for treating the Fu organs. Dazhui (GV 14), the meeting point of all Yang channels, lifts and reinforces Yang Qi, especially when moxibustion is done. Yang Qi arises to resist pathogens, thus her symptoms stop.

CASE II: LOU BAICENG'S MEDICAL RECORD

1. General data

Zhang, female, 42 years old.

2. Chief complaint

Loose stools for nearly one year.

3. History of present illness

She began to have loose stools 2–3 times a day because of improper food.

4. Present symptoms

Loose stools with undigested food in it, abdominal distention, tiredness, and poor appetite. Sallow complexion, listlessness.

5. Tongue and pulse

Tender tongue with white coating, soft thready pulse.

6. Differentiation and analysis

Her loose stools are caused by the weakness of Spleen and Stomach in transportation and transformation. Tender tongue with white coating and soft thready pulse are the signs of Spleen deficiency.

7. Diagnosis

TCM: Diarrhoea (Spleen and Stomach deficiency).

Western medicine: Diarrhoea.

8. Treating principle

Strengthen the Spleen, harmonize the Stomach, stop diarrhoea.

9. Prescription

Pishu (BL 20), Tianshu (ST 25), Zusanli (ST 36).
   Reinforcing with lifting and thrusting.

10. Effect

After 3 treatments, the stools were not loose. Six treatments made the stools completely normal. The follow-up after half a year found no recurrence.

11. Essentials

Back-Shu point, Pishu (BL 20), and Tianshu (ST 25), Front-Mu point, the places where the Qi of Spleen and Large Intestine is infused, together with Zusanli (ST 36), the He-Sea point, are to strengthen the Spleen, harmonize the Stomach, and regulate the Qi of Stomach and intestines to stop diarrhoea.

CASE III: MENG HONG'S MEDICAL RECORD

1. General data

Liu, male, 2 years old.

2. Chief complaint

The mother said that the boy had diarrhoea for 1 week.

3. History of present illness

One week ago, he suddenly had a fever of 39.2°C, diarrhoea for more than 10 times a day, red lips, dry mouth, irritability, thirst with preference for drinking water, sweating, coarse breathing, yellow scanty urine. He was diagnosed with acute enteritis and treated with Chinese and Western medicine, his body temperature was getting normal but the diarrhoea continued, and tenesmus also appeared.

4. Present symptoms

Diarrhoea, crying before discharging stools, yellow watery stools with stinking smell, tiredness, irritability.

5. Tongue and pulse

Light red tongue, thin yellow sticky coating; soft weak rapid pulse.

6. Differentiation and analysis

Damp Heat diarrhoea. The Stomach Qi failed to descend, retention of food caused vomiting. The Spleen failed to carry out transportation and transformation, the Damp accumulated, so diarrhoea resulted. *Plain Questions (Su Wen)* says: 'When

Damp is accumulated, there appears diarrhoea'. No matter whether the diarrhoea is of the Heat type or Cold type, Damp is always part of the combination. The high fever, rapid pulse and thin yellow tongue-coating were all the manifestations of Heat. Therefore this was a Damp Heat diarrhoea in syndrome differentiation.

7. Diagnosis

TCM: Diarrhoea (Damp Heat type).

Western medicine: Diarrhoea.

8. Treating principle

Clear Heat, dissolve Damp.

9. Prescription

Tianshu (ST 25), Zusanli (ST 36), Xiawan (CV 10), Pishu (BL 20), Gongsun (SP 4), Neiguan (PC 6).

 Acupuncture with medium stimulation, without retaining of needles, once a day.

10. Effect

After 2 treatments in succession, the child was getting better in spirit, his thirst was relieved, frequency of defecation changed to 4–5 times a day. Five treatments made all the symptoms disappear.

11. Essentials

Babies are quite delicate in constitution; improper feeding can damage the Spleen and Stomach, and careless nursing causes invasion of pathogenic factors. Quick needling without retention of needles is the method for infants.

SUMMARY

Diarrhoea refers to abnormal frequency and liquidity of faecal discharges, including enteritis, intestinal tuberculosis, colitis, and intestinal dysfunctions, etc. The acute case, if prolonged, may develop into a chronic one.

Main points: Zhongwan (CV 12), Tianshu (ST 25), Dachangshu (BL 25), Zusanli (ST 36).

Dazhui (GV 14), Quchi (LI 11) and Hegu (LI 4) are added for the diarrhoea caused by exogenous pathogenic factors; Qihai (CV 6) added for Cold Damp; Neiting (ST 44), Yinlingquan (SP 9) and Hegu (LI 4) added for Damp Heat; Zhangmen (LR 13) and Taibai (SP 3) added for the Spleen deficiency; Shenshu (BL 23), Mingmen (GV 4), Taixi (KI 3), Guanyuan (CV 4), and Baihui (GV 20) added for the Kidney deficiency.

SECTION NINE • CONSTIPATION

CASE I: YANG JIEBIN'S MEDICAL RECORD

1. General data

Wang, male, 40, first visited on March 17, 1964.

2. Chief complaint

Constipation for 2 months.

3. History of present illness

Two months ago he had diarrhoea due to improper food. After the diarrhoea ceased, he was constipated instead.

4. Present symptoms

The bowel movements were once every 3–4 days with scanty dry stools in the shape of sheep's faeces, accompanied by abdominal fullness, poor appetite, and clear urine. Tenderness in the Tianshu (ST 25) region.

5. Tongue and pulse

Slightly red tongue, thin yellow sticky coating, deep forceful pulse.

6. Differentiation and analysis

The constipation here is due to improper food, causing Heat to accumulate in Yangming. The Dryness of the intestines and Qi stagnation make the transportation of faeces difficult, so the stools become as dry as sheep's faeces. Deep forceful pulse indicates the dry stools in intestines.

7. Diagnosis

TCM: Constipation (Qi stagnation and intestinal Dryness).

Western medicine: Constipation.

8. Treating principle

Remove the obstruction in the intestines, circulate Qi, moisten the intestines.

9. Prescription

Zhigou (TE 6), Tianshu (ST 25), Dachangshu (BL 25), Zhaohai (KI 6).

Treatment was given once a day with the needles retained for 30 minutes and manipulated once every 3 minutes.

10. Effect

After 1 treatment, the bowel movements seemed to come. After 3 treatments, the stools became soft and discharged normally every day in the morning with mucus in them. After 4 treatments, the bowel movements changed to become normal.

11. Essentials

The treating principle for this case is to remove the obstruction in the intestines by circulating Qi and moistening the faeces. Tianshu (ST 25) and Dachangshu (BL 25) dredge the intestines directly. Zhigou (TE 6), a distal point, promotes Qi circulation of Triple Burner to smooth the intestines. Zhaohai (KI 6) replenishes the Kidney Water to produce Essence and Blood to reinforce Yin to moisten the Dryness for moving the faeces.

CASE II: LOU BAICENG'S MEDICAL RECORD

1. General data

Du, female, 50 years old.

2. Chief complaint

Having difficulties in passing stools for 2 years.

3. History of present illness

Constipation without clear inducement.

4. Present symptoms

Her stools were difficult to discharge, with a movement once every 3–5 days and now even 7–8 days. She had abdominal distention and poor appetite.

5. Tongue and pulse

Moistened tongue-coating, wiry pulse.

6. Differentiation and analysis

Qi circulation of intestines and Stomach is obstructed. The transmitting function of the Large Intestine is disturbed. There exists constipation.

7. Diagnosis

TCM: Constipation (Qi stagnation in intestines).

Western medicine: Constipation.

8. Treating principle

Circulate Qi, remove obstruction, smooth stools.

9. Prescription

Dachangshu (BL 25), Daheng (SP 15), Zhigou (TE 6).
   Reducing by lifting-thrusting, once every day.

10. Effect

One hour after acupuncture each time she could pass stools, although only a little. She was asked to try to pass stools at a regular time in order to cooperate with the treatment. With 10 treatments, her stools became normal.

11. Essentials

Dachangshu (BL 25) is to circulate the stagnated Qi. Daheng (SP 15) is to promote the Spleen in transportation for moving the stools. Zhigou (TE 6) is to smooth the Qi circulation of Triple Burner. The pathology of modern medicine holds that weakened peristalsis is the cause of constipation. The mild reducing with lifting-thrusting is used to strengthen the peristalsis. If strong reducing is given, peristalsis will be inhibited.

SUMMARY

Constipation, difficult in passing stools over 3 days, includes excess and deficiency syndromes. The excess refers to the obstruction of pathogenic factors in the intestines, while the deficiency to the non-moisture of intestines failing to move the stools. To remove the obstruction and to moisten the intestines are the principles to follow in the treatment.

Main points: Tianshu (ST 25), Dachangshu (BL 25), Zusanli (ST 36), Zhigou (TE 6).

For abdominal distention, add Zhongwan (CV 12) and Qihai (CV 6). For excess Heat in intestines, add Quchi (LI 11), Hegu (LI 4) and Ciliao (BL 32). For Qi and Blood deficiency, add Pishu (BL 20) and Shenshu (BL 23).

SECTION TEN • LONG BI (URINATION DISTURBANCE)

CASE I: LU SHOUYAN'S MEDICAL RECORD

1. General data

Liu, a 51-year-old man, visited on December 7, 1962.

2. Chief complaint

Having frequent and difficult urination for more than 10 years.

3. History of present illness

He had lumbar vertebra fracture in 1950. Thereafter, he had frequent urination with turbid urine and not well-formed stools.

4. Present symptoms

Frequent, scanty, and turbid urine, loose stools. Throbbing felt below the umbilicus, soft abdomen, soreness and distention on pressure in the region of Mingmen (GV 4) and Yaoyangguan (GV 3).

5. Tongue and pulse

Swollen tongue, thick sticky coating. Thready wiry rapid pulse, Chi pulse weak and superficial, right Taixi (KI 3) pulse deep and weaker than that of left, Chongyang (ST 42) pulse extremely strong, Taichong (LR 3) pulse wiry and full.

6. Differentiation and analysis

The Bladder is the organ which stores urine, and with normal Qi activities, urination is normal; when abnormal, difficult urination will appear, known as Long-dysuria.

Triple Burner is the passage through which the Water travels, and when obstructed, difficult urination will occur, known as Bi-retention.

Plain Questions (*Gu Kong Lun*) says: 'Governor Vessel…along the penis down…is diseased, producing difficult urination, haemorrhoid and enuresis.'

This patient had a lumbar vertebral fracture which damaged the Governor Vessel, the Qi of which is deficient, the Lower Burner is poorly nourished, the Qi activities of the Bladder fail to function well in discharging urine, and together with Damp Heat invasion at this time, Long-dysuria is formed. The Chi pulse is weak and Taixi (KI 3) pulse deep and weak, meaning Kidney deficiency and the Lower Burner poorly nourished. Wiry rapid pulse means Heat. Turbid urine means Damp Heat moving downward.

7. Diagnosis

TCM: Long (deficiency complicated with excess).

Western medicine: Dysuria.

8. Treating principle

Replenish Kidney Yang, reinforce the Kidneys and the Governor Vessel, clear Damp Heat, clear obstruction of the Water passage.

9. Prescription

Zhongji (CV 3), Qihai (CV 6), Yingu (KI 10), Taixi (KI 3), Gaohuang (BL 43), Shuidao (ST 28), Sanyinjiao (SP 6), Yaoyangguan (GV 3), Pangguangshu (BL 28), Sanjiaoshu (BL 22), Weiyang (BL 39).

Reinforcing-reducing by lifting and thrusting the needle was adopted.

Weiyang (BL 39), Pangguangshu (BL 28), Sanyinjiao (SP 6), Sanjiaoshu (BL 22) and Shuidao (ST 28) were reduced. The others were reinforced. The needles were retained for 15 minutes. Once a day, 12 treatments as 1 course.

10. Effect

11. Essentials

Reduce Weiyang (BL 39), Lower He-Sea of Triple Burner, and Pangguangshu (BL 28) and Sanjiaoshu (BL 22) to clear Heat of Triple Burner and remove Damp Heat of Bladder. Reduce Shuidao (ST 28) and Sanyinjiao (SP 6) to induce diuresis.

Reinforce Yingu (KI 10), He-Sea Water point, Taixi (KI 3), Yuan-Source point, Gaohuang (BL 43), from here the Foot-Shaoyin Channel enters into the Kidneys and connects with the Bladder, Qihai (CV 6), the sea of Yuan-Source originating Qi, to replenish Kidney Yang. Reinforce Yaoyangguan (GV 3) to tonify Yang of the Governor Vessel. Reinforce Zhongji (CV 3), Front-Mu of the Bladder, to strengthen its Qi activities.

The pathological condition of this patient is deficiency complicated with excess, so reduce the Back-Shu to decrease the pathogenic Heat in the Bladder, and reinforce Front-Mu to promote Kidney Yang. This is a treating method in which there is Reducing within Reinforcing.

CASE II: YANG YONGXUAN'S MEDICAL RECORD

1. General data

Wang, a 20-year-old man.

2. Chief complaint

Retention of urine for 2 days.

3. History of present illness

He had mental illness and badly injured his left foot by jumping down from a building, leading to an amputation. After the operation, he suffered from urine retention and abdominal distention.

4. Present symptoms

Retention of urine, distending pain in the lower abdomen.

5. Tongue and pulse

Cun and Guan pulse strong, Chi pulse thready.

6. Differentiation and analysis

Plain Questions (*Xuan Ming Wu Qi*) says: 'The Bladder is disordered, causing Long.' Lower Burner Qi activities dysfunctions and Damp Heat accumulation blocking the Bladder are conditions of excess. This patient's retention of urine with fullness in the lower abdomen is caused by the failure of Qi of the Shanzhong region to descend. The sudden onset of his urine retention is caused by Heat. His pulse describes the upper excess and lower deficiency.

7. Diagnosis

TCM: Bi (upper excess and lower deficiency).

Western medicine: Retention of urine.

8. Treating principle

Reduce the excess and reinforce the deficiency.

9. Prescription

Pianli (LI 6), Lieque (LU 7). Right side: Ququan (LR 8), Yinlingquan (SP 9), Taixi (KI 3).

   Reinforcing-reducing by rapid and slow insertion and withdrawal of the needle was adopted. Taixi (KI 3) was reinforced and the others were reduced.

10. Effect

Three hours after acupuncture, the urination became smooth. More treatments were given to consolidate the effect.

11. Essentials

Professor Yang treated him with reducing Taiyin and Jueyin and reinforcing Shaoyin to make Qi smooth for urine to pass without difficulties.

CASE III: CAO HUAIREN'S MEDICAL RECORD

1. General data

Zhang, a 28-year-old man.

2. Chief complaint

Dysuria for 2 days and retention for 1 day.

3. History of present illness

He had a common cold for 10 days and had difficulty in passing urine.

4. Present symptoms

Dysuria. Only 40ml of urine was discharged in 8 hours and then it stopped, without even a drop. An insufferable distending pain in his lower abdomen made him sweat and his extremities were cold.

Examination: The Bladder was full.

5. Tongue and pulse

6. Differentiation and analysis

The urine retention follows his common cold owing to the exogenous pathogenic factors causing obstruction of the Lungs in dispersing, thus, the Water passage is blocked, resulting in not a single drop being passed.

7. Diagnosis

TCM: Bi (pathogenic factor blocked the Lungs in dispersing).

Western medicine: Retention of urine.

8. Treating principle

Promote the Lungs in dispersing, regulate the Lower Burner.

9. Prescription

Lieque (LU 7), Taiyuan (LU 9), Guanyuan (CV 4), Zhaohai (KI 6).

Lieque (LU 7) and Taiyuan (LU 9) were punctured with needle retained for 10 minutes. Guanyuan (CV 4) and Zhaohai (KI 6) were punctured with strong stimulation without retaining.

10. Effect

About 10 minutes later, the urine was discharged and his pain stopped.

11. Essentials

Taiyuan (LU 9), Yuan-Source of the Lung Channel, Lieque (LU 7) and Zhaohai (KI 6), Confluent points, are to disperse Lung Qi. Guanyuan (CV 4), a meeting point of Conception Vessel and the three foot Yin channels, is the important point for urine retention, just as it is said in *Zhenjiu Zisheng Jing* (*Experience on Acupuncture and Moxibustion*): 'The point Guanyuan (CV 4) is indicated in diseases with urine retention.' And Zhaohai (KI 6), together with Guanyuan (CV 4), is to promote the Lower Burner Qi activities.

SUMMARY

Long Bi (urination disturbance) is a urinary disease, dysuria or complete retention, caused by Damp Heat in the Lower Burner, Kidney Yang deficiency or traumatic injury.

Main points: Zhongji (CV 3), Sanyinjiao (SP 6), Ciliao (BL 32).

Yinlingquan (SP 9) and Pangguangshu (BL 28) are used for Lower Burner Damp Heat. Shenshu (BL 23) and Guanyuan (CV 4) are used for Kidney Yang deficiency, with moxibustion added. Sanjiaoshu (BL 22) and Qihai (CV 6) are used for traumatic injury.

In the treatment of Bi-retention of urine, if the routine points are not effective enough, Zuwuli (LR 10) is always responsible because the Foot-Jueyin Liver Channel 'goes along the medial aspect of the thigh, enters into the perineum, curves around the genitals and arrives in the lower abdomen.'

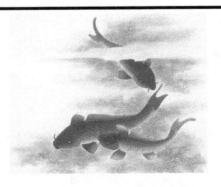

SECTION ELEVEN • LIN ZHENG (URINATION DISTURBANCE)

CASE I: YANG JIASAN'S MEDICAL RECORD

1. General data

Anonymous 71-year-old man, visited on August 26, 1996.

2. Chief complaint

Frequent urination.

3. History of present illness

He was diagnosed with prostatic hypertrophy because of the frequent urination. Medication was not helpful. He was referred for an operation. He refused as he had a pacemaker, so came for acupuncture.

4. Present symptoms

He had urination once every hour in the daytime and 6–7 times a night, accompanied by a distending pain in his lower abdomen.

5. Tongue and pulse

Tongue normal, coating thin white, pulse deep thready.

6. Differentiation and analysis

Prostatic hypertrophy, a common disease seen in old men, manifested as dripping urination with increased frequency in mild cases and urine retention in serious cases, falls into the category of Lin Zheng and Long Bi in Traditional Chinese Medicine. The causative factors are Kidney Qi deficiency, Qi activities stagnation, failure of the Bladder in opening and closing, retained Damp transforming into Heat, and Damp Heat staying in the Lower Burner, resulting in a complicated case with both excess and deficiency.

7. Diagnosis

TCM: Lin (dysuria caused by Qi dysfunction, deficiency syndrome).

Western medicine: Prostatic hypertrophy.

8. Treating principle

Reinforce Yuan-Source Qi, regulate Qi circulation.

9. Prescription

Lieque (LU 7), Zhaohai (KI 6), Sanyinjiao (SP 6).

Medium stimulation was adopted. Once every other day.

10. Effect

The frequency was lowered, 2 times a night. Ten treatments made his urination as regular as normal.

Two weeks later, he came again and said that 1 week after the acupuncture, the frequency was increased to 4–5 times a night and now he had headache, dizziness, tiredness, and poor appetite as well.

Treatment: Lieque (LU 7), Zhaohai (KI 6), Sanyinjiao (SP 6), Fengchi (GB 20), Baihui (GV 20), Hegu (LI 4).

He urinated 2–3 times a night. His headache and dizziness were relieved. In total he was treated for 1 month, about 15 times, urination at night was kept to 1–2 times and occasionally 3 times, although some discomfort still existed in the lower abdomen. The follow-up was carried out 3 months after the end of treatment and found his condition steady.

11. Essentials

Professor Yang holds that the treatment is aimed at reinforcing Yuan Qi and regulating the Qi circulation of the Triple Burner. The basic points are Lieque (LU 7) and Zhaohai (KI 6). The former is the Luo-Connecting point and at the same time a Confluent point, confluent with Conception Vessel, dispersing the Lung Qi to unobstruct Water passage on one hand, and on the other hand, reinforcing and regulating Kidney Qi, indicated in 'frequent but scanty urine'. Zhaohai (KI 6) is to regulate and reinforce Kidney Qi to promote Qi activities of the Bladder. For the deficiency syndrome, Sanyinjiao (SP 6), Shenshu (BL 23) and Pangguangshu (BL 28) should be used to reinforce Kidney Qi. For the Damp Heat syndrome, which is characterized as painful urination, Yanggu (SI 5) and Guanyuan (CV 4) are used to clear Heat and dissolve Damp.

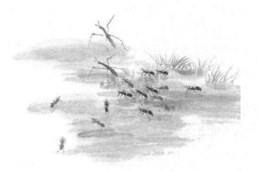

SECTION TWELVE • OEDEMA

CASE I: LU SHOUYAN'S MEDICAL RECORD

1. General data

Xu, a 54-year-old woman.

2. Chief complaint

Oedema of the whole body.

3. History of present illness

Her oedema started from the lower limbs and gradually involved the abdominal region and face.

4. Present symptoms

Whole body oedema, listlessness with cold limbs, fullness in epigastrium and abdomen, poor appetite, loose stools, scanty urine.

5. Tongue and pulse

Pale swollen tongue, white moistened coating, deep thready pulse.

6. Differentiation and analysis

Poor appetite, scanty urine, loose stools, deep thready pulse, pale swollen tongue imply Spleen and Kidney Yang deficiency. According to the manifestations of pulse and symptoms of the patient, it is a Yin oedema in nature caused by Spleen and Kidney Yang deficiency.

7. Diagnosis

TCM: Oedema (Spleen and Kidney Yang deficiency).

Western medicine: Oedema.

8. Treating principle

Warm Yang to strengthen the Spleen, circulate Qi to induce diuresis.

9. Prescription

Feishu (BL 13), Pishu (BL 20), Shenshu (BL 23), Qihai (CV 6), Shuifen (CV 9).

Moxibustion was applied to Shuifen (CV 9) for 5–10 minutes. The other points were reinforced. Warming-needle moxibustion was applied to Pishu (BL 20) and Shenshu (BL 23) after the needles were manipulated lifting-thrusting and rotating. Qihai (CV 6) was punctured with lifting-thrusting but without retaining the needle.

10. Effect

On the second visit, her oedema was greatly relieved, by half, and all her symptoms were better although she still had loose stools, increased urine, and a pale tongue with white coating, and deep thready pulse. The above-mentioned points plus Yinlingquan (SP 9) were applied. Yinlingquan (SP 9) was reinforced first and then reduced and warming-needle moxibustion done to it.

On the third visit, her oedema was almost completely resolved. Her appetite improved and she felt energetic. There was no more abdominal distention. Urine and stools were normal. Tongue was slightly pale, coating thin white. For warming Yang to strengthen the Spleen to consolidate the good effect, Pishu (BL 20), Shenshu (BL 23), Qihai (CV 6) and Zusanli (ST 36) were all reinforced, Pishu (BL 20) and Shenshu (BL 23) without retaining of needles, and warming-needle moxibustion to all other points.

11. Essentials

Professor Lu selected Feishu (BL 13) to circulate Lung Qi, Pishu (BL 20) to strengthen Spleen to control Water, Shenshu (BL 23) to reinforce the Kidneys to warm Yang, Qihai (CV 6) to replenish Yuan-Source Qi, and did moxibustion to Shuifen (CV 9) to induce diuresis to relieve the oedema. On the second visit, Yinlingquan (SP 9), the Water point of the Earth Channel, is reinforced to strengthen the Earth, and reduced to control the Water. Reinforcing and reducing are organically combined with each other by Professor Lu, therefore, the urine is increased and oedema ceases. On the third visit, the pathogenic factors are removed but the anti-pathogenic Qi is weak; strengthening the Earth to control Water is the right principle to follow to cure her oedema successfully.

CASE II: ZHENG YIZHONG'S MEDICAL RECORD

1. General data

Ren, a 21-year-old girl, visited on February 9, 1960.

2. Chief complaint

Puffy face and oedema in her feet, repeated lumbar pain.

3. History of present illness

Half a year ago she was admitted into the hospital for pyelitis and discharged when improved. Later on she had repeated occurrences of oedema, especially when exposed to cold.

4. Present symptoms

Puffy face and oedema in her feet, lumbar pain and frequent and urgent urination.

Examination: Urine: protein (+), WBC (+), platycyte (+), RBC 1–4.

5. Tongue and pulse

Light red tongue, thin white coating, deep and a somewhat slow pulse.

6. Differentiation and analysis

7. Diagnosis

TCM: Oedema (Kidney Qi deficiency).

Western medicine: Oedema.

8. Treating principle

Warm and reinforce Mingmen.

9. Prescription

Moxibustion was done to Shenshu (BL 23) once a day, 30 minutes each time.

10. Effect

After one treatment, the oedema was obviously better. After 10 treatments, the symptoms disappeared and the urine became normal. One year later, the follow-up found no recurrence.

11. Essentials

The prolonged pathological condition leads to Kidney Qi deficiency, Mingmen Fire weakness, failing to distribute Water in a correct way, producing a Cold deficiency. Moxibustion to Shenshu (BL 23) is very effective to warm and reinforce Mingmen to activate the Bladder for diuresis to treat oedema.

SUMMARY

Occurrence of oedema is attributed to hypofunction of the Lungs, Spleen and Kidneys, so that Water is out of control, running abnormally to the skin. Yin and Yang, exterior and interior, deficiency and excess should be clearly differentiated for setting up the treating principle.

Invasion of Wind Damp is usually related to Yang oedema, characterized by quick onset, from face and head to the whole body. Endogenous factors usually induce Yin oedema due to Yang Qi insufficiency characterized by slow onset, from feet or eyelids gradually to the whole body.

Main points for Yang oedema: Hegu (LI 4), Quchi (LI 11), Lieque (LU 7), Feishu (BL 13).

Main points for Yin oedema: Pishu (BL 20), Shenshu (BL 23), Qihai (CV 6), Shuifen (CV 9), Yinlingquan (SP 9).

Renzhong (GV 26) for facial oedema. Pianli (LI 6) for upper limbs. Sanyinjiao (SP 6) and Zulinqi (GB 41) for lower limbs, and especially for serious and prolonged cases, thick needles are used to puncture to eliminate Water.

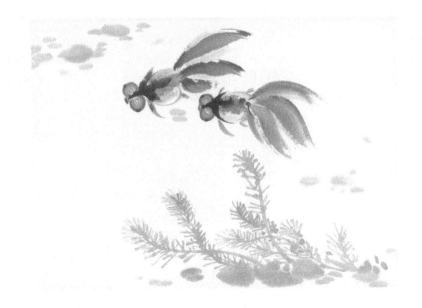

SECTION THIRTEEN • XIAO KE

CASE I: WANG FAXIANG'S MEDICAL RECORD

1. General data

Zhao, a 49-year-old woman, visited on March 7, 1995.

2. Chief complaint

Pain of lower limbs for 3 weeks.

3. History of present illness

She suffered from diabetes for 3 years, and 3 weeks ago she began to have pain in her lower extremities.

4. Present symptoms

Pain in her lower extremities, dry mouth, thirst, tiredness, irritability, dizziness and tinnitus.

Examination: Fasting Blood-glucose 14mmol/L, glucose in urine (+++).

5. Tongue and pulse

Dark tongue, thready pulse.

6. Differentiation and analysis

The pain caused by Xiao Ke is owing to hypofunction of the Zang Fu organs resulting in deficiency of Qi and Blood and Body Fluid insufficiency leading to poor nourishment of the limbs. In nature it is mainly a deficiency but is complicated by stasis excess.

7. Diagnosis

TCM: Xiao Ke (Qi Yin deficiency, obstruction of channels).

Western medicine: Diabetes II.

8. Treating principle

Reinforce Qi, replenish Yin, activate Blood circulation to remove obstruction of channels.

9. Prescription

Pishu (BL 20), Shenshu (BL 23), Weizhong (BL 40), Zusanli (ST 36), Chengshan (BL 57), Sanyinjiao (SP 6), Taixi (KI 3), Rangu (KI 2).

Arrival of Qi is essential. Reinforce Zusanli (ST 36), and other points with even method. Once every day, 15 treatments as 1 course.

10. Effect

After 1 course of treatment, her pain and thirst were greatly reduced, and fasting Blood-glucose 8mmol/L. After 1 more course, her pain and all symptoms disappeared. The follow-up found she was in a steady condition.

11. Essentials

In this case the patient's lower limb pain was caused by diabetes. The treatment should be focused on the Spleen and Kidneys. As *Zhen Jiu Da Cheng* (*Great Compendium of Acupuncture and Moxibustion*) summarized: Xiao Ke (diabetes) is all because of 'Kidney Water exhaustion, Water and Fire disharmony, and dysfunction of both Spleen and Kidneys.' Pishu (BL 20), Shenshu (BL 23), Zusanli (ST 36), Sanyinjiao (SP 6), Taixi (KI 3) and Rangu (KI 2) are used for this patient to treat the root cause and Chengshan (BL 57) and Weizhong (BL 40) for relieving the pain.

SUMMARY

Xiao Ke, diabetes in modern medicine, relates to the Upper, Middle and Lower Burner, that is, all five Zang organs, especially Spleen and Kidneys. In the beginning, the pathological condition is of Heat that exhausts Body Fluid, manifesting as Yin deficiency and dry Heat, symptomized by thirst and overeating, because the Body Fluid is less and the Stomach Fire is brought on. In addition, this is accompanied by Spleen and Kidney deficiency. The urine smells sweet due to the Spleen deficiency with the food Essence incompletely absorbed down directly to the Bladder. The increased urine is the outcome of Kidney Qi failure to control. In the middle stage, Qi exhaustion follows Yin deficiency; therefore, there is exhaustion of both Qi and Yin. At the same time, stasis occurs because Qi is weak in circulating Blood. The Zang Fu dysfunctions extend in severity and complications start. In the late stage, Qi and Yin deficiency gets worse and Blood stasis is aggravated, with the result that the manifestations of Yin and Yang as both deficient and with more organs diseased. That is why diabetes in the late stage is always complicated in pathogenesis and has a lot of complications.

The treating principles, depending on the individual conditions, include clearing Heat; moistening the Dryness; reinforcing Qi; replenishing Yin; strengthening the Kidneys to consolidate the root; activating Blood to remove obstruction of the channels; cooling Blood and promoting its circulation, etc.

Main points: Front: Rangu (KI 2), Taixi (KI 3), Sanyinjiao (SP 6), Zusanli (ST 36), Neiguan (PC 6).

Back points: Pishu (BL 20), Shenshu (BL 23), Geshu (BL 17).

Yuji (LU 10) is added for thirst; Neiting (ST 44) for voracious appetite; Guanyuan (CV 4) for polyuria; Weizhong (BL 40), Chengshan (BL 57), Kunlun (BL 60) penetrating to Taixi (KI 3) for pain or numbness of the lower limbs; Taichong (LR 3) and Renying (ST 9) for hypertension; Tianshu (ST 25), Zhigou (TE 6) and Fenglong (ST 40) for constipation; Tianshu (ST 25), Shangjuxu (ST 37) and Xiajuxu (ST 39) for diarrhoea; Jingming (BL 1) and Taichong (LR 3) for eye diseases; Shenmen (HT 7) and Neiguan (PC 6) for palpitations; Shenmen (HT 7) and Sanyinjiao (SP 6) for insomnia; Zhongwan (CV 12) and Neiguan (PC 6) for fullness in the chest; Shanzhong (CV 17) and Neiguan (PC 6) for chest pain; Hegu (LI 4) and Fuliu (KI 7) for sweating; Houxi (SI 3) and Yinxi (HT 6) for night sweating; Quchi (LI 11) and Xuehai (SP 10) for itching; Ligou (LR 5) for perineal itching; Dahe (KI 12), Guanyuan (CV 4) and Taichong (LR 3) for impotence; and moxibustion at Guanyuan (CV 4) and Shenque (CV 8) for deficiency Cold.

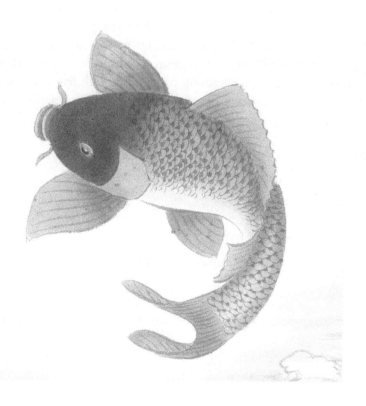

SECTION FOURTEEN • PALPITATIONS

CASE I: LU SHOUYAN'S MEDICAL RECORD

1. General data

Li, a man, aged 50.

2. Chief complaint

Palpitated subjectively.

3. History of present illness

He was disappointed because of defeat in his work before he got palpitations.

4. Present symptoms

Palpitations. With fear he couldn't sleep. Flushed face.

5. Tongue and pulse

Chi pulse thready weak, Cun pulse beating hard.

6. Differentiation and analysis

According to *Internal Classic* that 'over thinking and not satisfied' are the causes of depression. If prolonged, transformation to Fire and production of Phlegm, exhaustion of Yin Blood, and Phlegm stirred up by Fire to disturb the Heart will take place, in which the Blood fails to nourish the Heart, thus the Mind stored in the Heart is out of dependence, causing palpitations with fear and poor sleep. The patient is suffering from Phlegm Fire developed from Qi stagnation disturbing the Mind stored in the Heart, and this is the cause of his palpitations.

7. Diagnosis

TCM: Palpitations (Phlegm Fire disturbing Heart).

Western medicine: Palpitations.

8. Treating principle

Relax the chest, relieve depression, dissolve Phlegm, calm the Mind.

9. Prescription

Xinshu (BL 15), Juque (CV 14), Guanyuan (CV 4), Neiguan (PC 6), Fenglong (ST 40), Xingjian (LR 2).

    Reinforcing-reducing was done by means of lifting-thrusting. Guanyuan (CV 4) was reinforced, Neiguan (PC 6) reduced first and then manipulated to circulate Qi to the chest, Xinshu (BL 15) reduced first and reinforced (the technique *Yin Zhong Yin Yang*), and other points reduced.

10. Effect

Three treatments relieved his palpitations greatly and he was without fear thereafter. After 1 month he was treated again to consolidate the effect.

11. Essentials

Professor Lu selected Neiguan (PC 6) and Juque (CV 14) to relax the chest to relieve depression and calm the Mind, reduced Xingjian (LR 2) to soothe the Liver to remove Qi stagnation, reduced Neiguan (PC 6) to circulate Qi inside the chest and as a result achieved the immediate effect. Lu has his own knack in this method. Xinshu (BL 15) is reduced first to remove Fire and reinforced to astringe deficient Yang, which is known as *Yin Zhong Yin Yang*. Guanyuan (CV 4) is reinforced to replenish Essence to nourish Heart. Fenglong (ST 40) is reduced to dissolve Phlegm so as not to disturb the Heart. In this way, the palpitations are greatly relieved with 3 treatments and cured within 1 month.

YIN ZHONG YIN YANG: REDUCE FIRST AND THEN REINFORCE
Manipulate the needle at deep and shallow levels in the following way:

The needle is inserted to the deep level first and manipulated to reduce with 6 times of quick lifting and slow thrusting and then lifted to the shallow level and manipulated to reinforce with 9 times of quick thrusting and slow lifting. It is applied to treat the disease with Heat first and then Cold.

This is a technique opposite to **Yang Zhong Yin Yin** (see p.174). Both of them are indicated in complicated syndromes where there is deficiency and excess at the same time.

CASE II: CHENG XINNONG'S MEDICAL RECORD

1. General data

Wu, woman, aged 48, visited on May 11, 1992.

2. Chief complaint

Palpitations with shortness of breath for 4 years.

3. History of present illness

She went to have treatment in a hospital and was not found to have any organic disease.

4. Present symptoms

Palpitations, shortness of breath, insomnia, forgetfulness, dizziness, tinnitus, back soreness, dry stools. Less menstrual flow in irregular cycles, in dark colour and with clots. Lustreless complexion.

5. Tongue and pulse

Red tongue, small and with cracks, white coating, deep thready wiry pulse.

6. Differentiation and analysis

Blood deficiency gives rise to Fire, disturbing the Mind stored in the Heart, thus palpitations, shortness of breath and insomnia. Red small tongue and with cracks, and less menstrual flow imply Yin deficiency with internal Fire.

7. Diagnosis

TCM: Palpitations (Yin deficiency with Fire).

Western medicine: Palpitations.

8. Treating principle

Replenish Yin to reduce Fire, tranquillize Heart to calm the Mind.

9. Prescription

Juque (CV 14), Shanzhong (CV 17), Xinshu (BL 15), Shenshu (BL 23), Daling (PC 7), Neiguan (PC 6), Shenmen (HT 7), Sanyinjiao (SP 6), Taixi (KI 3), Taichong (LR 3).

Xinshu (BL 15) and Shenshu (BL 23) were punctured with quick needling; Sanyinjiao (SP 6) and Taixi (KI 3) with the reinforcing method; other points with even method.

10. Effect

After 1 course of treatment, she was relieved of palpitations and shortness of breath. With 2 more courses, although not in succession, for consolidation, she was kept in a steady condition with only occasional palpitations.

11. Essentials

Xinshu (BL 15), the Back-Shu, Juque (CV 14), the Front-Mu, Neiguan (PC 6), the Luo-Connecting, Shanzhong (CV 17), Influential point of Qi, function together to reinforce Qi to produce Blood to nourish the Heart to stop palpitations, and with other points in combination, to replenish Yin to reduce Fire and tranquillize the Heart to calm the Mind.

CASE III: ZHOU YUNXIAN'S MEDICAL RECORD

1. General data

He, female, 75 years old, a professor of China Central Academy of Fine Arts.

2. Chief complaint

Palpitations with precordial pain for 2 months.

3. History of present illness

Two months ago, she began to have precordial pain, about 10 times every day. The pain was stabbing in nature and accompanied with palpitations, shortness of breath, fullness in the chest, and tiredness all over the body. ECG showed left ventricular hypertrophy, S-T segment and T wave changes, as well as occasional ventricular premature beats. She was admitted in hospital and treated with both Chinese and Western medicines. She was discharged when her pathological condition got better.

4. Present symptoms

Precordial pain became occasional, but premature beats were frequent. A Western doctor advised her to install a pacemaker, but she refused the suggestion. She came for acupuncture treatment. Her appetite was normal, sleep good, urine and stools normal. BP: 130/86mmHg.

5. Tongue and pulse

Pale tongue, some purple spots on the tip and borders of the tongue, thin white coating; intermittent pulse with 5–6 missed beats per minute.

6. Differentiation and analysis

Because of the Heart Qi deficiency, the Blood circulation was getting slower, thus the Blood stasis of the Heart resulted in precordial pain. The Heart Qi was deficient causing palpitations and intermittent pulse. Qi deficiency failed to nourish the tongue, so pale tongue. Purple spots on the tongue indicated the Blood stasis.

7. Diagnosis

TCM: Heart pain.

Western medicine: Coronary heart disease.

8. Treating principle

Reinforce the Heart Qi, activate Blood circulation, dissolve Blood stasis. Select points mainly from the Heart and Pericardium meridians. Use Back-Shu and Front-Mu points.

9. Prescription

Xinshu (BL 15), Jueyinshu (BL 14), Geshu (BL 17), Shanzhong (CV 17), Juque (CV 14), Qihai (CV 6), Neiguan (PC 6), Zusanli (ST 36), Sanyinjiao (SP 6). Even method.

10. Effect

After 1 treatment, the attacks of her precordial pain were greatly reduced. One course of treatment made the pain basically stop. Her ventricular premature beats were significantly decreased with 2 courses of treatment.

11. Essentials

This is a case of Heart Qi deficiency and Heart Blood stagnation. The combination of Back-Shu and Front-Mu points, Xinshu (BL 15) and Juque (CV 14), Jueyinshu (BL 14) and Shanzhong (CV 17), is good at treating heart diseases. Geshu (BL 17) is to activate Blood and dissolve stasis. Qihai (CV 6) reinforces and circulates Qi. The Luo-Connecting point of the Pericardium Meridian, Neiguan (PC 6), one of the Confluent points, is effective for Heart and chest diseases, and here, promotes Blood circulation too. Sanyinjiao (SP 6) is to conduct Blood and to treat the heart diseases as well.

SUMMARY

Palpitations, known as Jing Ji in Chinese medicine, are treated with the Back-Shu and Front-Mu points in combination.

Main points: Xinshu (BL 15), Juque (CV 14), Shenmen (HT 7), Neiguan (PC 6).

For those who are with Heart Blood deficiency, add Pishu (BL 20) and Weishu (BL 21) to promote Blood production; for Yin deficiency with Fire, add Ganshu (BL 18), Taixi (KI 3), Shenshu (BL 23) and Taichong (LR 3) to replenish Yin to smooth the Liver and communicate between the Heart and Kidneys; for Yang deficiency with Damp retention, add Guanyuan (CV 4), Shanzhong (CV 17) and Zusanli (ST 36) to strengthen the Spleen to dissolve Damp; for getting frightened all of a sudden, add Sishencong (EX-HN1) and Yintang (EX-HN3) to tranquillize and calm the Mind.

SECTION FIFTEEN • BU MEI (INSOMNIA)

CASE I: LU SHOUYAN'S MEDICAL RECORD

1. General data

Li, a man, aged 33.

2. Chief complaint

Difficulty in falling asleep for half a year.

3. History of present illness

His sleep problem became worse recently.

4. Present symptoms

Difficulty in falling asleep, and complicated by dizziness, tinnitus, dry throat, irritability, seminal emission and lumbar soreness.

5. Tongue and pulse

Red tongue, little coating, thready rapid pulse.

6. Differentiation and analysis

The Heart is the house of the Mind and the Kidneys the house of Essence. The dizziness, tinnitus, seminal emission and lumbar soreness are the signs of deficiency of Kidney Essence; dry throat and irritability are those of Yin deficiency with Fire; red tongue and rapid pulse mean Fire flaring up.

7. Diagnosis

TCM: Insomnia (disharmony between Heart and Kidney).

Western medicine: Insomnia.

8. Treating principle

Strengthen Water to control Fire, harmonize Heart and Kidneys.

9. Prescription

Xinshu (BL 15), Shenshu (BL 23), Shenmen (HT 7), Sanyinjiao (SP 6).

Moxibustion with 3 grain-sized cones was done at Xinshu (BL 15). Lifting-thrusting needling without retaining was done at other points. Shenshu (BL 23) and Sanyinjiao (SP 6) were reinforced; Shenmen (HT 7) reduced.

10. Effect

Second visit: His condition was improved. Red tongue, thready pulse.

Jueyinshu (BL 14), Shenshu (BL 23), Sanyinjiao (SP 6), Taixi (KI 3), Shenmen (HT 7), Neiguan (PC 6).

Moxibustion with 3 grain-sized cones was done at Jueyinshu (BL 14). Lifting-thrusting needling without retaining was done at other points. Shenshu (BL 23), Sanyinjiao (SP 6) and Taixi (KI 3) were reinforced; Shenmen (HT 7) and Neiguan (PC 6) reduced.

Third visit: He was able to have deep sleep and felt much stronger. His dizziness, tinnitus, dry throat and irritability disappeared. Red tongue, little coating, thready pulse. The treating principle was still to harmonize Heart and Kidneys assisted by reinforcing and regulating the Spleen and Stomach to produce Blood to tranquilize the Mind to consolidating the effect.

Neiguan (PC 6), Shenmen (HT 7), Sanyinjiao (SP 6), Pishu (BL 20), Zusanli (ST 36), Taixi (KI 3).

Lifting-thrusting needling without retaining was done. Neiguan (PC 6) and Shenmen (HT 7) were reduced; other points reinforced.

11. Essentials

Professor Lu treated him with the principle of strengthening Water to control Fire and harmonize Heart and Kidneys. Moxibustion with 3 cones done at Xinshu (BL 15) was to drive the Fire out. Reduce Shenmen (HT 7) to clear Heart Fire to tranquilize the Mind. Reinforce Shenshu (BL 23) and Sanyinjiao (SP 6) to strengthen Water to control Fire. On the second visit, moxibustion with 3 cones at Jueyinshu (BL 14) was to reduce Heart Fire, reduce Neiguan (PC 6) to tranquilize the Mind, and reinforce Taixi (KI 3) to replenish Water. On the third visit, moxibustion was not used, but with Pishu (BL 20) and Zusanli (ST 36) added to strengthen Spleen and Stomach to produce Blood to calm the Mind. Three treatments cured his half a year's insomnia successfully.

CASE II: XIAO SHAOQING'S MEDICAL RECORD

1. General data

Li, a lady, aged 67, visited on October 24, 1994.

2. Chief complaint

Insomnia for more than 30 years, worse for 1 year.

3. History of present illness

One year ago, her insomnia became worse because of the death of her husband. She couldn't sleep without hypnotics. She began to have indigestion with diarrhoea after a cholecystectomy in 1992.

4. Present symptoms

Difficulty in falling asleep, dream-disturbed sleep, accompanied by dizziness, dull expression, depression. Overthinking with anxiety and poor appetite. Loose stools.

5. Tongue and pulse

Pale tongue, white sticky coating, wiry rolling pulse.

6. Differentiation and analysis

This patient is generally overthinking. Especially with the emotional depression, her stagnated Liver Qi is worse and attacking the Middle Burner, the Qi of which is disturbed by the cholecystectomy, hence the Spleen and Stomach are weak, so Phlegm is produced. The stagnated Liver Qi and Phlegm disturb the Heart, causing restlessness of Mind, thus poor sleep.

7. Diagnosis

TCM: Insomnia (Phlegm retention with Qi stagnation, restlessness of Mind).

Western medicine: Insomnia.

8. Treating principle

Dissolve Phlegm, relieve stagnation, tranquillize the Heart, calm the Mind.

9. Prescription

Baihui (GV 20), Yintang (EX-HN3), Dingshen (Extra), Shenmen (HT 7), Jiangshi (PC 5), Zusanli (ST 36), Fenglong (ST 40), Sanyinjiao (SP 6), Taichong (LR 3).

Even method was adopted, the needles retained for 20 minutes and manipulated every 10 minutes. Once every day.

10. Effect

On the second visit she said that she felt better after needling, but still did not sleep well. The same treatment was given to her. On the third visit, she said she slept for 5 hours without taking hypnotics. After 1 course of treatment, she could sleep about 10 hours. The nightmares stopped. Her appetite improved. Her pulse was a bit slow but forceful and her tongue and coating tended towards normal.

11. Essentials

Professor Xiao used Yintang (EX-HN3) and Dingshen (Extra) in combination with Baihui (GV 20) to clear obstruction of the Governor Vessel to wake up the Mind; used Shenmen (HT 7) and Jiangshi (PC 5) to calm the Mind for resourcefulness; used Zusanli (ST 36), Sanyinjiao (SP 6) and Fenglong (ST 40) to strengthen the Spleen to dissolve Phlegm; used Taichong (LR 3) to soothe the Liver to regulate Qi.

The successful treatment is derived from the principle of dissolving Phlegm, regulating stagnated Qi, and calming the Mind stored in the Heart.

> **DINGSHEN**
>
> Dingshen (Extra) is located at the conjunction of the lower and middle one third of the philtrum. Pinch the skin, insert a 3 cun filiform needle horizontally about 2.5 cun with an angle of 15° quickly to the subcutaneous level. It produces very strong soreness and distention. After a while, the patient will feel relaxed and can even fall asleep quickly. This is Professor Xiao's established point for insomnia with irritability. Xiao uses it to treat mental disorders such as epilepsy and so on and gets good results too.

CASE III: CHENG XINNONG'S MEDICAL RECORD

1. General data

Wu, a man, aged 59, visited on September 12, 1992.

2. Chief complaint

Poor sleep over 30 years.

3. History of present illness

In the last 3 years, he couldn't sleep at all without hypnotics. Two years ago, his blood test showed a higher bilirubin and he was diagnosed with gastrointestinal dysfunction.

4. Present symptoms

Difficulty in falling asleep, dream-disturbed sleep, especially when tired. Epigastric fullness, poor appetite, diarrhoea after drinking milk, soreness in lumbar region, frequent flatulence, bowel movements 2–3 times a day.

5. Tongue and pulse

Purplish tongue, tip red, white coating, wiry pulse.

6. Differentiation and analysis

The Spleen dominates transportation and transformation of food Essence and sends the essential substance upward to nourish. When it is too weak to function well, the Heart will lack nourishment. The Stomach receives food and sends the roughly digested food down. When its Qi goes up instead of going down normally, the Mind stored in the Heart will be disturbed, thus causing insomnia.

7. Diagnosis

TCM: Insomnia (disharmony between Spleen and Stomach).

Western medicine: Insomnia.

8. Treating principle

Strengthen Spleen, harmonize Stomach, rest the Heart, calm the Mind.

9. Prescription

Zhongwan (CV 12), Tianshu (ST 25), Qihai (CV 6), Neiguan (PC 6), Shenmen (HT 7), Zusanli (ST 36), Sanyinjiao (SP 6), Taixi (KI 3).
 Qihai (CV 6) and Zusanli (ST 36) were reinforced; others even method.

10.Effect

With 4 courses of treatment, his Spleen and Stomach symptoms were greatly relieved and his sleep was better. Hypnotics dosage was half reduced. Another 4 courses, although intermittent, made him sleep 6–8 hours each night without taking hypnotics any more. He was cured.

11.Essentials

Zhongwan (CV 12), Tianshu (ST 25), Qihai (CV 6) and Zusanli (ST 36) are selected to promote the Spleen in transportation and transformation and harmonize the Stomach in digestion; Neiguan (PC 6), Shenmen (HT 7) and Sanyinjiao (SP 6) are the established points for insomnia; Neiguan (PC 6), Luo-Connecting, Shenmen (HT 7), Yuan-Source, Sanyinjiao (SP 6), the meeting point of the Spleen, Liver and Kidney channels are to rest the Heart and calm the Mind. Taixi (KI 3) and Shenmen (HT 7) harmonize the Heart and Kidneys.

CASE IV: ZHOU YUNXIAN'S MEDICAL RECORD

1. General data

Wang, female, 45 years old, a finance manager.

2. Chief complaint

Insomnia for 5 years, worse in the recent 6 months.

3. History of present illness

Because the patient had responsibility for financial management in a company, she had mental tension. Gradually she had difficulty in falling asleep and awakened from sleep. Every night she could only sleep for 3–4 hours or could not sleep at all. Therefore she had to take sleeping pills every day, from 1 to 4 tablets. Later she took herbal medicine, but this was not effective either. She came for acupuncture treatment.

4. Present symptoms

In the recent 6 months, her irritability and anxiety became aggravated, so her insomnia was aggravated. Dream-disturbed sleep caused her tiredness, poor memory, palpitations and poor appetite. Urine and stools were normal. Menstrual flow was less than before.

5. Tongue and pulse

Red swollen tongue, toothmarks, little and dry coating; string-taut thready pulse, a little rapid.

6. Differentiation and analysis

The work pressure is the cause of Liver Qi stagnation, so she has irritability, hot temper, and anxiety. The prolonged Qi stagnation is transformed into Fire, disturbing the Mind stored in the Heart, so she has dream-disturbed sleep and palpitations. The Liver overacts on the Spleen, leading to the poor Blood production, and anxiety exhausts the Heart Blood, the Mind stored in the Heart becomes lacking in nourishment, so her insomnia gets worse. The Heart and Spleen deficiency results in tiredness, listlessness, and poor memory. Red swollen tongue with dry little coating and toothmarks indicates Spleen Qi deficiency and Heart Yin deficiency. String-taut thready rapid pulse shows the Liver stagnation causing Heat and Qi and Yin deficiency too.

7. Diagnosis

TCM: Insomnia.

Western medicine: Anxiety.

8. Treating principle

Soothe the Liver, clear Heat, nourish the Heart, calm the Mind. Select points mainly from the Liver, Heart, and Pericardium meridians, and use Governor Vessel points and Back-Shu points.

9. Prescription

Baihui (GV 20), Sishencong (EX-HN1), Shenmen (HT 7), Neiguan (PC 6), Sanyinjiao (SP 6), Zusanli (ST 36), Qihai (CV 6), Taichong (LR 3), Ganshu (BL 18), Xinshu (BL 15), Pishu (BL 20).
   Even method.

10. Effect

Six treatments seemed not to have very much effect. After 7 treatments she began to have better sleep, so she was relaxed during the daytime and getting better in spirits. After that she went to bed at 10 o'clock in the evening and could sleep to 5 o'clock in the morning, and even if awakened during the night, she could fall asleep again. Totally she was treated for 15 times.

11. Essentials

Liver Qi stagnation, Heat Yin deficiency, Spleen Qi deficiency.

Baihui (GV 20) and Sishencong (EX-HN1) for calming the Mind. Neiguan (PC 6), Shenmen (HT 7), Sanyinjiao (SP 6), and Xinshu (BL 15) for nourishing the Heart and calming the Mind. Ganshu (BL 18) and Taichong (LR 3) for soothing the Liver and clearing Heat so to nourish the Liver. Zusanli (ST 36) and Qihai (CV 6) for strengthening the Spleen to reinforce Qi and Blood. The Heart Yin is nourished sufficient, calming the Mind is realized, therefore she could sleep well.

SUMMARY

'Yang enters into Yin, you sleep. Yang comes out of Yin, you wake up.' Zhang Jingyue: 'Sleep depends on Yin that nourishes the Mind. The Mind rests well, you sleep well. The Mind is restless, you can't sleep well.' The restlessness of the Mind results from the invasion of pathological factors or poor nourishment. Heart and Spleen deficiency, Yin deficiency with Fire, Liver and Gallbladder Fire and disharmony of the Stomach are common causes of insomnia. The treating principle is to rest the Heart and calm the Mind. The stimulation of acupuncture should not be strong, avoiding disturbing the Mind.

Main points: Shenmen (HT 7), Neiguan (PC 6), Sanyinjiao (SP 6).

Xinshu (BL 15) and Pishu (BL 20) are added for Heart and Spleen deficiency; Xinshu (BL 15), Shenshu (BL 23), Taixi (KI 3) added for Yin deficiency with Fire, or select Zhaohai (KI 6) to regulate the Qiao-Heel channels; Ganshu (BL 18), Danshu (BL 19), Xingjian (LR 2), Wangu (GB 12) added for Liver and Gallbladder Fire; Weishu (BL 21), Zhongwan (CV 12), Zusanli (ST 36) are added for disharmony of the Stomach.

SECTION SIXTEEN • HEADACHE

CASE I: CHENG XINNONG'S MEDICAL RECORD

1. General data

Li, male, aged 52, first visited on November 22, 1985.

2. Chief complaint

Paroxysmal headache at the right parietal region for 4 days.

3. History of present illness

He began to have the headache on the top of his head due to being busy at work.

4. Present symptoms

The unendurable headache lasted seconds with an interval of 10–30 minutes each time, accompanied by dizziness, palpitations, poor sleep, bitter taste in mouth, hot temper, irritability, and dry stools.

5. Tongue and pulse

Border and tip of his tongue red, yellow coating in the middle, wiry pulse.

6. Differentiation and analysis

His busy work causes the Liver Fire to flare up. The stagnated Qi of Liver transforms into Fire and it is likely to transmit to Gallbladder because of their exterior–interior relation. This is the reason for his dizziness, bitter taste in mouth, hot temper and irritability. Yellow coating and wiry pulse imply the Fire of Liver and Gallbladder.

7. Diagnosis

TCM: Headache (Liver Fire rushing upward).

Western medicine: Angioneurotic headache.

8. Treating principle

Clear Liver and Gallbladder Fire, remove obstruction of channels, stop pain.

9. Prescription

Baihui (GV 20), Fengchi (GB 20), Neiguan (PC 6), Hegu (LI 4), Taichong (LR 3), Yanglingquan (GB 34). Right side: Shuaigu (GB 8). Ashi.

10. Effect

He just came with the onset of the headache. Acupuncture was applied and his headache stopped. On the following day, he said he only had 2 episodes of head-ache with mild pain. It stopped completely with 3 treatments. Two more treatments of acupuncture were applied to consolidate the effect. The follow-up found no recurrence.

11. Essentials

Hegu (LI 4), Taichong (LR 3), Yanglingquan (GB 34) are selected to clear the Fire of Liver and Gallbladder; Fengchi (GB 20) to eliminate Wind blocked in channels; Ashi to stop pain; Baihui (GV 20) to clear Fire by bringing it down; Neiguan (PC 6) to rest the Heart and calm the Mind. The pain is stopped because the Liver is restored in keeping the free flow of Qi, the Fire is cleared away, and the obstruction of the channels is removed.

CASE II: SUN LIUHE'S MEDICAL RECORD

1. General data

Anonymous male, aged 37.

2. Chief complaint

A jumping pain in the forehead for months.

3. History of present illness

Every day the jumping pain started after breakfast without clear inducing factors.

4. Present symptoms

Jumping pain in the forehead after breakfast and getting gradually worse, becoming better after lunch and stopped slowly. Dry stools.

5. Tongue and pulse

Red tongue, thin yellow coating, surging pulse.

6. Differentiation and analysis

The pain is in the forehead and starts at Mao which is the flowing time of Yangming Large Intestine Channel, indicating Yangming excess Heat syndrome. Dry stools and surging pulse are the typical symptoms of Yangming excess Heat.

7. Diagnosis

TCM: Yangming headache (excess Heat).

Western medicine: Angioneurotic headache.

8. Treating principle

Reduce Heat to stop pain.

9. Prescription

Neiting (ST 44), Hegu (LI 4).

10. Effect

He was cured with 1 week of treatment.

11. Essentials

Neiting (ST 44), a lower point for upper disease, is selected to bring down the Heat, and the Ying-Spring point, to clear Yangming Heat; Hegu (LI 4), Yuan-Source point, to be reduced to clear Heat to stop pain. This is the combination of upper and lower points.

 If the stabbing pain is in the forehead, in the evening or irregular, dark purple tongue, hesitant pulse, this is the Blood stasis syndrome of headache. Hegu (LI 4), Shoumian (Extra, points on the forehead along the affected channel), Geshu (BL 17), Xuehai (SP 10), Weizhong (BL 40) are selected, with Neiyingxiang (Extra) added for serious cases. Of the points, Hegu (LI 4) and Shoumian (Extra) are selected according to the channel differentiation and others according to syndrome differentiation. Geshu (BL 17), Xuehai (SP 10), Weizhong (BL 40) activate Blood circulation to remove Blood stasis; Neiyingxiang (Extra), the important point for Yangming headache, especially for the serious case, is pricked with a #26 or 28 needle to the root of the nose to bleed 3–5ml dark Blood.

CASE III: SUN LIUHE'S MEDICAL RECORD

1. General data

Anonymous male, aged 26.

2. Chief complaint

Temporal headache after traumatic injury.

3. History of present illness

His headache was stabbing in nature and not relieved by half a month's acupuncture at Fengchi (GB 20), Waiguan (TE 5) and points in the temporal region in the hospital of his hometown.

4. Present symptoms

Stabbing headache.

5. Tongue and pulse

Blood spots on the tongue, wiry hesitant pulse.

6. Differentiation and analysis

This is the Blood stasis syndrome of Shaoyang headache after trauma. Blood spots on the tongue and wiry hesitant pulse imply Blood stasis as well.

7. Diagnosis

TCM: Shaoyang headache (Blood stasis).

Western medicine: Traumatic headache.

8. Treating principle

Activate Blood circulation, remove Blood stasis, stop pain.

9. Prescription

Fengchi (GB 20), Zulinqi (GB 41), Xuehai (SP 10), Geshu (BL 17).

When puncturing Fengchi (GB 20), after the heaviness and distention appeared, the needle was rotated with the thumb forward to direct the needling sensation to the temporal region.

10. Essentials

For this Blood stasis syndrome of Shaoyang headache, Fengchi (GB 20) is selected to activate Blood circulation; Zulinqi (GB 41), the Wood point of the Wood Channel, to clear the Heat of the Gallbladder to stop pain; Xuehai (SP 10) and Geshu (BL 17) to remove Blood stasis to stop pain.

If the headache is characterized by a sensation like being wrapped with bandages and is accompanied by dizziness and nausea and vomiting, it is the Phlegm retention syndrome of Shaoyang headache. Touwei (ST 8) penetrating to Jiaosun (TE 20) may be adopted with 3 cun inserted, and the needling sensation should be led to the temporal region. Touwei (ST 8) is indicated in Damp and Phlegm, and Jiaosun (TE 20) is a local point; Zhongwan (CV 12) and Neiguan (PC 6) to regulate Qi, dissolve Phlegm, eliminate Damp, and remove obstruction of channels.

CASE IV: SUN LIUHE'S MEDICAL RECORD

1. General data

Anonymous female, aged 42.

2. Chief complaint

Hollow-like headache at the top of the head for 2 years.

3. History of present illness

Her hollow-like headache at the top of the head lasted more than 2 years, frequent acupuncture treatment was not effective for her.

4. Present symptoms

Hollow-like headache at the top of the head, worse when the head was moved. Poor sleep.

5. Tongue and pulse

6. Differentiation and analysis

Hollow-like headache at the top of the head is indicative of Liver and Kidney Yin deficiency.

7. Diagnosis

TCM: Jueyin headache (Yin deficiency of Liver and Kidneys).

Western medicine: Headache.

8. Treating principle

Reinforce Liver and Kidneys, remove obstruction, stop pain.

9. Prescription

Yongquan (KI 1), Taixi (KI 3), Baihui (GV 20).

10. Effect

Several times of treatment cured her. But 1 year later she had the headache again. The same treatment was applied and it was effective again.

11. Essentials

For the headache on the top of the head caused by Liver and Kidney Yin deficiency, Yongquan (KI 1) is selected to replenish Kidney Water to reinforce the mother of

Liver, Taixi (KI 3) is to replenish Yin of the Liver and Kidneys, and Baihui (GV 20) to bring the channel Qi up to the affected area. All three points are exactly opposed to Yin deficiency of Liver and Kidney and affected channels, thus there is an immediate effect, just as *Zhou Hou Ge* (*A Handbook of Points in Verse*) says: 'For the headache on the top with difficulties in opening eyes, puncture Yongquan (KI 1) to keep fit.'

CASE V: HU JINSHENG'S MEDICAL RECORD

1. General data

Hua, female, 30 years old, from Inner Mongolia.

2. Chief complaint

Headache with repeated attacks for 20 years.

3. History of present illness

From the year when she was 10 years old, she began to have headaches because she was attacked by Wind Cold on the evening of Spring Festival in Celebration Party. Medication stopped her headache. But later, whenever she was exposed to Wind Cold or when the weather changed, she would experience the onset of her headache which would only be relieved by painkillers. The suffering had lasted for 20 years already. CT scanning and other examinations didn't find any abnormalities. Various kinds of treatment, herbs and drugs, didn't help much.

4. Present symptoms

The headache lasted for several hours every day. It was on the top of her head, a little to the left side, started with a jumping feeling and then changed to distending pain, accompanied by irritability, hot temper, and nausea. The pain changed her manner, she became irritable and excited, quarrelled with people often, and used to have the notion of making light of her life. She felt tired all over the body after the headache, had sweating, insomnia with dream-disturbed sleep, and this was accompanied by discomfort in the epigastric region, large quantity of menstrual flow with Blood clots, and distending pain in the lower abdomen.

5. Tongue and pulse

Dark tongue with Blood spots on it, toothmarks on the borders, thin white coating; deep thready and string-taut pulse.

6. Differentiation and analysis

At the beginning, it was the Wind Cold that caused her Shaoyang headache. The pain lasting for 20 years made the Zang Fu organs become involved. The irritability, hot temper, and string-taut pulse were the manifestations of Liver Yang hyperactivity. Insomnia with dream-disturbed sleep, and thready pulse indicated the Heart Blood deficiency owing to the Mind stored in the Heart being poorly nourished. Discomfort in the epigastric region, nausea, and tiredness were the result of dysfunctions of the Spleen and Stomach. The fixed location of her headache and Blood clots in the menstrual flow and dark tongue with Blood spots on it showed the excess nature of disease. In this complicated case, the Liver, Gallbladder, Heart, Spleen and Stomach were all involved, and together with the Blood stasis, presenting a pathological condition of both deficiency and excess.

7. Diagnosis

TCM: Headache (invasion of Wind Cold, prolonged to Blood stasis).

Western medicine: Neurovascular headache.

8. Treating principle

Dispel Wind Cold, remove obstruction of meridians and collaterals.

9. Prescription

Acupuncture on Baihui (GV 20), Fengchi (GB 20), Shuaigu (GB 8), Taiyang (EX-HN5), Waiguan (TE 5), Neiguan (PC 6), Hegu (LI 4), Xuehai (SP 10), Sanyinjiao (SP 6), Zulinqi (GB 41), Taichong (LR 3), Ashi.

Moxibustion to dispel Wind Cold. Bloodletting to remove Blood stasis.

10. Effect

In the first course of treatment, acupuncture was applied and moxibustion was done at the left side of the top of her head, each time for 30 minutes. After 5 treatments, she was getting sensitive to the moxibustion warmth, and her headache was becoming relieved. In the second course, bloodletting with the three-edged needle at Ashi points and Taiyang (EX-HN5) was given twice a week. After 4 times of bloodletting, her headache was much relieved. Although the headache on the left or right side appeared alternatively, it was mild only. The above-mentioned treatment was carried out for 6 courses, which consisted of 3 courses of moxibustion, 6 times of bloodletting, 60 times of acupuncture, after which her headache stopped and other symptoms improved. The treatment lasted for 3 months in all.

11. Essentials

Her headache which was caused by invasion of Wind Cold was not cured quickly, so the pathogenic factors stayed in the meridians and collaterals, resulting in repeated attacks, especially on Wind Cold days. This is known as 'head Wind' or 'thunder head Wind', a serious condition of headache. In the Wind Cold days, the Wind Cold in the meridians and collaterals will be stirred up, causing the headache attack; this is exactly the characteristics of 'head Wind'. The meridians and collaterals are blocked by the Wind Cold, and if prolonged, Blood stasis will occur. TCM says that 'prolonged pain enters the collaterals' which is just the result of Blood stasis from the prolonged pain. Analyzed from the relation of exterior and interior, this case is a complicated one, showing the changes from, at the beginning the invasion of Wind Cold to the meridians and collaterals, to the later prolonged involvement of the Zang Fu organs, the Liver, Gallbladder, Heart, Spleen and Stomach.

CASE VI: LIU TAOXIN'S MEDICAL RECORD

1. General data

A female, 28, first visited in December 1999.

2. Chief complaint

Headache for 1 year.

3. History of present illness

Headache for 1 year. It became worse in spring and even worse because of whip-lash syndrome due to a car accident in summer time. The most aching area was in the occipital-nape region and next was in the vertex region. Aching referred to the ears. Dizziness might accompany it. She also felt dazed and her left Jingming (B 1) area felt cold. She was allergic to all kinds of light such as sunlight, lamplight and candlelight and was confined to dark rooms almost all the time. She was allergic to the smell in her house and the smell in a new house still made her nauseous. Low spirits because of the trouble.

She felt tired and was afraid of cold. Her sacral region was always cold.

She preferred warm food and drinks. Her sleep was OK. Her bowel movement and urination were normal. Menses normal.

No treatment in Western medicine.

4. Present symptoms

Headache; muddle-headed; heavy of head; cold sensation in left Jingming (B 1) area; lustreless face.

5. Tongue and pulse

White tongue-coating; fairly slow and deep pulse.

6. Differentiation and analysis

Deficiency of Yang Qi producing Cold which moved to the head.

Deficiency of Yang Qi resulted in preference for warm food and drinks, aversion to cold, fatigue, cold sacral region, white tongue-coating and fairly slow and deep pulse. Pathogenic Cold was produced internally and went up to affect the Bladder Meridian and Liver Meridian causing headache and cold sensation in the left eye region.

7. Diagnosis

TCM: Taiyang headache and Jueyin headache.

Western diagnosis: Headache requiring further examination.

8. Treating principle

To reinforce Yang Qi with warmth to disperse Cold and stop headache.

9. Prescription

Moxibustion to Baihui (Du 20), Shenshu (BL 23) and Yongquan (K 1).

Moxibustion to Baihui (Du 20) could warm local Yang Qi to disperse Cold and moxibustion to Shenshu (BL 23) could reinforce primary Yang. The lowest point Yongquan (KI 1) echoing the highest point Baihui (Du 20) could treat disorders at the vertex. Yongquan (KI 1) was selected also because the aching at the occipital-nape region was severe and the Kidney Meridian and Bladder Meridian were exteriorly–interiorly related.

10. Effect

Second visit: Headache reduced greatly after last treatment and the patient felt very happy. She told the doctor that she forgot to mention something during her first visit and she did not know if it was significant.

The story was that she came from Iceland and when she was there one evening she opened the Window for ventilation when her friends left. She felt tired and lay down to take a short rest. She fell asleep. She was frozen, with frost covering her hair and unable to move when she woke up. She decided that she would not die like this and tried very hard to move. She did not know how long it was before she fell from the bed, crawled to the bathroom and managed to turn on the hot water and she survived. Headache started then.

This was very important information which not only told the cause of her problem but also explained why she was so afraid of light. Generally speaking patients suffering from excess of Yin due to Yang deficiency liked anything Yang such as light but this case was an exceptional one because the Cold was so severe that it rejected Yang in an extreme way. What was more was that this extra information corrected the previous differentiation of syndromes although the therapeutic effect had been good. Previous differentiation of syndromes regarded this case as an excess due to deficiency (root cause) but actually deficiency was caused by excess (injury of Yang due to extremely strong Cold). The same points were used but the order was changed to apply moxibustion to Yongquan (KI 1) first and then Shenshu (BL 23) and then Baihui (Du 20) so as to make warmth going upwards.

Third visit: Almost all symptoms disappeared.

Fourth treatment: Cure achieved after 4 treatments.

11. Essentials

The routine order of moxibustion in ancient times was to operate on Yang regions first, and then Yin regions (upper part of the body first and then lower part of the body; back and lower back first and then chest and abdomen etc.). Nowadays, more doctors prefer to prescribe one point in the upper part of the body and another one in the lower part of the body so as to guide Fire Qi down. This patient had an exceptional condition of the worst Cold-injured area in the head so that the doctor changed the order of operation and it worked miraculously. This experience showed that the clinical treating method was very elastic and the therapeutic effect was everything.

SUMMARY

The head is the place where all the Yang channels meet, and clean Yang Qi of the six Fu organs and the Essence of the five Zang organs all flow upward to it. In any case of derangement of Qi and Blood leading to obstruction of channels in the head, no matter whether caused by exogenous or endogenous factors, headache will be the outcome.

Exogenous headache is manifested as quick onset and non-stop pain with the neck and back involved. Wind Cold headache is characterized by aversion to wind and cold and superficial tight pulse; Wind Heat headache by a distending pain, fever and superficial rapid pulse; Wind Damp headache by a bandage-wrapped sensation and accompanied by heaviness and tiredness of the body and limbs, and soft pulse.

Endogenous headache is manifested as slow onset and accompanied by dizziness. Headache due to upsurge of Liver-Yang, including Liver Fire and Liver Wind, relates to Kidney deficiency failing to irrigate Wood and Blood deficiency failing to nourish Liver, manifesting a wiry pulse. Headache due to deficiency of Qi and Blood manifests as a dull pain with dizziness, becoming worse when tired, and the pulse is thready weak.

For treatment, the reducing method is adopted for excess syndrome while the reinforcing method is adopted for deficiency syndrome.

Main points: Baihui (GV 20), Fengchi (GB 20), Taiyang (EX-HN5), Hegu (LI 4).

Frontal headache is involved with the Yangming Channel, and known as Yangming headache; Touwei (ST 8), Yintang (EX-HN3) and Zanzhu (BL 2) should be added.

Occipital headache is involved with the Taiyang Channel, and known as Taiyang headache; Tianzhu (BL 10), Houxi (SI 3) and Kunlun (BL 60) should be added. For an intractable case of occipital headache, Zhiyin (BL 67) should be added, as it is said in *Zhou Hou Ge* (*A Handbook of Points in Verse*): 'Puncture Zhiyin (BL 67) for the diseases of head and face.'

Migraine is the headache involved with the Shaoyang Channel, and known as Shaoyang headache; Shuaigu (GB 8), Waiguan (TE 5) and Zulinqi (GB 41) should be added.

Parietal headache is involved with the Jueyin Channel, and known as Jueyin headache; Tongtian (BL 7) and Taichong (LR 3) should be added.

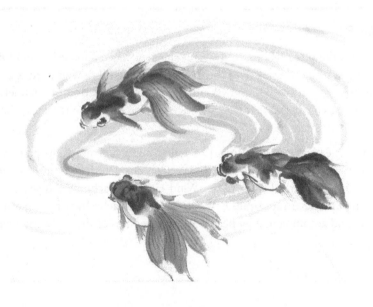

SECTION SEVENTEEN • XUAN YUN (DIZZINESS)

CASE I: CHENG XINNONG'S MEDICAL RECORD

1. General data

Xia, male, 62. May 27, 1985.

2. Chief complaint

Dizziness and nausea for 20 days.

3. History of present illness

Twenty days ago, he felt suddenly dizzy and nauseous and could not open his eyes. Diagnosed 'cerebral arteriosclerosis', he was treated with medication in a hospital. He was better after treatment.

4. Present symptoms

He felt dizzy, heavy in the head, could not open his eyes and his ears were obstructed. Generally he was in a hot temper. He had a bitter taste in his mouth, dry stools, poor appetite, and thirst without desire to drink.

5. Tongue and pulse

Dark red tongue, yellow and slightly thick coating, wiry pulse.

6. Differentiation and analysis

'All the Wind diseases and dizziness are due to the Liver disorders.' This patient's problem is caused by the stagnant Liver Qi transforming into Fire, Spleen deficiency leading to Damp retention in the Middle Burner, clean Yang failing to ascend. As Zhu Danxi said: 'Without Phlegm, there will not be dizziness. Phlegm is brought up by Wind.' Bitter taste in mouth, yellow thick coating, and wiry pulse also imply the Phlegm Heat.

7. Diagnosis

TCM: Dizziness (Phlegm Damp retention in Middle Burner).

Western medicine: Cerebral arteriosclerosis.

8. Treating principle

Pacify Liver, subdue Yang, dissolve Phlegm, regulate Middle Burner.

9. Prescription

Baihui (GV 20), Fengchi (GB 20), Taiyang (EX-HN5), Hegu (LI 4), Taichong (LR 3), Yanglingquan (GB 34), Zusanli (ST 36), Fenglong (ST 40), Sanyinjiao (SP 6).

Taichong (LR 3) and Yanglingquan (GB 34) were reduced. Moxibustion was done at Sanyinjiao (SP 6). Even method was used on the other points.

10. Effect

The patient said that with moxibustion at Sanyinjiao (SP 6), he felt the warmth going from his abdomen up to his chest and then down to the lower abdomen. After waking up after noon, he was thirsty and drank 5 cups of water and his dizziness was greatly relieved. With 30 treatments, all his symptoms were relieved. He felt especially better with covering on the abdomen and back to keep the warmth.

11. Essentials

Baihui (GV 20), located in the middle of the top of the head, entering into the brain, brings clean Yang up and disperses Qi and Blood. Hegu (LI 4) and Taichong (LR 3) reduce Liver Fire. Fengchi (GB 20) helps Taiyang (EX-HN5) to subdue the flared Yang in the head. Yanglingquan (GB 34) clears Liver Fire. Zusanli (ST 36) and Sanyinjiao (SP 6) reinforce the Middle Burner and strengthen Spleen and Stomach. Fenglong (ST 40) dissolves Phlegm. The dizziness was cured by treatment for a month.

CASE II: CHENG XINNONG'S MEDICAL RECORD

1. General data

Wang, female, 32. April 9, 1992.

2. Chief complaint

Dizziness for more than 1 month.

3. History of present illness

She was diagnosed with 'vestibular neuritis' in a hospital.

4. Present symptoms

She had dizziness, nausea, vomiting, poor appetite, insomnia, neck pain, constipation, postdated menstruation with little flow, and sallow complexion.

5. Tongue and pulse

Pale tongue with tooth prints on the border, white coating slightly sticky, wiry pulse, Chi pulse weak.

6. Differentiation and analysis

The Spleen and Stomach are the production source of Qi and Blood. The Spleen sends the clean upward. When the clean Qi is not ascending, there will be dizziness. The Stomach sends the turbid downward. When the turbid Qi is not descending, there will be nausea, vomiting and constipation. Derangement of the Stomach causes insomnia. The late period with little menstrual flow is because the Middle Burner is weak, not able to produce enough Qi and Blood.

7. Diagnosis

TCM: Dizziness (Qi and Blood deficiency).

Western medicine: Vestibular neuritis.

8. Treating principle

Strengthen Spleen, harmonize Stomach, ascend clear Yang, descend turbid Qi.

9. Prescription

Dazhui (GV 14), Fengchi (GB 20), Tianzhu (BL 10), Taiyang (EX-HN5), Zanzhu (BL 2), Shanzhong (CV 17), Zhongwan (CV 12), Neiguan (PC 6), Pishu (BL 20), Zusanli (ST 36), Fenglong (ST 40), Sanyinjiao (SP 6), Gongsun (SP 4).

The reinforcing method for Pishu (BL 20) and Zusanli (ST 36). Even method for other points.

10. Effect

Her dizziness was relieved with 2 courses of treatment. After another 2 courses for consolidation, she was cured.

11. Essentials

'Without deficiency, there will be no dizziness.' Reinforcing Pishu (BL 20) and Zusanli (ST 36) is to strengthen the Spleen and Stomach to send the clean Yang upward to the head to stop dizziness.

CASE III: JI XIAOPING'S MEDICAL RECORD

1. General data

Zhang, female, 42 years old, came on May 5, 2002 for the first visit.

2. Chief complaint

Dizziness, nausea, vomiting for 3 weeks.

3. History of present illness

Recently, because her hard work gave her big mental pressure, and she had to manage the housework too, 3 weeks ago she began to have tinnitus, dizziness, nausea, and vomiting. When it was severe, she felt everything around her turning, and she could not get out of bed. Beijing Chaoyang Hospital diagnosed her with Meniere's disease and prescribed her medicines for anti-dizziness, and Vitamin B6, B12, and oryzanol. After taking medication for 2 weeks, although getting better, she still had dizziness and vomiting, and could not work. Her friend introduced her to come for acupuncture treatment.

4. Present symptoms

Dizziness, nausea, vomiting, feeling everything around her turning, not able to stand steadily, walking only with the help of holding onto things, tinnitus with a sound in low pitch.

5. Tongue and pulse

Pale swollen tongue with teeth prints on borders, white sticky coating; string-taut and rolling pulse.

6. Differentiation and analysis

The cause of her pathological condition is anxiety and overwork damaging the Spleen Qi. The Spleen Qi deficiency causes her sallow complexion, poor appetite, and tiredness and heaviness all over the body. Phlegm Damp resulted from the Spleen Qi deficiency obstructs the Stomach. Nausea and vomiting are induced by the non-descending of Stomach Qi. Spleen is the Earth and Liver the Wood. When the Spleen is weak, the Liver will overact on it. A Liver Wood preponderance produces internal Wind, giving rise to dizziness and tinnitus. Pale swollen tongue with teeth prints on borders and white sticky coating is the manifestation of Phlegm Damp caused by the Spleen deficiency. White sticky coating and rolling pulse indicate Damp. String-taut pulse means Liver disease and rolling pulse is the sign of Phlegm Damp.

In short, this is the Spleen Qi deficiency, Phlegm Damp retention, and the onset of Liver Wind.

7. Diagnosis

TCM: Dizziness.

Western medicine: Meniere's disease.

8. Treating principle

Strengthen the Spleen and Stomach, dissolve Phlegm Damp, stop Liver Wind, remove obstruction of the meridians and collaterals.

9. Prescription

Zusanli (ST 36), Yinlingquan (SP 9), Sanyinjiao (SP 6), Fenglong (ST 40), Taichong (LR 3), Tinggong (SI 19), Shuaigu (GB 8), head Wangu (GB 12).

Even method, retaining the needles for 30 minutes, 3 times a week.

10. Effect

After 3 treatments, her vomiting stopped and her dizziness was relieved. Seven treatments cured her. She could work normally again.

11. Essentials

Meniere's disease is a disease of the eye, ear, nose and throat department. Western medicine thinks that it is caused by a build up of fluid in the inner ear. But in TCM it is due to Spleen deficiency. The Spleen and Stomach are closely related to each other. The Stomach is involved in Spleen disease, so there is nausea and vomiting. The relation between the Spleen and Liver is that of Earth and Wood. The Liver is involved in Spleen deficiency, so there is dizziness and tinnitus.

In this case, TCM theory in the relation between Zang and Fu, and Zang and Zang is applied in differentiation; at the same time, the important concept of TCM, whole body regulation and local treatment, is applied in treatment. The use of Zusanli (ST 36), Yinlingquan (SP 9), Sanyinjiao (SP 6), Fenglong (ST 40), and Taichong (LR 3) is to strengthen the Spleen and Stomach, dissolve Damp, and stop the Liver Wind for the regulation of the whole body, while the use of Tinggong (SI 19), Shuaigu (GB 8), and head Wangu (GB 12) is to remove obstruction of the meridians and collaterals in the ear for the local treatment.

Whole body regulation and local treatment and application of differentiation of syndrome according to the theory of Zang Fu ensure the good result of treatment.

CASE IV: HU JINSHENG'S MEDICAL RECORD

1. General data

Dong, male, 32 years old.

2. Chief complaint

Dizziness, nausea, sweating, and poor sleep for 3 years.

3. History of present illness

The patient worked 10 hours every day. He felt tired and got dizziness since the summer of 2006. During an attack of dizziness it seemed that everything around him was turning. This dizziness occurred once every month.

4. Present symptoms

Recently, his dizziness was getting worse and more frequent. The accompanied symptoms were nausea, vomiting, accelerated heartbeats, and tiredness. The dizziness lasted about 1 hour each time. In 2006, he was diagnosed with Meniere's disease in Western medicine. Herbal treatment, acupuncture, and Western medicine were not very effective for him. Now the frequent onset of dizziness made him very tired and his appetite poor. His urine and stools were normal.

5. Tongue and pulse

Light red tongue with toothmarks, white coating slightly sticky; deep weak pulse.

6. Differentiation and analysis

The dizziness in this patient is caused by deficiency. The location of the disease is in the Heart, Spleen, and Stomach. The nature of the disease is deficiency. Deficiency of Qi refers to the Spleen Qi deficiency, so he has tiredness, poor appetite, pale tongue with toothmarks, and weak pulse. Deficiency of Blood refers to the Heart Blood deficiency, so he has accelerated heartbeats and poor sleep. With the Spleen Qi deficiency, the water metabolism is getting disturbed, resulting in the appearance of Phlegm Damp blocking the Middle Burner, resulting in the failure of clear Yang to ascend and turbid Yin to descend. The brain is therefore lacking nourishment because of the failure of clear Yang to ascend. The dizziness is caused by the turbid Qi disturbing the brain because of its failure to descend. Qi deficiency fails to produce Blood, and Blood deficiency fails to moisten and nourish the brain. This causes dizziness.

7. Diagnosis

TCM: Dizziness.

Western medicine: Meniere's disease.

8. Treating principle

Strengthen the Spleen, dissolve the Damp, calm the Mind.

9. Prescription

Acupuncture: Baihui (GV 20), Fengchi (GB 20), Taiyang (EX-HN5), Hegu (LI 4), Taichong (LR 3), Zusanli (ST 36), Fenglong (ST 40), Sanyinjiao (SP 6). Vertigo-auditory area (of scalp-acupuncture).

Moxibustion and TDP lamp: Shenque (CV 8) area.

Once a day, 30 minutes each time, 10 times as 1 course.

10. Effect

His dizziness was relieved after 3 treatments. His dizziness and nausea and vomiting stopped after 10 treatments. All the symptoms got better after 20 treatments.

11. Essentials

Dizziness here is caused by the dysfunction of the Spleen in transportation and transformation, retention of Damp in the Middle Burner, and misting of the brain. Damp has the same nature as Water, pertaining to Cold. The treating principle given by *Synopsis of Prescriptions of the Golden Chamber* (*Jin Gui Yao Lue*) for Phlegm Damp is to 'warm and dissolve'. The pathological condition of this patient is the retention of Water Damp, so moxibustion is used to warm and dissolve it. Shenque (CV 8) is the place of Yuan-Source Qi, through the warmth of moxibustion the Water Damp can be steamed and dispersed. In addition, moxibustion can help the Spleen to carry out its transportation and transformation function well. The Spleen is the Yin-Earth, the moxibustion warmth helps the Spleen Yang Qi for a better function in transforming and transporting Water Damp. The Vertigo-auditory area of scalp-acupuncture is very effective for dizziness, and especially good for Meniere's disease.

SUMMARY

Xuan, blurred vision, Yun, dizziness. The mild case can be relieved by closing one's eyes, and the serious case has an illusion of bodily movement with a rotatory sensation like sitting in a sailing boat or moving car, and can even be accompanied by vomiting. Dizziness is explained as derangement of the equilibrium of the senses in Western medicine. Clinically, it is commonly seen in hypertension, neurasthenia, Meniere's disease, labyrinthitis, hypotension, etc. The ancient doctors attributed it to Wind, Phlegm and deficiency. This is evidence of three syndromes in clinical treatment.

Main points: Baihui (GV 20), Fengchi (GB 20), Zusanli (ST 36), Taichong (LR 3).

In the case of Liver Yang upsurge with manifestation of dizziness, tinnitus, distending pain in head, and hot temper, Taixi (KI 3), Xingjian (LR 2), Ganshu

(BL 18) and Shenshu (BL 23) should be added. Xingjian (LR 2) and Ganshu (BL 18) pacify Liver to subdue Yang. Taixi (KI 3) and Shenshu (BL 23) produce Water to soften Wood.

In the case of Phlegm Damp retention in the Middle Burner with symptoms of headache like the head being wrapped with bandages, fullness in chest, nausea and vomiting, Touwei (ST 8), Neiguan (PC 6), Zhongwan (CV 12), Fenglong (ST 40) should be added. Touwei (ST 8) clears the Phlegm Heat of Yangming and the other points strengthen the Spleen to dissolve Phlegm and remove retention in the Middle Burner.

In the case of Qi and Blood deficiency characterized by dizziness, blurred vision, pale complexion, tiredness, Guanyuan (CV 4), Zusanli (ST 36) and Sanyinjiao (SP 6) should be added. Zusanli (ST 36) and Sanyinjiao (SP 6) replenish Qi and Blood; and Guanyuan (CV 4) strengthens the Yuan-Source Qi.

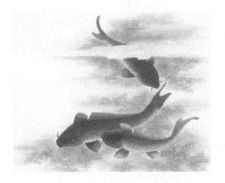

SECTION EIGHTEEN • FACIAL PAIN

CASE I: LU SHOUYAN'S MEDICAL RECORD

1. General data

Guo, male, 42. October 16, 1963.

2. Chief complaint

His right cheek and temporal region were painful.

3. History of present illness

He suffered from facial pain some years ago and cured by the tapping therapy of Seven-star needle. Recently he had a recurrence because of tiredness.

4. Present symptoms

The pain in the right side of the face, especially worse on the lateral side of the nostril and in reponse to warmth, started every day in the evening. His stools were not well formed.

5. Tongue and pulse

Swollen red tongue, white sticky coating, soft and a bit slow and wiry pulse.

6. Differentiation and analysis

The patient getting his pain due to tiredness, his stools, pulse and tongue are all the signs of Spleen deficiency with Damp produced, only the slightly wiry pulse and red tongue indicate deficiency Fire retained in the interior. It is said that the deficiency Fire may be stirred up by tiredness. The patient is a mental worker, hard work made his Heart Blood exhausted, so Heart Fire stirs up Liver Yang, bringing Damp and disturbing the Yangming Channel. This explains why he always has an onset of pain after noon when deficiency Yang is floating.

7. Diagnosis

TCM: Facial pain (Damp retained in Yangming).

Western medicine: Trigeminal neuralgia.

8. Treating principle

Clear Liver, reduce Heat, dissolve Damp, remove retention.

9. Prescription

Taiyang (EX-HN5), Yingxiang (LI 20), Yifeng (TE 17), Jiache (ST 6), Zhongwan (CV 12), Hegu (LI 4), Zusanli (ST 36), Yinlingquan (SP 9), Xingjian (LR 2).

The reinforcing method for Zusanli (ST 36) and Zhongwan (CV 12). The reducing method for the rest. Once every other day.

10. Effect

Four treatments cured him.

11. Essentials

Yangming is distributed on the cheek. 'Facial diseases are attributed to Stomach.' Therefore, the combination of Fire flaring up to the face and the Qi of the Yangming Channel being blocked may result in facial pain. Clinically, it is common in patients in old age, especially those who have Yin deficiency with Fire. Some young patients with Yangming Fire flaring up or who have overeaten spicy greasy food may also suffer from facial pain.

Professor Lu differentiated and found out the cause clearly, treated Biao-symptom with the principle to clear Liver and reduce Heat and treated Ben-cause with the strategy to dissolve Phlegm and remove the retention in Yangming. Hence, the patient was quickly cured after only 4 treatments.

CASE II: CHENG XINNONG'S MEDICAL RECORD

1. General data

Wang, male, 55. September 2, 1986.

2. Chief complaint

Paroxysmal pain in the right orbital region for 2 months.

3. History of present illness

His paroxysmal pain in the right orbital region lasted for 2 months. The pain began when washing his face or when the face was touched, and had no after-effects.

4. Present symptoms

The paroxysmal pain was electronic shock-like in nature, once every 2 to 3 days or a week, lasting about 1 minute each time.

5. Tongue and pulse

Red tongue, thin coating, wiry pulse.

6. Differentiation and analysis

The pain is due to Liver and Stomach excess Fire blocked in Yangming and Shaoyang channels. The orbital region and the cheek are the attributed areas of Yangming and Shaoyang channels. Wiry pulse indicates a painful syndrome.

7. Diagnosis

TCM: Facial pain (Liver and Stomach excess Fire).

Western medicine: Trigeminal neuralgia.

8. Treating principle

Remove obstruction of channels, reduce Fire, stop pain.

9. Prescription

Baihui (GV 20), Sibai (ST 2), Yangbai (GB 14), Taiyang (EX-HN5), Sizhukong (TE 23), Zanzhu (BL 2), Yuyao (EX-HN4), Waiguan (TE 5), Hegu (LI 4).

Taiyang (EX-HN5) penetrating to Sizhukong (TE 23), Zanzhu (BL 2) penetrating to Yuyao (EX-HN4). Other points were reduced.

10. Effect

With 5 treatments, the pain stopped gradually.

11. Essentials

Baihui (GV 20) clears the Fire and regulates Qi and Blood. Hegu (LI 4) and Waiguan (TE 5) disperse Qi of Shaoyang. Others are local points to activate Blood, remove blockage of channel to stop pain.

CASE III: LIU JIAYING'S MEDICAL RECORD

1. General data

Wang, male, 53 years old, a cadre.

2. Chief complaint

Facial pain on the left side for 2 months.

3. History of present illness

The patient began to have toothache on the left lower side in July 2005. He had a tooth extraction but the pain still continued. The neurologist diagnosed him with primary trigeminal neuralgia (the second and third branches). Treated by point block therapy and medication, his symptoms basically disappeared. Twenty days ago, the facial pain on the left side started again owing to his common cold. He came for the first visit on July 5, 2008.

4. Present symptoms

His facial pain was aggravated gradually. It was paroxysmal, like electric shock and knife cutting. Attacking 15–20 times every day, each time lasting several seconds to 1 minute, induced by washing his face, cleaning his teeth, yawning, eating, and speaking, it was accompanied by thirst and constipation.

Examination: listlessness, sallow and painful complexion, tenderness at the starting point in the distribution area of the second and third branches of trigeminal nerve on the left side.

5. Tongue and pulse

Red tongue, yellow coating; rolling rapid pulse.

6. Differentiation and analysis

The pathogenic Wind Heat invaded the facial region when he had a common cold. The circulation of Qi and Blood in the local area was obstructed.

7. Diagnosis

TCM: Facial pain.

Western medicine: Primary trigeminal neuralgia (II-III branches).

8. Treating principle

Dredge the meridians and collaterals, dispel Wind, stop pain.

9. Prescription

Sibai (ST 2), Xiaguan (ST 7), Dicang (ST 4), Quanliao (SI 18), Hegu (LI 4), Taichong (LR 3), Neiting (ST 44).

All the facial points were punctured with deep insertion and penetrating method. The electro-stimulation with the intensity the patient could endure was applied to the tender spots and Neiting (ST 44) of the opposite side, once a day. Retaining time of the needles was 25 minutes each time. Ten times made 1 course.

10. Effect

With 3 treatments, his pain was greatly relieved, and the frequency of attacks decreased to 5–6 times a day. Two courses of treatment made the pain completely disappear. One year follow-up found no relapse.

11. Essentials

It was the invasion of Wind Heat to the facial region. Sibai (ST 2), Dicang (ST 4), Quanliao (SI 18) and Xiaguan (ST 7) on the distribution area of the trigeminal neuralgia were selected to dredge the local meridians and collaterals to remove the obstruction. Hegu (LI 4), the Yuan-Primary point of Hand-Yangming Meridian, for all kinds of facial diseases, is combined with Taichong (LR 3) to dispel Wind and stop pain. Neiting (ST 44) clears the Wind Heat of the Yangming Meridian.

SUMMARY

Facial pain is a kind of severe pain occurring in transient paroxysms with abrupt onset like an electric shock, cutting, burning and intolerable, lasting seconds to minutes, in a frequency of several times a day. It is referred to as trigeminal neuralgia in Western medicine. Mostly it occurs between the ages of 40 and 60 in women. In acupuncture, retaining of needles is adopted. For secondary cases, treatment should be aimed at its primary cause.

Main points: Fengchi (GB 20), Xiaguan (ST 7), Hegu (LI 4).

Yangbai (GB 14) penetrating to Yuyao (EX-HN4), Sizhukong (TE 23) penetrating to Yuyao (EX-HN4) for orbital pain; Sibai (ST 2) penetrating to Juliao (ST 3) for infraorbital pain; Jiache (ST 6) penetrating to Dicang (ST 4) for lower gum pain.

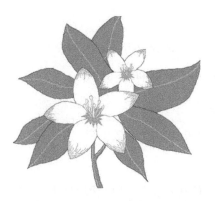

SECTION NINETEEN • FACIAL PARALYSIS

CASE I: CHENG XINNONG'S MEDICAL RECORD

1. General data

Hu, female, 33. December 7, 1987.

2. Chief complaint

Facial paralysis of right side for 4 days.

3. History of present illness

Six days ago, she felt a distending pain in the right mastoideum with the mendibular region involved and took Banlangen Chongji (Radix Isatidis Infusion). Four days ago when she got up in the morning she began to have muscle paralysis on the right side of her face, deviation of the mouth and incomplete closure of the eye. She had acupuncture twice in a hospital.

4. Present symptoms

Paralyzed facial muscles and headache on the right side, dream-disturbed sleep, poor appetite, and normal stools and urine.

Examination: Disappearance of wrinkles on the right side, incomplete closure of the eyelid, dropping of the angle of the mouth, inability to frown.

5. Tongue and pulse

Red tongue, white coating, cracks in the middle of tongue, deep wiry pulse.

6. Differentiation and analysis

Invasion of Wind and blockage of channels cause the muscles to be poorly nourished, thus they are paralyzed. Obstruction of Qi and Blood causes the mastoid pain and headache.

7. Diagnosis

TCM: Facial paralysis (invasion of Wind, blockage of channels).

Western medicine: Peripheral facial paralysis.

8. Treating principle

Dispel Wind, activate Blood, remove obstruction of channels.

9. Prescription

Baihui (GV 20), Fengchi (GB 20), Taiyang (EX-HN5), Chengjiang (CV 24), Zusanli (ST 36), Sanyinjiao (SP 6), Hegu (LI 4), Taichong (LR 3).

Right side: Quanliao (SI 18), Yangbai (GB 14), Jingming (BL 1), Sibai (ST 2), Yingxiang (LI 20), Dicang (ST 4), Jiache (ST 6).

The needle was inserted 0.8–1.5 cun into Jingming (BL 1) without retaining. Dicang (ST 4) penetrated to Jiache (ST 6). Even method for the other points.

10. Effect

Fourteen treatments cured her.

11. Essentials

Baihui (GV 20) regulates Yin and Yang to circulate Qi and Blood. Fengchi (GB 20) dispels Wind, driving the pathogenic factor out. Taiyang (EX-HN5) disperses the exterior pathogenic Wind. Zusanli (ST 36), Sanyinjiao (SP 6), Hegu (LI 4) and Taichong (LR 3) activate the anti-pathogenic Qi to regulate Qi and Blood of whole body. The others dispel Wind and remove obstruction of the channels. When Wind is dispelled, the channels become unobstructed, and the muscles are well nourished, paralysis is cured.

CASE II: CHENG XINNONG'S MEDICAL RECORD

1. General data

Li, male, 50. October 29, 1982.

2. Chief complaint

Deviation of mouth and eye on the right side for 1 day.

3. History of present illness

One day ago, he felt tight on the right side of his face due to exposure to Wind and his mouth and eye deviated.

4. Present symptoms

Tightness of the right side of the face, deviation of mouth to the left side, incomplete closing of the right eye. Appetite normal, urine and stools normal.

5. Tongue and pulse

Slightly red tongue, yellow thick coating, wiry pulse.

6. Differentiation and analysis

The facial region is the distributed area of the Yangming and Shaoyang channels. The pathogenic Wind invades on the occasion of the deficiency of the channels, the Qi of which is blocked, the muscles lack nourishment and become paralyzed.

7. Diagnosis

TCM: Facial paralysis (invasion of exogenous Wind).

Western medicine: Peripheral facial paralysis.

8. Treating principle

Dispel Wind, activate Blood, remove obstruction of channels.

9. Prescription

Baihui (GV 20), Fengchi (GB 20), Hegu (LI 4). Right side: Yangbai (GB 14), Sibai (ST 2), Quanliao (SI 18), Dicang (ST 4), Jiache (ST 6).

Dicang (ST 4) penetrated to Jiache (ST 6). Even method for other points.

10. Effect

With 2 weeks' treatment, he was clinically cured.

11. Essentials

For the treatment, the principles should be to activate Blood, dispel Wind, and re-move obstruction of the channels. The points of Yangming and Shaoyang channels are selected.

CASE III: YANG JIEBIN'S MEDICAL RECORD

1. General data

Luo, male, 16. March 5, 1995.

2. Chief complaint

Deviation of mouth and eye to the left side for 2 months.

3. History of present illness

Two months ago he began to have deviation of mouth and eye to the left side, numbness of the facial region, and hypogeusia. With treatment of Chinese and Western medicine and acupuncture, there was no improvement.

4. Present symptoms

The right eye was deviated and the angle of the mouth dropped, numbness and twitch of facial muscles, disappearance of wrinkles, inability to frown and blow out the cheek, palpebral fissure of 1.5cm, nasolabial groove becoming shallow, philtrum deviating to the left side, tenderness in mastoid region.

5. Tongue and pulse

Dark red tongue, thin white coating, wiry thready pulse.

6. Differentiation and analysis

This case of facial paralysis is caused by weak defence, disharmonious Ying and Wei, Wind Cold invasion, obstructed channels, muscular malnutrition, resulting in paralysis.

7. Diagnosis

TCM: Facial paralysis (invasion of exogenous Wind).

Western medicine: Peripheral facial paralysis.

8. Treating principle

Remove obstruction of channels, strengthen body resistance to dispel pathogens.

9. Prescription

Main points: Conjunctiva of right eye, buccal mucosa.

Accompanied points:

- Dicang (ST 4) penetrating to Jiache (ST 6), Yangbai (GB 14), Qiuhou (EX-HN7), Yingxiang (LI 20), Renzhong (GV 26), Hegu (LI 4).

- Heliao (LI 19) penetrating to Quanliao (SI 18), Yizhong (Extra), Chengqi (ST 1), Zusanli (ST 36), Lieque (LU 7).

Conjunctiva of right eye and buccal mucosa were pricked for bleeding. Even method for other points. Cupping for 5–10 minutes at Xiaguan (ST 7) after needling. Once every day or every other day.

10. Effect

The symptoms were obviously relieved after 1 course of treatment. Luo was clinically cured with 15 treatments.

11. Essentials

Plain Questions (*Tiao Jing Lun*) says: 'For the disease in Blood, treat the collaterals.' Pricking to cause bleeding is aimed at removing obstructions of Qi and Blood and dispelling Wind. Professor Yang applied the bleeding and cupping after needling. The muscles are warmed and nourished. The paralysis is cured via unobstructing the channels and regulating Qi and Blood.

> **PRICKING CONJUNCTIVA AND BUCCAL MUCOSA FOR BLEEDING (AFFECTED SIDE)**
>
> Pricking conjunctiva: Expose the conjunctiva, disinfect with sterilized cotton ball dipped in physiological saline, prick the tarsus 5-7 times with a #28 filiform needle or a thin three-edged needle until there is a little bleeding.
>
> Pricking buccal mucosa: The patient is asked to open his mouth to expose the buccal mucosa. Disinfect with alcohol cotton ball. Prick the buccal mucosa with a three-edged needle 15cm in length once every 0.5cm in distance, until there is a little bleeding.

CASE IV: YANG JIEBIN'S MEDICAL RECORD

1. General data

Song, male, 34.

2. Chief complaint

Deviation of mouth and eye of the left side.

3. History of present illness

Two years ago, he had facial paralysis on the left side due to invasion of Wind Cold. With acupuncture, physical therapy, and medication, his symptoms were relieved but not cured. Recently it became worse because of tiredness and being caught in the rain.

4. Present symptoms

Deviation of mouth and eye of the left side.

Examination: Left frontal wrinkles disappeared, left mimetic paralysis, inability to frown, blow out the cheek, and show the teeth or whistle, incomplete closure of eyelids, left nasolabial groove becoming shallow, philtrum deviating to the right side, leaking of water when drinking, and pain in the mastoid region.

5. Tongue and pulse

Slight red tongue, thin white coating, deep thready pulse.

6. Differentiation and analysis

Two years ago he had a facial paralysis, and this time it was induced by tiredness and being caught by rain and became worse because of the invasion of Wind Cold blocked in the facial region, stagnation of Qi and Blood causing malnutrition of muscles.

7. Diagnosis

TCM: Facial paralysis (channels and collaterals being blocked by Qi and Blood stagnation).

Western medicine: Peripheral facial paralysis.

8. Treating principle

Remove obstructions, activate Blood, regulate Ying and Wei.

9. Prescription

Left side: Conjunctiva and buccal mucosa. Dicang (ST 4), Jiache (ST 6), Yangbai (GB 14), Yuyao (EX-HN4), Yingxiang (LI 20), Sibai (ST 2). Both sides: Hegu (LI 4), Zusanli (ST 36).

Conjunctiva and buccal mucosa were pricked with filiform needle for bleeding, 2–4, facial points were punctured each time with the penetrating method. Dicang (ST 4) to Jiache (ST 6), Yangbai (GB 14) to Yuyao (EX-HN4), Sibai (ST 2) to Yingxiang (LI 20). Moxibustion was applied for 5 minutes after needling. Perpendicular insertion at Hegu (LI 4) and Zusanli (ST 36), even method.

Once every day, 10 times as 1 course.

10. Effect

He was better 1 month later and clinically cured after half a year's treatment in successive treatments.

11. Essentials

Pricking the conjunctiva and buccal mucosa for bleeding is to activate Blood circulation, and remove obstruction of the channels. Moxibustion after needling Dicang (ST 4), Jiache (ST 6), Yangbai (GB 14), Yuyao (EX-HN4), Yingxiang (LI 20), Hegu (LI 4), and Zusanli (ST 36) is to regulate Qi and Blood and harmonize Ying and Wei to nourish the muscles. For stubborn cases of facial paralysis, self massage and functional exercises can help to improve the recovery because of the patient's subjective efforts.

CASE V: YANG JINHONG'S MEDICAL RECORD

1. General data

Li, male, 65 years old.

2. Chief complaint

Deviation of mouth and eye for 2 months.

3. History of present illness

In the morning of June 6, 2009 he all of a sudden had discomfort on the left side of his face, incomplete closing of the eye, running tears, failure to frown, close the eye, raise the eyebrow, blow out the cheek, and show the teeth, disappearance of nasolabial groove, deviation of the mouth to the right side, pain in the mastoid region, and headache. His movement was without difficulty. He went to Dongfang Hospital. A CT scan of the skull didn't find anything wrong. He was treated with antiviral drugs iv. and B1 and B12 im. for 2 weeks, and acupuncture and herbal medicine, but the result was not very effective. Now his symptoms were disappearance of wrinkles, incomplete closing of the eye, running tears, conjunctival redness, drooping of the angle of the mouth, and salivation. Appetite was normal and urination and defecation normal.

4. Present symptoms

Disappearance of wrinkles, incomplete closing of the eye, drooping of the angle of the mouth.

5. Tongue and pulse

Swollen pale tongue, white sticky coating; string-taut tense pulse.

6. Differentiation and analysis

Constitutionally he has retention of Phlegm Damp and Qi and Blood stagnation. Now he is affected by pathogenic Wind Cold, which blocks the Yangming and Shaoyang, causing malnutrition of these meridians, thus resulting in deviation of mouth and eye.

7. Diagnosis

TCM: Deviation of mouth and eye.

Western medicine: Peripheral facial paralysis (left side).

8. Treating principle

Dispel Wind Cold, dissolve Damp, warm and remove obstruction of meridians, regulate Qi and Blood.

9. Prescription

Fengchi (GB 20), Yangbai (GB 14), Zanzhu (BL 2), Jingming (BL 1), Taiyang (EX-HN5), Sibai (ST 2), Xiaguan (ST 7), Dicang (ST 4), Yingxiang (LI 20), Renzhong (GV 26), Chengjiang (CV 24), Hegu (LI 4), Zusanli (ST 36), Fenglong (ST 40), Taichong (LR 3).

Yangbai (GB 14) penetrating to Yuyao (EX-HN4), Dicang (ST 4) penetrating to Jiache (ST 6).

The reducing method for Fenglong (ST 40), the reinforcing method for Zusanli (ST 36), even method for others. Retain needles for 30 minutes.

Electric stimulation for Zanzhu (BL 2) and Yangbai (GB 14), Dicang (ST 4) and Xiaguan (ST 7), dense-disperse wave.

Moxibustion with ginger as isolation for 3 facial points, 3 cones each time.

The first 5 treatments were applied once every day, and later every other day. In total, 20 treatments.

10. Effect

Remarkably effective. Wrinkles appeared, eyes could be closed, cheek could blow out, but the angle of the mouth was still a little bit deviated to the right side.

11. Essentials

This patient was in old age and with a history of hypertension and diabetes, and at the early stage of facial paralysis he didn't have acupuncture treatment regularly, prolonging the course of the disease.

The effect of moxibustion with ginger as isolation and electric stimulation for warming and removing obstruction of meridians is good for those patients who have a prolonged course with slow recovery.

CASE VI: LIU ZHAOHUI'S MEDICAL RECORD

1. General data

Liu, female, 28 years old, came on April 16, 1996.

2. Chief complaint

Deviation of eye and mouth and motor impairment of facial muscles on the right side for 1 day.

3. History of present illness

She was busy running about recently throughout 1 week. Two days before the onset of the condition, she was waiting for somebody in the cold weather for 1 hour and on the following day in the morning came home by aeroplane on a flight lasting nearly 9 hours. Because of her tiredness, she slept for 6 hours in the plane, with her head exposed to the cold wind in the air conditioning. Then the condition started.

4. Present symptoms

The patient was in good health generally, fully conscious with normal movement of four limbs and trunk. Her mouth deviated to the left side. The facial muscles of the right side were paralyzed with the drop of mouth angle and shallow nasolabial groove. When she raised her eyebrow, the wrinkles of the right side disappeared. The right eyebrow was lower than the left one, the palpebral fissure became bigger, and the tears were running. Bell's sign: right side (+), left side (-); blowing out the cheek: right side (+), left side (-). She was accompanied with headache and mastoid tenderness on the right side.

5. Tongue and pulse

The tongue was light red with thin white coating. The pulse was superficial and tight.

6. Differentiation and analysis

From the history it was clear that the invasion of Wind Cold attacked the facial meridians and collaterals, making the Qi and Blood obstructed and the facial muscles deprived of nourishment.

7. Diagnosis

TCM: Facial paralysis (Wind Cold syndrome, obstruction of Wind Cold in the meridians and collaterals of the facial region).

Western medicine: Peripheral facial paralysis.

8. Treating principle

Dispel Wind Cold, warm and remove obstruction of meridians, regulate Qi and Blood.

9. Prescription

Moving moxibustion with four moxa-sticks of Huatuo Brand bundled up was applied up and down and left and right at the affected side with the mastoid region included until the skin became red. The endurable Heat was left to penetrate into the muscles as much as possible. The treatment was done twice a day, 20 minutes each time.

10. Effect

By the third day, the symptoms had stopped developing. By the fifth day, the patient began to feel better. Her right eye could be closed completely, the wrinkles began to appear, the nasolabial groove of the affected side became deeper. The muscular movement of the facial region such as chewing and smiling were better. By the tenth day, the patient was basically cured.

Examination: The mouth was not deviated. Both eyes could open and close at the same time. The wrinkles of the left and right sides were basically the same. The nasolabial grooves of two sides were nearly the same in depth. Blowing out the cheek (-). Bell's test (-). The facial movement was normal. One more week of treatment was applied to consolidate the effect, once every other day. In total 13 treatments were given and the facial paralysis was cured without any sequalae left. There was no relapse in the follow-up at half a year.

11. Essentials

From the history it was clear that the invasion of Wind Cold attacked the facial meridians and collaterals, making the Qi and Blood obstructed and the facial muscles deprived of nourishment. The moxibustion functions to dispel Wind and Cold to treat the exterior syndrome, warm the meridians and collaterals, and activate Qi and Blood to remove the obstruction. The patient was invaded by exogenous Wind Cold, being the exterior excess syndrome. The strong moxibustion in the way of up-down and left-right movement is the reducing method, making the skin pores open and driving out the pathogenic factor. *The Great Compendium of Acupuncture and Moxibustion* says: 'The reducing method of moxibustion is to blow the ignited moxa rapidly and to make the point open.' The good result of the treatment originates from the reducing moxibustion being applied directly to the affected area.

SUMMARY

Facial paralysis, known as deviation of mouth and eye in Chinese medicine, without motor impairment of the extremities and loss of consciousness, is mostly caused by invasion of Wind in the facial region, or Phlegm retention in the channels, causing malnutrition of the facial muscles, or is secondary to tympanitis or herpes. Points of the Yangming channels of hand and foot are mainly selected and the even method adopted in treatment.

Main points: Fengchi (GB 20), Yifeng (TE 17), Sibai (ST 2), Quanliao (SI 18), Dicang (ST 4), Jiache (ST 6), Waiguan (TE 5), Hegu (LI 4).

Add Taiyang (EX-HN5) for headache; add Yangbai (GB 14) and Zanzhu (BL 2) for inability to frown; puncture Jingming (BL 1) as deep as 0.8–1.5 cun without retaining for incomplete closure of eyelid; add Yingxiang (LI 20) for inability to raise nose; add Renzhong (GV 26) for philtrum deviation; add Juliao (ST 3) for inability to show the teeth ; add Taichong (LR 3) for twitching of mouth and eyes; add Wangu (GB 12) for mastoid pain; add Fenglong (ST 40) for profuse Phlegm.

SECTION TWENTY • STROKE

CASE I: LU SHOUYAN'S MEDICAL RECORD

1. General data

Chen, male, 45. May 29, 1963.

2. Chief complaint

Left arm numbness.

3. History of present illness

He used to have Windstroke. Three months ago he had Windstroke again. Now the symptoms were getting better and the blood pressure tended towards normal, but the left shoulder, elbow, wrist, and fingers had numbness and contracture.

4. Present symptoms

Numbness of the left arm, contracture of the wrist and fingers, motor impairment, accompanied by dizziness, migraine on the right side, palpitations, nausea, preference for warmth and dislike of Cold.

5. Tongue and pulse

The right Cun and Guan pulse was wiry rolling and Chi big, the left pulse soft small and wiry. Pulse of Hanyan (GB 4) region: right stronger than left. Pulse of Chongyang (ST 42) region: strong. Pulse of Taichong (LR 3) region: wiry thready. Pulse of Taixi (KI 3) region: even. Thin slippery coating.

6. Differentiation and analysis

This patient is nearly 50 years old, his Kidney Qi is declining, Water less and Wood more, he is overweight, in constitution of Qi deficiency and Phlegm Damp. With hard mental working, the internal Fire flares up, bringing Phlegm Damp upward and obstructing the channels and collaterals. The Cunkou pulse: the right side bigger than the left; Hanyan pulse: the right side stronger than the left, means right excess and left deficiency.

7. Diagnosis

TCM: Windstroke with channels and collaterals being attacked (Water deficiency and Wood excess).

Western medicine: Stroke.

8. Treating principle

Replenish Water to soften Liver.

9. Prescription

- Hanyan (GB 4), Fengchi (GB 20), Taichong (LR 3), Fenglong (ST 40), Taixi (KI 3), Fuliu (KI 7).

  Taixi (KI 3) and Fuliu (KI 7), the reinforcing method. Other points, even method.

- Jianyu (LI 15), Binao (LI 14), Shousanli (LI 10), Hegu (LI 4), Waiguan (TE 5), Baxie (EX-UE9). Right side was reduced and left side reinforced.

Manipulation: Mainly rotating, secondarily lifting-thrusting.

Twelve times as 1 course.

10. Treatment

After the first course, 2 weeks for rest. After the second course, 2 weeks for rest. Then the third course. When the left and right Cunkou pulses were balanced, use the second group of points on the left side only, the reducing method, to dispel pathogenic factors to strengthen the resistance. Washing the affected extremity with herbal medicine was used in combination with acupuncture.

11. Essentials

Professor Lu reduced the right side and reinforced the left side to balance Yin and Yang.

Point group 1 aims to treat the root cause of his disease. Reduce Hanyan (GB 4) and Fengchi (GB 20) to reduce the upward flowing deficient Yang to clear the turbidity of the head. Reduce Taichong (LR 3) to pacify Liver to subdue Yang. Reduce Fenglong (ST 40) to dissolve Phlegm. Reinforce Taixi (KI 3) and Fuliu (KI 7) to replenish Water to moisten Wood.

Point group 2, selected mostly from the affected channels, aims to remove obstruction of the channels and collaterals to balance Yin and Yang. Because the right Cunkou pulse is bigger than that of left side, so reduce the right and reinforce the left.

CASE II: YANG JIASAN'S MEDICAL RECORD

1. General data

Zhu, male, 58. August 4, 1986.

2. Chief complaint

Weakness on the right side of the body for 6 days.

3. History of present illness

Six days ago, due to emotional depression, he began to have stiffness of tongue, right arm numbness, and right side body weakness. Administered herbal medicine, his condition was controlled, without pathological development.

4. Present symptoms

Distension in the head, dizziness, weakness of the right side of his body, especially the right arm, slurring of speech, stiffness of tongue, distention and Dryness of eyes, dry mouth but without desire to drink, and difficulty in falling asleep.

Examination: BP not steady, 130–150/80–110mmHg.

5. Tongue and pulse

Dark red tongue, white moistened coating, wiry pulse slightly rolling.

6. Differentiation and analysis

This is a syndrome of Yin deficiency and Yang hyperactivity transformed into Wind blocking in the brain, manifested as weakness of right side of his body, especially the right arm, slurring of speech, stiffness of tongue, and wiry rolling pulse. Distention and Dryness of eyes, and dry mouth but without desire to drink are the signs of Yin deficiency. It is the syndrome of upper excess and lower deficiency.

7. Diagnosis

TCM: Windstroke (attack on channels and collaterals) (Liver Yang transformed into Wind).

Western medicine: Stroke.

8. Treating principle

Replenish Yin, subdue Yang, calm the Mind.

9. Prescription

Qianding (GV 21), Houding (GV 19), Baihui (GV 20), Tongtian (BL 7), Fengchi (GB 20), Hegu (LI 4), Lieque (LU 7), Zhigou (TE 6), Juegu (GB 39), Taichong (LR 3).

Qianding (GV 21), Houding (GV 19), Baihui (GV 20), Tongtian (BL 7) were reinforced with mild stimulation; Lieque (LU 7), Zhigou (TE 6), Juegu (GB 39),

Taichong (LR 3) reinforced with medium stimulation; others reduced with medium stimulation.

10. Effect

Three months' treatment made the numbness of the right side of his body disappear and his speech basically returned to normal.

11. Essentials

The principle of treatment for this syndrome of Yin deficiency and Yang hyperactivity transformed into Wind with upper excess and lower deficiency should be replenishing Yin, subduing Yang, and stopping Wind for clearing the upper part, and reinforcing the lower part, and calming the Mind.

The points on head, Qianding (GV 21), Houding (GV 19), Baihui (GV 20), Tongtian (BL 7) to replenish marrow, strengthen brain and calm the Mind; Fengchi (GB 20) to dispel Wind of Upper Burner; Hegu (LI 4) and Zusanli (ST 36) to remove obstruction of the intestines for the clean ascending and the turbid descending; Quchi (LI 11) and Zusanli (ST 36) to bring down the reversed Qi. Hegu (LI 4) and Taichong (LR 3), Yuan-Source points, to soften Liver to stop Wind, to replenish Yin to clear Heat; Lieque (LU 7) to induce Kidney Water to nourish genuine Yin, combined with Juegu (GB 39) to increase Kidney Essence; Juegu (GB 39) and Taichong (LR 3) to increase Liver and Kidney Essence. Thus, reinforce the lower and clear the upper.

CASE III: CHENG XINNONG'S MEDICAL RECORD

1. General data

Wang, female, 73. October 31, 1986.

2. Chief complaint

Weakness of the right limbs for 2 days.

3. History of present illness

Two days ago, the patient got angry with her family and suddenly had weakness of her right limbs and sluggish movement.

4. Present symptoms

She came with weakness of the right limbs and sluggish movement, irritability, dry mouth, poor appetite, sleep almost normal, no dizziness and tinnitus, shortness of breath on exertion, and sometimes incontinence of urine.

5. Tongue and pulse

Tongue tip red, dry yellow coating, deep thready pulse, Chi weak.

6. Differentiation and analysis

This patient is in old age with Liver and Kidney deficiency, Qi and Blood insufficiency, and anger made her Liver Qi stagnate, so the limbs lack nourishment and are sluggish in movement. With Kidney Yin deficiency, Body Fluid fails to distribute upward, so the mouth is dry. Yin deficiency leads to internal Heat, so red tongue, yellow coating, thready rapid pulse. Kidneys are deficient, and not receiving Qi, so there is shortness of breath on exertion. Bladder is out of control owing to Kidney Qi being not consolidated enough, so there is incontinence of urine. It is a syndrome of Liver and Kidney deficiency.

7. Diagnosis

TCM: Windstroke (channels and collaterals being attacked, Liver and Kidney deficiency).

Western medicine: Signal symptoms of stroke.

8. Treating principle

Reinforce Liver and Kidney, regulate Qi and Blood.

9. Prescription

Baihui (GV 20), Fengchi (GB 20), Guanyuan (CV 4), Hegu (LI 4), Taichong (LR 3), Zusanli (ST 36), Sanyinjiao (SP 6), Taixi (KI 3), Yongquan (KI 1). Right side: Jianyu (LI 15), Quchi (LI 11), Waiguan (TE 5), Yanglingquan (GB 34), Xuanzhong (GB 39).

Fengchi (GB 20) and Taichong (LR 3) were reduced; Guanyuan (CV 4), Zusanli (ST 36), Sanyinjiao (SP 6), and Taixi (KI 3) were reinforced; even method for others.

10. Effect

After 3 treatments, there was a great relief of the numbness and weakness of the right limbs and movement was free from sluggishness. Her condition was kept steady with 10 treatments. The follow-up found no recurrence. On July 6, 1987, she felt weakness in lower limbs. This was Kidney deficiency, 8 treatments cured her.

11. Essentials

Baihui (GV 20) is to regulate Yin and Yang to circulate Qi and Blood; Fengchi (GB 20) to dispel Wind; Taichong (LR 3) to pacify Liver to subdue Yang; Guanyuan (CV 4) to reinforce Yuan-Source Qi; Zusanli (ST 36) to strengthen the Middle

Burner; Sanyinjiao (SP 6) to replenish Yin to subdue Yang; Taixi (KI 3) to replenish Water to irrigate Wood; Yongquan (KI 1) to conduct Fire downward; Jianyu (LI 15), Quchi (LI 11), Waiguan (TE 5), Hegu (LI 4), Yanglingquan (GB 34), and Xuanzhong (GB 39) to remove obstruction of channels and balance Yin and Yang.

CASE IV: SHI XUEMIN'S MEDICAL RECORD

1. General data

Li, male, 56. April 10, 1992.

2. Chief complaint

Hemiplegia of the right side for 4 days.

3. History of present illness

He had hemiplegia of the right side for 4 days, couldn't walk without help.

4. Present symptoms

Hemiplegia of the right side, the right hand too weak to take anything, clear consciousness, slurred speech, dull expression.

Examination: Myodynamia of right limbs 2–3. Head CT showing 'cerebral infarction in the left basal region'.

5. Tongue and pulse

Pale tongue, white coating, wiry pulse.

6. Differentiation and analysis

He had hemiplegia due to the Liver and Kidney deficiency because of his old age.

7. Diagnosis

TCM: Windstroke (attack on channels and collaterals).

Western medicine: Cerebral infarction.

8. Treating principle

Restore consciousness and induce resuscitation, clear obstruction of channels and collaterals of brain, replenish Liver and Kidneys.

9. Prescription

Neiguan (PC 6), Renzhong (GV 26), Sanyinjiao (SP 6), Jiquan (HT 1), Chize (LU 5), Weizhong (BL 40).

The technique of restoring consciousness and inducing resuscitation was adopted. First bilateral Neiguan (PC 6) was needled perpendicularly 1–1.5 cun with lifting-thrusting and rotating for 1 minute, then Renzhong (GV 26) needled, 5 minutes after insertion, lifting-thrusting like sparrow picking until the patient was producing tears; Sanyinjiao (SP 6) was inserted 1–1.5 cun at the posterior border of tibia with a 45° angle and the needle lifting-thrusting to make the lower limb contract 3 times; Jiquan (HT 1) inserted 1–1.5 cun perpendicularly and with the needle lifting-thrusting to make the upper limb contract 3 times; Chize (LU 5) needled in the same way with Jiquan (HT 1); Weizhong (BL 40) inserted 1 cun with the patient in supine position and leg stretched and lifted, and with the needle lifting-thrusting to make the lower limb contract 3 times.

10. Effect

After the first treatment, he could come by himself with the help of a walking stick and said his right limbs were much stronger. One week of treatment in succession made his walk nearly normal.

11. Essentials

In the treatment of Windstroke, for the purpose of dispelling Wind and removing obstruction of the channels and collaterals, doctors of all generations always select points from the Yangming channels which are believed to be full of Qi and Blood. But Professor Shi put forward the theory that the brain obstruction with the Mind disturbed was the root pathogenesis based on the diagnosis of disease localization in Western medicine. He held that obstruction of the brain caused no-dependence of Mind which was stored in the Heart, so limbs were soft and speech slurred. Restoring consciousness and inducing resuscitation should be the principle for treatment. And in line with the theory of Liver and Kidney Yin deficiency given by doctors of previous generations, he treated Windstroke with restoring consciousness and inducing resuscitation as the main principle, and unobstructing channels of the brain and replenishing Liver and Kidneys as supplementary.

Main points: Neiguan (PC 6), Renzhong (GV 26), Sanyinjiao (SP 6).

Supplementary points: Jiquan (HT 1), Chize (LU 5), Weizhong (BL 40).

Neiguan (PC 6), Luo-Connecting point, connecting with Yinwei Channel, nourishes the Heart, calms the Mind, circulates Qi and Blood; Renzhong (GV 26), a meeting point of the Governor Vessel which enters the brain and Yangming channels, restores consciousness and induces resuscitation; Sanyinjiao (SP 6), the meeting point of the three Yin channels of foot, replenishes Kidney Essence to fill up marrow. When the brain marrow is ample, the Mind has its dependence for nourishment; Jiquan (HT 1), Chize (LU 5), Weizhong (BL 40) are those on joints where the

Channels' Qi converges, strong in circulating channel Qi to improve the movement of limbs.

Added points: Fengchi (GB 20), Yifeng (TE 17), Wangu (GB 12) for dysphagia; Jinjin Yuye (EX-HN12) for aphasia; Hegu (LI 4) for inability to move fingers; others accordingly.

Manipulation of added points: Fengchi (GB 20), Yifeng (TE 17), Wangu (GB 12) were punctured towards the Adam's apple with a 2–2.5 cun insertion, reinforced by rotating needle with small amplitude and high frequency for half a minute; Hegu (LI 4) punctured towards Sanjian (LI 3) to the lower border of the second metacarpal bone with reducing of lifting-thrusting, making the index finger contracted; Jinjin Yuye (EX-HN12) pricked for bleeding.

Professor Shi stressed that the technique for each point should be done very strictly, thus good therapeutic results can be achieved. Many patients with channels and collaterals attacked get an immediate effect. And the shorter the duration of the disease, the better the effect.

CASE V: BO ZHIYUN'S MEDICAL RECORD

1. General data

Sun, male, 65.

2. Chief complaint

Motor impairment of right limbs and slurring of speech for 8 months, worse for 2 days.

3. History of present illness

Without obvious reasons he began to have motor impairment of right limbs, especially the arm. The head CT showed cerebral infarction of left temporal lobe. With treatment his symptoms were relieved. Two days ago, he was hospitalized again when his motor impairment became worse and he couldn't speak.

4. Present symptoms

Motor impairment of right limbs, oedema of the right arm in distal region, able to walk with the help of a walking stick, slurring of speech, salivation, no headache, nausea and vomiting.

Examination: Head CT scan showing 'big patch of shadow in the left temporal lobe, latent image of low density in the right corona radiata region', giving the impression of 'remote infarct focus of the left temporal lobe, ischaemic change of the right corona radiata region.'

5. Tongue and pulse

Pale tongue, white sticky coating, deep rolling pulse.

6. Differentiation and analysis

The Wind Phlegm blocking in the channels and collaterals is manifested as oedema of the right arm in distal region and salivation. Pale tongue, white sticky coating, deep rolling pulse are the signs of Phlegm turbidity.

7. Diagnosis

TCM: Windstroke (channels and collaterals being attacked) (Spleen and Kidney Yang deficiency).

Western medicine: Old cerebral infarction complicated with cerebral ischaemia.

8. Treating principle

Reinforce Spleen and Kidneys, dissolve Damp and Phlegm.

9. Prescription

Abdominal acupuncture.

Conduct Qi to its primary source: Zhongwan (CV 12), Xiawan (CV 10), Qihai (CV 6), Guanyuan (CV 4); abdominal Four Gates: Huaroumen (ST 24) and Wailing (ST 26), bilateral; Upper Rheumatism point, Upper Rheumatism Lateral point: Shenque (CV 8).

Conduct Qi to its primary source: insert needle to the Earth level. Abdominal Four Gates: insert needle to the human level. Rheumatism points: insert needle to the heaven level and triangular needling added. Moxibustion was done at Shenque (CV 8) for 40 minutes.

Once a day, 5 times a week, 10 times as 1 course.

10. Effect

After 10 treatments, the hand swelling greatly relieved, another 10 times, it completely disappeared, and there was no recurrence in 2 months.

11. Essentials

This patient was treated with the abdominal acupuncture invented by Professor Bo Zhiyun. It takes the Shenque (CV 8) regulating system as its theory. Shenque (CV 8) regulating system, formed in the embryo stage, the earliest regulating system of the human body and the mother of the channel system, distributes Qi and Blood to the whole body and regulates the human body macroscopically. Owing to the characteristics of the abdominal anatomical structure, the Shenque (CV 8) system bifurcates into two in the process of formation: one is located shallowly in the abdominal wall, regulating the whole body, known as the peripheral system; the other is located deep in the abdominal wall, regulating the viscera, named the visceral system. In abdominal acupuncture, the system of channels is a holo-image in the shape of a turtle, with Shenque (CV 8) as its centre, Zhongwan (CV 12) as the top, Guanyuan (CV 4) as the tail, and Daheng (SP 15) on the lateral. On the arm, the *Upper Rheumatism point* is located 0.5 cun superolateral to Huaroumen (ST 24), and the *Upper Rheumatism Lateral point* is 1 cun lateral to Huaroumen (ST 24). On the lower limbs, the *Lower Rheumatism point* is located 0.5 cun infralateral to Wailing (ST 26), and the *Lower Rheumatism Lower point* is 1 cun lateral to Daju (ST 27), with Shangqu (KI 17) as its neck, Siman (KI 14) as starting from the sacrococcyx. The abdominal Bakuo (the Eight Regions) system, taking the Houtian-acquired Bagua (the Eight Trigrams) as evidence, is to regulate the viscera. Of it, Zhongwan (CV 12) is Fire, Li, dominating Heart and Small Intestine; Guanyuan (CV 4) is Water, Kan, dominating Kidney and Bladder; the left *Upper Rheumatism point* is Earth, Kun, dominating Spleen and Stomach; the left Daheng (SP 15) is lake, Dui, dominating the Lower Burner; the left *Lower Rheumatism point* is heaven, Qian, dominating Lung and Large Intestine; the right *Upper Rheumatism point* is Wind, Xun, dominating Liver and Middle Burner; the right Daheng (SP 15) is thunder, Zhen, dominating Liver and Gallbladder; the right *Lower Rheumatism point* is mountain, Gen, dominating the Upper Burner. The points in each region have special therapeutic functions for their corresponding Zang Fu organs and play an important role in the balance of the internal organs.

In the theory of the traditional system of channels, Zhongwan (CV 12) is the Front-Mu of the Stomach and Influential point of the Fu organs; Xiawan (CV 10) is the meeting point of the Conception Vessel with the Foot-Taiyin Channel; Guanyuan (CV 4) is the Front-Mu point of the Small Intestine and the meeting point of the Conception Vessel with the three foot Yin channels, and same as Qihai (CV 6), a tonification point; Huaroumen (ST 24) and Wailing (ST 26), those of Foot-Yangming Channel. Therefore, puncturing Zhongwan (CV 12), Xiawan (CV 10), Qihai (CV 6), Guanyuan (CV 4) and the abdominal Four Gates (Huaroumen and Wailing) which have the function to *conduct Qi to its primary source* is to replenish Yang Qi of the Spleen and Kidneys, regulating Qi of the Spleen and Stomach, and strengthening the Spleen to dissolve Phlegm. When Yang Qi is strong, Water Damp is removed, when the Spleen is strong, Phlegm is without formation. In the recovery stage of cerebral apoplexy, Qi and Blood are consumed and deficient and the Spleen and Kidneys weak, mostly Qi deficiency. In the case of the actual patient here, his oedema of the right arm in the distal region means Qi deficiency that fails to circulate Water, and Phlegm retention in the collaterals. Abdominal acupuncture is more effective in regulating Qi and Blood to remove obstruction of channels in the affected area. Moxibustion is supplementary to promote Qi and Blood circulation. So the therapeutic effect is definitely reliable.

CONDUCT QI TO ITS PRIMARY SOURCE

It is composed of Zhongwan (CV 12), Xiawan (CV 10), Qihai (CV 6) and Guanyuan (CV 4). Of these, Zhongwan (CV 12) and Xiawan (CV 10) act on the Middle Burner, regulating the ascending and descending of Qi, because Hand-Taiyin Lung Channel originates from the Middle Burner, helping the Lungs in their function of descending; Qihai (CV 6) is the Sea of Qi, Guanyuan (CV 4) reinforces the Kidneys to consolidate the root and the Kidneys are related to Yuan-Source Qi in the congenital condition, which relies on nourishment from the acquired condition. In this way it is said to conduct Qi to its primary source. *Classic on Medical Problems (Si Nan)* says: 'Heart and Lungs exhale, Kidneys and Liver inhale.' These four points function well to treat the Heart and Lungs, regulate the Spleen and Stomach, and reinforce the Liver and Kidneys.

Abdominal Four Gates: These are composed of the bilateral Huaroumen (ST 24) and Wailing (ST 26). Of them, Huaroumen (ST 24) treats the upper portion of body and upper limbs, while Wailing (ST 26) treats the lower abdomen and lower limbs. They function to regulate Qi and Blood, circulate channel Qi up and down to the extremities, and distribute Zang Fu Qi to the whole body, indicated in whole body diseases. Used together with *Conducting Qi to the Kidneys* (primary source) or *Abdominal Heaven-Earth acupuncture*, they are very effective in clearing obstruction of the Fu organs.

Rheumatism points: Professor Bo's established points. The *Upper Rheumatism point* is 0.5 cun superolateral to Huaroumen (ST 24). The *Upper Rheumatism Lateral point* is 1 cun lateral to Huaroumen (ST 24). The *Lower Rheumatism point* is 0.5 cun infralateral to Wailing (ST 26). The *Lower Rheumatism Lower point* is 1 cun lateral to Daju (ST 27). They subdue swelling to stop pain, and used together with Daheng (SP 15), function to dispel Wind, lubricate joints, and remove Blood stasis. For treatment of shoulder and elbow, the Upper Rheumatism point may be used alone, and for lower limbs, the Lower Rheumatism point may be used alone.

CASE VI: YANG JIEBIN'S MEDICAL RECORD

1. General data

Li, female, 55.

2. Chief complaint

Her family said that she suddenly fell down and lost consciousness for half a day.

3. History of present illness

She suffered from blurred vision and dizziness for many years and sometimes numbness of the fingers. The diagnosis was hypertension. Today she was overworked, she fell down, lost consciousness, with Phlegm gurgling in her throat, left limbs paralyzed, staring eyes, and closed mouth.

4. Present symptoms

Unconsciousness, staring eyes, closed mouth, flushed face, Phlegm gurgling in throat, abrupt respiration.

Examination: BP 160/130mmHg

5. Tongue and pulse

Slightly red tongue, yellow sticky coating, rolling rapid pulse.

6. Differentiation and analysis

This is a case of Liver Yang transformed into Fire with Wind produced, Wind brought Phlegm Damp upward disturbing brain and flowing to the channels and collaterals, thus Windstroke, tense syndrome. Yellow sticky coating and rolling rapid pulse imply the Phlegm Heat misting the Heart, which is the cause of unconsciousness, staring eyes, and closed mouth.

7. Diagnosis

TCM: Windstroke (attack on Zang Fu organs, tense syndrome).

Western medicine: Stroke.

8. Treating principle

Promote resuscitation, pacify the Liver to stop Wind, resolve Phlegm, clear Fire.

9. Prescription

Five Centres, Renzhong (GV 26), Jing-Well points, Fenglong (ST 40), Hegu (LI 4), Taichong (LR 3).

'Five Centres' and Jing-Well points were pricked for bleeding; Renzhong (GV 26) punctured with a thick filiform needle and manipulated with sparrow picking method for 10 minutes; Fenglong (ST 40), Hegu (LI 4) and Taichong (LR 3) reduced heavily.

The needles were retained for 5 minutes and manipulated once every 5 minutes.

10. Effect

After the first time of treatment, her respiration tended towards normal and restlessness was relieved. On the following day, the same treatment was applied and her consciousness was restored. With another 3 treatments given in succession, her left limbs could move. Acupuncture was continued for 3 months, and her movement became normal again.

11. Essentials

For Windstroke, first-aid treatment should be given as quick as possible. In differentiation, flaccid or tense syndrome should be clearly diagnosed. In cases where the patient has staring eyes, mouth agape, clenched jaws, stiff limbs, coarse breathing, flushed face, and big floating pulse, it will be the Qi and Fire upward floating; if Phlegm is rattling in the throat, it will be excess tense syndrome. Promoting resuscitation and clearing Heat are the principles of treatment. Pricking to cause bleeding from the 'Five Centres' is important to save the patient from unconsciousness. Renzhong (GV 26, Hegu (LI 4)and Shixuan (EX-UE11) are to restore consciousness; Fenglong (ST 40) sends down and dissolves Phlegm; and Taichong (LR 3) pacifies Liver to stop Wind.

THE FIVE CENTRES

The Five Centres, created by Professor Yang Jiebin, are composed of Baihui (GV 20), bilateral Laogong (PC 8) and bilateral Yongquan (KI 1). Described as one brain centre, two palm centres and two sole centres, they restore consciousness and clear Heat very well.

SUMMARY

Windstroke is a commonly seen disease in acupuncture clinics. It is described as cerebrovascular accident in Western medicine. Its root cause is decline of anti-pathogenic Qi. The disease is in the brain and involves the Heart, Liver, Spleen, and Kidneys. The pathogenesis is genuine Qi deficiency and disorders of Qi and Blood, with retention of Wind, Fire, Phlegm, and stasis in the channels and collaterals.

In the first stage of Windstroke, 8 points from Yang channels are always selected: Jianyu (LI 15), Quchi (LI 11), Waiguan (TE 5), Hegu (LI 4), Huantiao (GB 30), Yanglingquan (GB 34), Xuanzhong (GB 39), Taichong (LR 3). Generally, the even method is adopted. Yang dominates movement. Points of the Yang channels are good to restore the movement of the limbs.

In the later stages, points of the Yin channels are selected as well, such as Chize (LU 5), Neiguan (PC 6), Sanyinjiao (SP 6), Taixi (KI 3) etc. to circulate Qi and Blood to balance Yin and Yang. Most patients will recover to varying degrees with several courses of treatment.

For numbness (Ma Mu) of limbs in the signal case, Waiguan (TE 5) and Houxi (SI 3) are used for the upper limbs, while Zhongdu (GB 32) and Xuanzhong (GB 39) are used for the lower limbs, to regulate the channels and remove obstructions. Zusanli (ST 36) and Sanyinjiao (SP 6) are selected in addition to replenish Qi and Blood because Qi deficiency is said to be the cause of Ma, and Blood deficiency the cause of Mu. The reinforcing method will be used. Usually it takes a long course of treatment in clinic.

SECTION TWENTY-ONE • LOWER BACK PAIN

CASE I: YANG YONGXUAN'S MEDICAL RECORD

1. General data

Mei, male, 46.

2. Chief complaint

Lower back pain due to sprain for 1 week.

3. History of present illness

He had strain for many years. Recently lower back pain started due to lumbar sprain. The pain was worse on cough and turning of the body. With the treatment of oral taking and external application of herbal medicine, his pain was not relieved. He came for acupuncture.

4. Present symptoms

Lower back pain with motor impairment. He looked tired.

5. Tongue and pulse

His tongue-coating was thin sticky and pulse thready and rolling.

6. Differentiation and analysis

This patient had an acute lumbar sprain with the Governor Vessel injured. Qi stagnation and Blood stasis caused the obstruction of channels and collaterals, resulting in pain.

7. Diagnosis

TCM: Lower back pain (Governor Vessel, the sea of Yang channels, being injured).

Western medicine: Acute lumbar sprain.

8. Treating principle

Remove obstruction, dispel Blood stasis.

9. Prescription

Shuigou (GV 26), Weizhong (BL 40), Qihaishu (BL 24).

The reducing method of rotating. Cupping after needling Qihaishu (BL 24). Once every other day.

10. Effect

He was getting better gradually and cured after 4 treatments.

11. Essentials

Acute lumbar sprain is commonly seen in the acupuncture department. *Yu Long Ge* (Jade Dragon in Verse) says to reduce Renzhong (GV 26) for spinal pain. Weizhong (BL 40) can be used to treat diseases of the lumbar region. Here, Shuigou (GV 26) is to regulate the reversed Qi of the Governor Vessel; Weizhong (BL 40) to regulate the Qi of the Bladder Channel; needling and cupping Qihaishu (BL 24) to warm and regulate Qi and Blood in the lower back. The pain is stopped when the obstruction is removed.

CASE II: RECORD IN *ACUPUNCTURE-MOXIBUSTION FOR DIFFICULT DISEASES*

1. General data

He, female, 50. January 18, 1999.

2. Chief complaint

Lower back pain for 8 months.

3. History of present illness

Repeated attacks of lower back pain. X-ray diagnosed her retrograde degeneration of lumbar vertebra.

4. Present symptoms

Her lower back pain became worse on exertion. Generally, she was afraid of cold, with cold extremities and increased urine.

Examination: Tenderness (+) at L4 and L5. Lifting-leg test (+).

5. Tongue and pulse

Pale tongue, white coating, thready pulse.

6. Differentiation and analysis

This is a patient with the retrograde degeneration of lumbar vertebra. It is lower back pain due to the Kidney deficiency. Being afraid of cold, cold extremities, and increased clear urine, pale tongue, white coating, and thready pulse imply Kidney Yang deficiency.

7. Diagnosis

TCM: Lower back pain (due to Kidney deficiency).

Western medicine: Degeneration of lumbar spine.

8. Treating principle

Strengthen Kidneys, circulate channel Qi.

9. Prescription

Shenshu (BL 23), Dachangshu (BL 25), Zhishi (BL 52), L2–5 Jiaji (EX-B2).

Shu Ci (Shu-point puncture) was applied. Cupping was done after needling. Once a day.

10. Effect

The pain was relieved after 6 treatments and cured after another 12 treatments.

11. Essentials

Shenshu (BL 23) is selected to reinforce the Kidneys; Dachangshu (BL 25) to strengthen the lumbus and knees and regulate the channel Qi in the lower back; Zhishi (BL 52) to replenish Kidney Yin and to strengthen the lumbus; L2–5 Jiaji (EX-B2), the important point for the retrograde degeneration of lumbar vertebra, is punctured deeply to 1.5 cun directly to the transverse process of lumbar vertebra. Cupping is good to promote the Blood circulation, regulate channel Qi in the local area. Qi and Blood circulation is improved, and the pain will be stopped.

SHU CI

Shu Ci (Shu-point puncture) is one of the needling methods mentioned in Internal Classic. It says: 'Shu Ci is to insert the needle as deep as to the bone for treating the Bone Bi (osseous pain) which is corresponding to the Kidneys.' This technique is developed in response to the diseases associated with the Kidneys, the organ in control of bones.

CASE III: CHENG XINNONG'S MEDICAL RECORD

1. General data

Li, male, 22. September 1, 1992.

2. Chief complaint

Pain in the back and lumbar region for 1 week.

3. History of present illness

The pain started owing to exposure to Wind after sweating.

4. Present symptoms

Pain in the back and lumbar region, a tense feeling in the back, aversion to wind, accompanied by irritability, insomnia, yellow urine, and constipation.

5. Tongue and pulse

Tongue tip red, cracks in the middle, white dry coating, superficial tight pulse.

6. Differentiation and analysis

The patient is constitutionally weak and his sweating causes the disharmony between Ying and Wei, on which, invasion of Wind Cold obstructs the channels and collaterals of the lower back, resulting in pain. The tense feeling in the back and aversion to wind are the signs of Wind Cold. The accompanying symptoms are the signs of Heat dispersing in the body stopped by Wind Cold.

7. Diagnosis

TCM: Lower back pain (disharmony between Ying-nutrient and Wei-defence).

Western medicine: Lumbago.

8. Treating principle

Dispel Wind and Cold, regulate Ying and Wei, remove obstruction of the channels, stop pain.

9. Prescription

Dazhui (GV 14), Fengchi (GB 20), Yaoyangguan (GV 3), Jianwaishu (SI 14), Shenshu (BL 23), Lieque (LU 7), Hegu (LI 4), Neiguan (PC 6), Shenmen (HT 7), Zusanli (ST 36), Sanyinjiao (SP 6), Taichong (LR 3), Neiting (ST 44).

Dazhui (GV 14), Fengchi (GB 20), Hegu (LI 4), Taichong (LR 3) and Neiting (ST 44) were reduced. Other points, even method.

10. Effect

Four treatments cured him.

11. Essentials

Clear the internal Heat, dispel the external Cold, regulate Ying-nutrient and Wei-defence systems, and remove obstruction of the channels and collaterals, then aim to stop pain.

CASE IV: CHENG XINNONG'S MEDICAL RECORD

1. General data

Li, male, 29. December 24, 1992.

2. Chief complaint

Lower back pain for 2 months.

3. History of present illness

Lower back pain without known reasons.

4. Present symptoms

A dull pain in the lower back, sometimes worse sometimes better, radiating to the sacral region, accompanied by yellow urine and frequent urination. Dark complexion without lustre.

5. Tongue and pulse

Purplish tongue with toothmarks on borders, white coating, rolling pulse, Chi pulse weak.

6. Differentiation and analysis

The Kidneys are located in the lower back region. When Kidney Qi is deficient, or Cold Damp invades, Qi and Blood will be obstructed in circulation, causing pain. The Kidneys control urine and stools, and their channel is externally–internally related with that of the Bladder. When the Qi activities of the Bladder mean that it is too weak to store urine, there will be frequent urination.

7. Diagnosis

TCM: Lower back pain (invasion of Cold Damp).

Western medicine: Lumbago.

8. Treating principle

Tonify Kidney Qi, dispel Cold Damp, remove obstruction of channels.

9. Prescription

Shenshu (BL 23), Yaoyangguan (GV 3), Mingmen (GV 4), Zhibian (BL 54), Weizhong (BL 40), Feiyang (BL 58), Zusanli (ST 36), Sanyinjiao (SP 6), Taixi (KI 3).

Moxibustion was applied at Shenshu (BL 23) and Yaoyangguan (GV 3). The reinforcing method was adopted at Mingmen (GV 4), Zusanli (ST 36) and Taixi (KI 3). Even method was adopted at the other points.

10. Effect

The lower back pain was greatly relieved after 4 treatments with a heavy sensation in the sacral region. All symptoms disappeared after 10 treatments.

11. Essentials

Taixi (KI 3), Shenshu (BL 23), Yaoyangguan (GV 3), Mingmen (GV 4), Zhibian (BL 54), and so on are used to reinforce the Kidney Qi and remove the obstruction of channels and collaterals, while Zusanli (ST 36) used for strengthen the acquired foundation.

CASE V: JI XIAOPING'S MEDICAL RECORD

1. General data

Anonymous male, 44 years old, German, came on January 30, 1995 for the first visit.

2. Chief complaint

Pain in lower back and legs for 15 years.

3. History of present illness

Pain in lower back and legs, sometimes worse sometimes better, aggravated when tired. X-ray and MRI examinations reported protrusion of the L4–L5 intervertebral disc. He had block therapy for more than 600 times that only alleviated his pain but did not cure it, so he came for acupuncture treatment.

4. Present symptoms

Pain in the right side of the lower back, buttocks, and the lateral side of the legs, aggravated when tired, numbness on the lateral side of the legs, small swellings at the Jiaji (EX-B2) areas of L4–L5 with severe tenderness radiating to the lateral side of the legs.

5. Tongue and pulse

Purple tongue with ecchymosis on it, white thick coating, string-taut and hesitant pulse.

6. Differentiation and analysis

The cause of his pathological condition is obstruction of meridian Qi. Huatuo Jiaji points are the distribution areas of the major collaterals of the Bladder Meridian. The buttocks and lateral side of the leg are the distribution areas of the Gallbladder Meridian. That is the obstruction of Bladder and Gallbladder Meridian Qi. Prolonged obstruction leads to Blood stasis. Swellings at the Jiaji (EX-B2) areas of L4–L5 with severe tenderness, purple tongue, and hesitant pulse are all the manifestations of Blood stasis. It can be seen that Qi obstruction and Blood stasis of the Bladder and Gallbladder meridians is the diagnosis for this case.

7. Diagnosis

TCM: Lower back and leg pain.

Western medicine: Protrusion of lumbar intervertebral disc, sciatica.

8. Treating principle

Remove obstruction of meridians and collaterals, circulate Qi and activate Blood.

9. Prescription

Shiqizhui (EX-B8), Jiaji (EX-B2) of L4 and L5, Dachangshu (BL 25), Weizhong (BL 40), Huantiao (GB 30) (right side), Yanglingquan (GB 34), Waiqiu (GB 36).
    The reducing method, retaining the needles for 20 minutes, twice a week.

10. Effect

After 3 treatments, his pain was greatly relieved, and 7 treatments later, his pain and numbness disappeared completely. One year follow-up found no relapse.

11. Essentials

His pain in the lower back and legs is the result of obstruction of the meridians and collaterals, without diseases of the Zang Fu organs. There are different methods of syndrome differentiation in TCM, including syndrome differentiation according to the theories of Eight Principles, Zang Fu, Meridians and Collaterals, etc. The patient has his pathological condition reflected in meridians and collaterals, not in Zang Fu, so the syndrome differentiation according to the theory of meridians and collaterals should be applied.

    In addition, TCM holds that prolonged Qi stagnation will cause Blood stasis. The 15 years' pain and with swelling and tenderness at the Jiaji area, purple tongue, and hesitant pulse of the patient here are all the manifestations of Blood stasis.

    The pathogenesis of this patient is Qi stagnation and Blood stasis. The correct differentiation brings out the success of treatment.

SUMMARY

Lower back pain can be found in invasion of exogenous pathogenic Wind Cold Damp, trauma due to sprain or contusion, known as the exogenous case; or Kidney deficiency caused by excessive sexual activity that consumes Essence and Qi or overwork that damages the Kidneys, known as the endogenous case. The lumbus houses the Kidneys. Kidney diseases cause lower back pain. Acupuncture is effective for lower back pain.

Main points: Shenshu (BL 23), Yaoyangguan (GV 3), Weizhong (BL 40).

Huantiao (GB 30), Chengshan (BL 57) and Kunlun (BL 60) are added for pain radiating to the lower extremities; Do bleeding at Weizhong (BL 40) for whose who are with Blood stasis due to traumatic injury; Renzhong (GV 26) is added for stiffness and pain in spine and back.

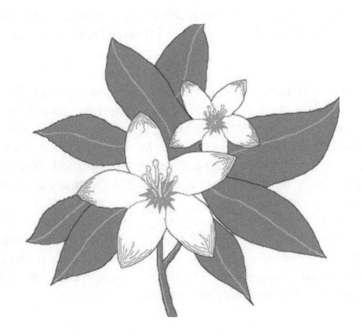

SECTION TWENTY-TWO • LUO ZHEN (TORTICOLLIS)

CASE I: YANG YONGXUAN'S MEDICAL RECORD

1. General data

Wang, male, 33.

2. Chief complaint

Pain in the nape for 3 days.

3. History of present illness

The day before yesterday, he slept on a pillow with a pillow-mat uneven on it. On the following day he got up with a stiff neck, seriously painful, and was unable to raise and turn his head.

4. Present symptoms

Neck pain with motor impairment.

5. Tongue and pulse

Thin sticky coating, a bit slow pulse.

6. Differentiation and analysis

The patient got his neck pain due to an awkward sleeping posture because of the pillow problem. The disturbance of local circulation of Qi and Blood blocked the channels.

7. Diagnosis

TCM: Luo Zhen (neck pain caused by an awkward sleeping posture) (disturbance of Qi and Blood).

Western medicine: Neck pain.

8. Treating principle

Dispel Wind Cold, warm channels, remove obstruction.

9. Prescription

Hegu (LI 4). Right side: Tianzhu (BL 10), Jianjing (GB 21), Fengmen (BL 12).

The reducing method of rotating was applied to Tianzhu (BL 10), Jianjing (GB 21) and Fengmen (BL 12). The reducing method of lifting-thrusting was applied to Hegu (LI 4). Moxibustion was applied to Jianjing (GB 21) after needling. Cupping was applied to Fengmen (BL 12) after needling.

10. Effect

One treatment cured him.

11. Essentials

For the treatment of neck pain, local points and cupping are effective. And the point Luozhen (Extra) punctured with the reducing method is also good. For serious pain, apply reducing to Kunlun (BL 60) and Xuanzhong (GB 39), or Lieque (LU 7) and Yanglao (SI 6). These are distal points but the therapeutic effect is very good too.

LUOZHEN

Luozhen (Extra) is located on the dorsum of the hand, between the second and third metacarpal bones, about 0.5 cun posterior to the metacarpophalangeal joint. Puncture perpendicularly or obliquely 0.5–1 cun. Indicated in neck pain and pain in shoulder and arm.

CASE II: CHENG XINNONG'S MEDICAL RECORD

1. General data

Liang, male, 34, visited on July 9, 1986.

2. Chief complaint

Pain in the left side of the neck for 2 days.

3. History of present illness

Two days ago, he began to have a pain in the left side of his neck owing to reading a book for a long time at night. The pain was gradually getting worse, causing motor impairment. With acupuncture and cupping, it was not getting better.

4. Present symptoms

Serious pain, motor impairment, tenderness along the Taiyang and Shaoyang channels in the local area.

5. Tongue and pulse

Pale tongue, slightly yellow coating, deep and a bit slow pulse.

6. Differentiation and analysis

Obstruction of Taiyang and Shaoyang channels with Qi and Blood stagnation is the cause of the neck pain for its location is along the distribution of these channels.

7. Diagnosis

TCM: Neck pain (due to improper position causing the Qi and Blood obstructed in channels and collaterals).

Western medicine: Torticollis.

8. Treating principle

Activate Blood, remove Blood stasis, soothe the muscles.

9. Prescription

Affected side: Tianzhu (BL 10), Houxi (SI 3), Fengchi (GB 20). The reducing method.

10. Effect

After acupuncture, the pain was stopped immediately and the neck could move freely.

11. Essentials

The points of the affected channels are selected. Tianzhu (BL 10) and Fengchi (GB 20) are good to regulate Qi and Blood, remove obstruction of these channels to stop pain; while the distal point, Houxi (SI 3), is used to circulate the Qi of Taiyang Channel. The combination of local and distal points stops the pain by removing the obstruction of channels.

SUMMARY

Torticollitis (Luo Zhen) here refers to wryneck with motor impairment caused by an awkward sleeping posture and attack of Wind Cold that leads to disturbance of Qi and Blood in the channels. In acupuncture treatment, the affected channels should be clearly found out.

Main points: Dazhui (GV 14), Tianzhu (BL 10), Juegu (GB 39), Houxi (SI 3).

Jianwaishu (SI 14) is added for pain involved in the shoulder and back, and cupping is applicable; Kunlun (BL 60) is added for difficulty in bending the head forward and backward; Zhizheng (SI 7) added for difficulty in turning the head to the left and right.

SECTION TWENTY-THREE • CERVICAL SPONDYLOSIS

CASE I: YANG JIASAN'S MEDICAL RECORD

1. General data

Liu, female, 65, first visited on April 4, 1987.

2. Chief complaint

Neck motor impairment with pain and snap for 1 year.

3. History of present illness

She had a neck pain with motor impairment. It became better with massage treatment, but not cured.

4. Present symptoms

Pain in the neck with snap, right hand numbness, dizziness, headache, nausea, and back heaviness.

Examination: Tenderness at C6 and C7. X-ray film showed a slightly straight cervical curvature, C4–7 hyperosteogeny, and narrowing of intervertebral space. Impression: Cervical spondylosis.

5. Tongue and pulse

Tongue tip red, coating thin yellow, pulse deep wiry.

6. Differentiation and analysis

The neck area is the Yang part of human body, easily attacked by pathogenic factors Wind, Cold, Heat, etc. If the Qi and Blood of the channels are blocked, then there will be pain and numbness.

7. Diagnosis

TCM: Bi syndrome (Wind and Cold blocking the channels of the neck region).

Western medicine: Cervical spondylosis.

8. Treating principle

Clear the upper part, reinforce the lower part.

9. Prescription

Fengchi (GB 20), Tianzhu (BL 10), C4–7 Jiaji (EX-B2), Lieque (LU 7), Houxi (SI 3).

Fengchi (GB 20) and Tianzhu (BL 10) were reduced with medium stimulation; even method with medium stimulation was used for the rest of points. The needles were retained for 20 minutes. Once every other day.

10. Effect

Ten treatments stopped all the symptoms.

11. Essentials

Fengchi (GB 20), Tianzhu (BL 10) and cervical Jiaji (EX-B2) dispel Wind and remove obstruction of channels to stop pain; Lieque (LU 7) connecting with Conception Vessel, Houxi (SI 3) with Governor Vessel, both extra channels originate from the Kidneys, the two points in combination regulate Yin and Yang, treating the root cause of cervical spondylosis at the same time as relieving pain.

CASE II: BO ZHIYUN'S MEDICAL RECORD

1. General data

Xu, female, 55, first visited on April 12, 1992.

2. Chief complaint

Neck motor impairment with soreness for 5 years.

3. History of present illness

Pain in the neck with motor impairment, sometimes worse sometimes better.

4. Present symptoms

Pain in the neck, motor impairment, shoulder muscles aching, numbness of the left arm radiating to the ring and small fingers. At night she was often waking up due to numbness and pain of the hands, which could be relieved with a little movement.

5. Tongue and pulse

6. Differentiation and analysis

Pain in the neck, shoulder muscles aching, numbness of the arm are the result of obstruction of Damp. As she is 55 years old, her Kidney Essence is deficient.

7. Diagnosis

TCM: Cervical spondylosis (Spleen and Kidney deficiency).

Western medicine: Cervical spondylosis.

8. Treating principle

Reinforce Spleen and Kidneys, remove obstruction of channels.

9. Prescription

Abdominal Heaven–Earth acupuncture: Zhongwan (CV 12), Guanyuan (CV 4), Shangqu (KI 17), Huaroumen (ST 24), the Upper Rheumatism point.

10. Effect

Twenty minutes after needling, the pain stopped and the neck could move freely. On the following day, she said that her pain was relieved during sleep, and her neck could move normally when she got up in the morning and the symptoms of the shoulder and the left arm were 70% less. The same treatment was applied for a total of 7 times, all symptoms disappeared.

11. Essentials

In abdominal acupuncture therapy, the location of points is in the shape of a turtle, a holo-image of whole body, with Zhongwan (CV 12) as top, Guanyuan (CV 4) as tail, Huaroumen (ST 24) as shoulder, and Shangqu (KI 17) located at the junction of neck and shoulder.

The 6 points, Zhongwan (CV 12), Guanyuan (CV 4), Shangqu (KI 17), Huaroumen (ST 24), form a prescription for the treatment of cervical spondylosis. The cervical hyperosteogeny is related to Kidney deficiency. Thus Guanyuan (CV 4) is used to reinforce the Kidneys. The incidence of cervical hyperosteogeny is rather high, but only some patients have symptoms, and most symptoms involve poor functions of the cervical muscles. The Spleen is the organ which dominates the muscles, so to reinforce the Spleen, Zhongwan (CV 12) is used. Huaroumen (ST 24) is used to circulate the channel Qi of the arms and head; Shangqu (KI 17) is used to treat the local area.

ABDOMINAL HEAVEN-EARTH ACUPUNCTURE

Zhongwan (CV 12) is the Front-Mu point of the Stomach, which is externally-internally related with the Spleen. The Spleen and Stomach are known as the Sea of Food Essence; Guanyuan (CV 4), also known as the Dantian, is the Front-Mu point of the Small Intestine, functioning to consolidate the Kidneys, reinforce Qi and restore Yang. They are used in combination with each other to tonify the Spleen and Kidneys.

RHEUMATISM POINTS

These are Professor Bo's established points. Of them, the Upper Rheumatism point is located 0.5 cun superolateral to Huaroumen (ST 24), and the Lower Rheumatism point is located 0.5 cun infralateral to Wailing (ST 26). They are good for relieving swelling and stopping pain, and used together with Daheng (SP 15), function to dispel Wind, lubricate joints, and remove Blood stasis. For treatment of the shoulder and elbow, the Upper Rheumatism point may be used alone, and for lower limb, the Lower Rheumatism point may be used alone.

CASE III: YANG JINHONG'S MEDICAL RECORD

1. General data

Kong, female, 47 years old.

2. Chief complaint

Pain of both upper extremities, weakness of the left arm, dysfunctions of the left wrist, palm and fingers for 3 months.

3. History of present illness

Three months ago, she began to have stabbing pain and numbness of the upper extremities after getting cold. The stabbing pain was accompanied by a feeling of an electric shock. The neck was especially stiff on the left side. With the development of the condition, she couldn't lift her left arm, and the motor impairment of the hand appeared. She went to Peking University Hospital and an MRI scan showed the lumbar intervertebral disc protruding and fusion of the L4–L5 vertebral bodies. After an operation, the right arm functions were restored in lifting and grasping although the strength was a little weak and the pain still existed; the left arm could lift but the wrist and fingers have pain and could not stretch. And she was very sensitive to Wind and Cold.

4. Present symptoms

Pain and numbness of the shoulders, arms and hands, inability of the wrist and fingers of the left hand to stretch and weakness in flexion.

5. Tongue and pulse

Light red tongue, thin white coating; string-taut thready pulse.

6. Differentiation and analysis

Constitutionally she was weak. The invasion of exogenous pathogenic Wind Cold and Damp obstructed the meridians and collaterals. Stagnated Qi and Blood circulation caused the pain, numbness and motor impairment of the extremities.

7. Diagnosis

TCM: Bi syndrome.

Western medicine: 1. cervical spondylosis, or 2. neuronal damage of radial nerve.

8. Treating principle

Dispel Wind Cold, promote circulation of Qi and Blood, stop pain.

9. Prescription

Baihui (GV 20), Fengchi (GB 20), Jianyu (LI 15), Naohui (TE 13), Shousanli (LI 10), Waiguan (TE 5), Hegu (LI 4), Baxie (EX-UE9), Ashi. Acupuncture with electro-stimulation for 30 minutes.

Warming-needle moxibustion for 3 points on the arm each time.

Once a day. Ten treatments later, once every other day. In total 30 treatments.

10. Effect

Effective. After 10 treatments, the pain was significantly relieved; after 20 times, the pain basically stopped, the muscle strength was reinforced and the flexion improved; after 30 treatments, the stretching of the wrist was considerably better.

11. Essentials

This is a difficult case. Warming-needle moxibustion functions to dispel Wind Cold and Damp to remove obstruction of the meridians and collaterals to stop pain, effective for serious cases of Wind Cold and Damp going into the interior.

SUMMARY

Cervical spondylosis is the manifestation of the retrogression of the cervical intervertebral disk, cervical hyperosteogeny and degeneration of connecting ligaments with the pathological changes caused by the pressed nerve roots, spinal cord and vertebral artery. According to Professor Yang Jiasan, the root cause of cervical spondylosis is Liver and Kidney deficiency, tendon and bone malnutrition, and at the same time, invasion of exogenous pathogenic Wind Cold causing non-smooth circulation of Qi and Blood, or Liver Yang hyperactivity causing Shaoyang Qi obstruction. In this case, stiffness and pain of neck and dizziness appears. With the development of the disease, the Spleen and Stomach, the acquired condition of the human body, will be involved, and numbness, muscular atrophy, and spasm of the tendons and muscles of the extremities appear, showing the pathological changes of Ben deficiency and Biao excess and lower part deficiency and upper part excess. Because it is rooted in Liver and Kidney deficiency, the lower, and manifested in neck and head, the upper, the treating principle is to reinforce the lower and clear the upper, with the points mainly selected from Yang channels.

Basic points: Fengchi (GB 20), Tianzhu (BL 10), Lieque (LU 7), Houxi (SI 3), and cervical Jiaji (EX-B2).

Supplementary points: Baihui (GV 20) for dizziness; Waiguan (TE 5) and Baxie (EX-UE9) for numbness of fingers.

Fengchi (GB 20), the meeting of Foot-Shaoyang and Yangwei channels, is good at dispelling the internal Wind upward disturbance and the external Wind invasion as well, so it is important in treating Wind; and, it is located in the nape, so is good to get the cervical joints free from motor impairment. Tianzhu (BL 10) dispels Wind Cold and removes obstruction of channels. As said in *Bai Zhen Fu* (*Treatment of Diseases in Verse*): 'Stiff neck with aversion to wind, Shugu (BL 65) and Tianzhu (BL 10) for treatment.'

Lieque (LU 7), the Luo-Connecting point of the Hand-Taiyin Lung Channel, connecting with the Conception Vessel, is used to disperse the Lungs and dispel pathogens, and regulate the Conception Vessel, treating pain of neck and head. *Si Zong Xue Ge* (Song of the Four Most Common Points) says: 'For diseases of head and neck, Lieque (LU 7) is the most common point to select.' And, the Conception Vessel pertains to the Kidneys, dominating Yin of the whole body, Lung Metal produces Kidney Water, reinforcing the mother for a deficiency syndrome, thus, Lieque (LU 7) is used to replenish the Yin of the Kidneys as well. Houxi (SI 3) is the Shu-Stream of the Hand-Taiyang Channel, connecting with the Governor Vessel. *Classic on Medical Problems* (*Liu Shi Ba Nan*) says: 'Shu-Stream points are indicated in the heavy sensation of the body and painful joints.' It is believed to be able to promote the circulation of Qi of channels of the back and clear the deficient Heat of the Upper Burner for subduing Wind Yang upward disturbance. The combination of Lieque (LU 7) and Houxi (SI 3) is to regulate the Conception and Governor vessels, that is, Yin and Yang.

Cervical Jiaji (EX-B2) points, are located 0.5 cun lateral to the lower border of the spinous process of the cervical vertebra, at the medial border of trapezius. Those 8 bilateral to C3–C7 are commonly used. Although not yet written in formal textbooks, they are commonly used in the clinic because of their good effect in removing obstructions of channels and stopping pain.

In this prescription, which is precisely made up with careful selection of points, Fengchi (GB 20) and Tianzhu (BL 10) mainly treat Biao in unobstructing channels by dispelling pathogenic factors, while Lieque (LU 7) and Houxi (SI 3) treat Biao on one hand in dispelling pathogenic factors and treat Ben on the other hand in reinforcing the lower and clearing the upper to regulate Yin and Yang; and Jiaji (EX-B2) directly acts on the affected area to circulate Qi and Blood.

SECTION TWENTY-FOUR • XING BI (WANDERING BI)

CASE I: LU SHOUYAN'S MEDICAL RECORD

1. General data

Wang, male, 22, first visited on April 30, 1963.

2. Chief complaint

A migrating pain in the joints of the 4 extremities for 2 months.

3. History of present illness

Migrating pain in the joints of the extremities occurred with unknown cause.

4. Present symptoms

Migrating pain, motor impairment of knee and wrist joints, accompanied with dizziness, listlessness, fullness in chest, palpitations, and scanty yellow urine.

5. Tongue and pulse

Swollen tongue, thin coating, wiry rapid pulse, Hanyan (GB 4) pulse strong.

6. Differentiation and analysis

Wandering Bi is mainly due to invasion by pathogenic Wind which is characterized by constant movement and changes. The patient here was invaded by Wind Cold Damp with an internal Water deficiency and Wood hyperactivity, in this case, the external Wind and internal Liver Wind give rise to migrating pain, resulting in wandering Bi. His palpitations and chest fullness are the outcome of pathogens entering the Heart.

7. Diagnosis

TCM: Wandering Bi (Water less and Wood hyperactive, Wind Yang floating).

Western medicine: Arthritis.

8. Treating principle

Replenish Yin, subdue Yang, dispel Wind, dissolve Damp.

9. Prescription

Baihui (GV 20), Fengchi (GB 20), Fengfu (GV 16), Dubi (ST 35), Xiyan (EX-LE5), Zhongzhu (TE 3), Hegu (LI 4), Xiaxi (GB 43), Taixi (KI 3), Taichong (LR 3).

Reinforcing and reducing through lifting-thrusting and rotating were applied.
Taixi (KI 3), the reinforcing method, other points, the reducing method, with
the needles retained for 10 minutes.

10. Effect

With four of the above-mentioned treatments, the dizziness and pain got better,
but the palpitations and fullness in chest still existed. Thready wiry rolling pulse.
The Hanyan (GB 4) and Chongyang (ST 42) pulses strong. The pathogenic factor
entering the Heart made the Mind stored in the Heart disturbed. In addition to
the previous method, the treatment aimed at calming the Mind was added. Points:
Fengchi (GB 20), Ximen (PC 4), Shenmen (HT 7), Zhongzhu (TE 3), Hegu (LI 4),
Taixi (KI 3) and Taichong (LR 3). Reinforcing and reducing of lifting-thrusting
and rotating were applied. Taixi (KI 3) was reinforced and other points reduced, the
needles retained for 10 minutes.

After 12 times of acupuncture, the pulse now was a little wiry and rapid, the left
side pulse bigger than the right one, Hanyan (GB 4) pulse even. The tongue-coating
was thin white. So Fengchi (GB 20), Ximen (PC 4), Hanyan (GB 4), Taichong
(LR 3) were used to consolidate the effect. The needles were retained for 10 minutes.

11. Essentials

Professor Lu punctured Baihui (GV 20), Fengchi (GB 20) and Fengfu (GV 16) with
the reducing method for dispelling Wind to subdue Yang, punctured Hegu (LI 4)
and Taichong (LR 3), the Four Gates, with the reducing method for subduing Wind
Yang, punctured Taixi (KI 3) with the reinforcing method for replenishing Kidney
Water to soften Liver Wood, and punctured Shenmen (HT 7), Ximen (PC 4) and
Neiguan (PC 6) with the reducing method to remove pathogenic factor invading
the Heart. In addition, some local points along the running course of affected channels are selected to stop pain. Twelve treatments in this way achieved a remarkable
effect.

CASE II: CHENG XINNONG'S MEDICAL RECORD

1. General data

Shang, male, 65, first visited December 6, 1991.

2. Chief complaint

Migrating pain in the right arm for 1 week.

3. History of present illness

Migrating pain in the right arm radiating to the shoulder and back.

4. Present symptoms

The arm pain is moving, radiating to the shoulder and back, accompanied by dizziness, a slight numbness in the left cheek, poor sleep.

5. Tongue and pulse

Swollen purple tongue, thin yellow coating, thready wiry pulse.

6. Differentiation and analysis

The pathogenic Wind Cold and Damp, with the Wind as the most severe of the three, block in channels and collaterals, there is a migrating pain. The dizziness, facial numbness, and poor sleep are the manifestation of Qi and Blood deficiency resulting from the blockage of channels and collaterals by pathogenic factors.

7. Diagnosis

TCM: Wandering Bi (anti-pathogenic Qi weak, pathogenic Qi invading).

Western medicine: Scapulohumeral periarthritis.

8. Treating principle

Dispel Wind Cold, remove obstruction of channels.

9. Prescription

Fengchi (GB 20), left side: Quanliao (SI 18), Jiache (ST 6), Jianyu (LI 15), Jianliao (TE 14), Quchi (LI 11), Waiguan (TE 5), Hegu (LI 4), Houxi (SI 3).
    Acupuncture with even method.

10. Effect

After 4 times of acupuncture the pain was relieved, and after 10 times, the patient was cured.

11. Essentials

Reinforce the anti-pathogenic Qi, to treat Qi and Blood deficiency, and reduce pathogenic Qi, to dispel Wind Cold and remove obstruction of channels, at the same time.

SECTION TWENTY-FIVE • ZHUO BI (FIXED BI)

CASE I: LU SHOUYAN'S MEDICAL RECORD

1. General data

Chu, male, 30, first visited on June 7, 1963.

2. Chief complaint

Pain in the joints of the extremities for many years.

3. History of present illness

Pain in the joints of the extremities for many years, accompanied by numbness in the lower back.

4. Present symptoms

Numbness and soreness in the right extremities, the right hand not able to grasp, soreness in the lower back, seminal emission, weakness in the lower extremities, dizziness, poor appetite, and loose stools twice a day.

5. Tongue and pulse

Red tongue, sticky coating, Cunkou pulse soft and a bit slow, Taixi (KI 3), Chongyang (ST 42) and Taichong (LR 3) pulses thready, Hanyan (GB 4) pulse big.

6. Differentiation and analysis

Fixed Bi is mainly due to invasion by pathogenic Damp which is characterized by heaviness. The patient here is invaded mainly by Damp, manifested as pain in the joints of the extremities, numbness and weakness in the lower back and lower extremities, poor appetite, and loose stools. The signs of Kidney deficiency are soreness in the lower back and seminal emission. Dizziness and red tongue plus Hanyan (GB 4) pulse big means deficient Yang floating upward. It is the syndrome of Liver, Spleen and Kidney deficiency, Damp formation together with Liver Yang hyperactivity.

7. Diagnosis

TCM: Fixed Bi (Spleen deficiency, Damp retention, Liver and Kidney deficiency).

Western medicine: Arthritis.

8. Treating principle

Replenish Water, inhibit Wood, strengthen Earth, transport Damp.

9. Prescription

Fengchi (GB 20), Hanyan (GB 4), Taixi (KI 3), Xingjian (LR 2), Shenshu (BL 23), Zusanli (ST 36), Pishu (BL 20), Yinlingquan (SP 9).

Right side: Quchi (LI 11), Shousanli (LI 10), Yanglingquan (GB 34), Juegu (GB 39), Baxie (EX-UE9).

Reinforcing and reducing through lifting-thrusting and rotating were applied.

Taixi (KI 3), Shenshu (BL 23), Zusanli (ST 36) and Pishu (BL 20) were reinforced, others reduced, the needles retained for 10 minutes.

10. Effect

11. Essentials

Moxibustion can be applied, but this patient has a deficient Yang floating upward, not the indication of moxibustion, so acupuncture alone adopted.

Fengchi (GB 20) and Hanyan (GB 4) are selected to clear the floating Yang; Taixi (KI 3), Shenshu (BL 23), Zusanli (ST 36), Pishu (BL 20) to reinforce Spleen and Kidneys; Xingjian (LR 2) reduced to reduce the Liver Fire; Yinlingquan (SP 9) reduced to dissolve Damp; and those points on the right extremity to remove obstruction of channels and collaterals to eliminate Bi.

CASE II: CHENG XINNONG'S MEDICAL RECORD

1. General data

You, male, 26, first visited on August 31, 1992.

2. Chief complaint

Pain and heaviness in both knees for half a year.

3. History of present illness

He said that his pain was due to invasion of Wind Cold.

4. Present symptoms

The pain was accompanied with heaviness in both knees. The epigastric distending pain was worse on intake of cold food. Loose stools. Soreness in lower back. Dark complexion.

5. Tongue and pulse

Toothprints on borders of tongue, white slippery coating, wiry rolling pulse, Chi pulse weak.

6. Differentiation and analysis

Invasion of Cold and Damp is the cause of a heavy pain in the knees, Cold Damp damages the Spleen which dislikes the Damp, leading to poor transportation and transformation, resulting in epigastric distending pain and loose stools. Dark complexion, lower back pain, and Chi pulse weak are the signs of Kidney deficiency.

7. Diagnosis

TCM: Fixed Bi (Cold Damp invasion).

Western medicine: Gonitis.

8. Treating principle

Dispel Cold, eliminate Damp, remove obstruction of channels, stop pain, warm Stomach, strengthen Spleen.

9. Prescription

Fengchi (GB 20), Xiyan (EX-LE5), Dubi (ST 35), Heding (EX-LE2), Yinlingquan (SP 9), Yanglingquan (GB 34), Zusanli (ST 36), Sanyinjiao (SP 6), Xuanzhong (GB 39), Kunlun (BL 60), Tianshu (ST 25), Zhongwan (CV 12), Guanyuan (CV 4).

Zhongwan (CV 12) and Guanyuan (CV 4) were applied with moxibustion. Other points, even method.

10. Effect

After 5 acupuncture treatments, the pain in the knees and distending pain in the epigastrium was relieved. After 10 times, the distending pain in the epigastrium was greatly relieved and the heavy pain in the knees cured.

11. Essentials

Moxibustion at Zhongwan (CV 12) and Guanyuan (CV 4) functions to strengthen the Yuan-Source Qi and reinforce the Kidneys to dispel Cold and eliminate Damp, warm the channels and collaterals to stop pain, and warm the Stomach and promote the functions of the Spleen.

> **HEDING**
> Heding (EX-LE2), located in the depression of the midpoint of the superior patellar border, is indicated in knee pain, crane-knee syndrome (arthroncus of knee), and flaccidity of lower limbs, etc.

CASE III: WEI LIXIN'S MEDICAL RECORD

1. General data

Hussein, male, 37 years old, Bangalese.

2. Chief complaint

Knee joint swelling and pain for more than 6 months, especially the right knee.

3. History of present illness

Six months ago, the knee joints began to be painful, worse on rainy days. Physiotherapy and medication didn't relieve the pain much. He came for acupuncture treatment.

4. Present symptoms

Knee joint swelling, friction in the joint, motor impairment in the right knee joint, tenderness and rope-like nodules felt on the medial side of knee joints, soreness, heaviness, fixed pain and numbness in the knee joints. Appetite and sleep were normal. X-ray examination showed joint space narrower and the right knee joint soft tissue shadow full. Erythrocyte sedimentation rate (ESR) and antistreptolysin O (ASO) were normal.

5. Tongue and pulse

Pale tongue, white sticky coating; soft weak retarded pulse.

6. Differentiation and analysis

Swelling and pain of knee joints, especially on rainy days, relates to Damp. Soreness, heaviness, and fixed pain is thought to be in accordance with the heavy and turbid nature of Damp. Pale tongue, white sticky coating, and soft weak retarded pulse indicates not only Damp but also Spleen deficiency. Damp affects the Spleen, the deficiency of which produces Damp. Because Damp is characterized by viscosity and stagnation, so the pathological condition is prolonged without relief.

7. Diagnosis

TCM: Fixed Bi.

Western medicine: Knee osteoarthritis complicated with synovitis.

8. Treating principle

Strengthen the Spleen, dissolve Damp, remove obstruction of meridians and collaterals.

9. Prescription

Heding (EX-LE2), Neixiyan (EX-LE4), Dubi (ST 35), Yinlingquan (SP 9), Yanglingquan (GB 34), Zusanli (ST 36), Xuehai (SP 10), Liangqiu (ST 34), Ashi.
  Acupuncture and moxibustion.

10. Effect

One course of treatment made the swelling disappear and greatly relieved the pain. Two courses of treatment cured the pain.

11. Essentials

The climate of Bangladesh is humid, so those people with a weak constitution are likely to be attacked by pathogenic Damp. The influence of geographical conditions should be taken into consideration in the treatment. This is an important point but one easily neglected in clinical practice.

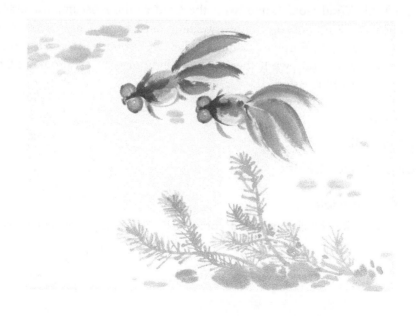

SECTION TWENTY-SIX • TONG BI (PAINFUL BI)

CASE I: CHENG XINNONG'S MEDICAL RECORD

1. General data

Zhao, male, 23, first visited on December 2, 1987.

2. Chief complaint

Pain in the left lower limb for 3 months, worse for about 20 days.

3. History of present illness

Three months ago, he got a distending pain in the left calf from taking a shower after sweating. About 20 days ago, since the weather was getting cold, he began to have a pain in the posterior aspect of the left lower limb.

4. Present symptoms

The pain was in the posterior aspect of the left lower limb, worse at night and made better by warmth, worse on exertion, and accompanied with the contracture of the lower limb. Herbal medication and Antifan didn't relieve the pain. His appetite was normal.

5. Tongue and pulse

Purplish tongue, white coating, wiry tight pulse.

6. Differentiation and analysis

The pathogenic Wind Cold Damp, with the Cold as the most important aspect, invade when the skin pores open after sweating and when taking a shower. Thus painful Bi is the result. Purplish tongue implies the Blood stasis comes from the Cold stagnated in the body, while the wiry pulse indicates pain syndrome, and tight pulse means the Cold invasion.

7. Diagnosis

TCM: Painful Bi.

Western medicine: Arthritis.

8. Treating principle

Remove obstruction of channels and collaterals, activate Blood circulation, stop pain.

9. Prescription

Baihui (GV 20), Dazhui (GV 14), Fengchi (GB 20), Yaoyangguan (GV 3), Shenshu (BL 23), Sanyinjiao (SP 6). Left side: Huantiao (GB 30), Ciliao (BL 32), Weizhong (BL 40), Chengshan (BL 57), Kunlun (BL 60).

Fengchi (GB 20), Dazhui (GV 14), Weizhong (BL 40) and Kunlun (BL 60) were reduced; other points, even method; moxibustion applied to Yaoyangguan (GV 3). Once a day.

10. Effect

He came with a serious pain with motor impairment of the left lower limb, and by taking 4 Antifan tablets he could sleep at night. Six times of acupuncture treatment as mentioned above relieved his pain greatly. The motor impairment was basically cured. Without analgesic, a slight pain was still present at night, but the contracture of the lower limb disappeared. His pulse was wiry and tongue light red. The same treatment was given for a total of 12 times, and his symptoms stopped. He was asked to take care of himself well, especially not to carry heavy loads, and avoid exposure to Wind Cold. Two months later, the follow-up found no recurrence.

11. Essentials

For the Painful Bi, Dazhui (GV 14), Fengchi (GB 20), Sanyinjiao (SP 6) are used to dispel the pathogenic factors, plus local points, to remove obstruction of channels and collaterals. Even after he is cured he needs to take good care in daily life, to avoid being attacked again.

JIANNEILING

Jianneiling (Extra), with the arm naturally down, is located midway between the end of the anterior axillary fold and Jianyu (LI 15). It functions to dispel Wind, remove obstruction of channels and clear collaterals, indicated in hemiplegia, shoulder pain with inability to lift the arm, and pain in the medial aspect of the upper arm. Method: puncture perpendicularly 1-1.5 cun or penetrating 2-3 cun to Jianzhen (SI 9).

CASE II: CHEN YUELAI AND ZHENG KUISHAN'S MEDICAL RECORD

1. General data

Xiao, female, 32, first visited on December 5, 1999.

2. Chief complaint

Pain in the left lower limb for 1 month, worse for 1 week.

3. History of present illness

One month ago, she suddenly felt a pulling pain in the left lower limb from below the buttocks down to foot dorsum along the posterior lateral side, worse on walking, exposed to cold and tiredness. The hospital diagnosed her sciatic neuritis and prescribed her Brufen and Fenbid. Bed rest and medication didn't relieve her much.

4. Present symptoms

The pain was in the left lower extremity. When walking, the toes of the left foot touched the ground first. Tenderness at the spinous processes of lumbar vertebra (-), jaw-chest test (-), tenderness at the posterior aspect of thigh and the course of sciatica nerve (+), straight lifting leg test (+), CT scan showed no abnormality of lumbosacral vertebra.

5. Tongue and pulse

Red tongue, thin white coating, wiry thready pulse.

6. Differentiation and analysis

This is a Bi syndrome with Cold Damp retention in channels and collaterals.

7. Diagnosis

TCM: Painful Bi (Cold Damp retention).

Western medicine: Sciatic neuritis.

8. Treating principle

Remove obstruction of channels and collaterals, stop pain.

9. Prescription

Shenshu (BL 23), Zhibian (BL 54), Weizhong (BL 40), Kunlun (BL 60).

Wen Tong Fa (warming and unobstruting method) was adopted. Puncture Shenshu (BL 23) first, let the needling sensation go to Zhibian (BL 54) and keep it for 1 minute; then puncture Zhibian (BL 54), let the sensation go to Weizhong (BL 40) or foot dorsum and keep it for 1 minute; then puncture Weizhong (BL 40), let the sensation go to Kunlun (BL 60) and keep it for 1 minute; then puncture Kunlun (BL 60), let the sensation go to foot dorsum and keep it for 1 minute. Retention of the needle at each point was 20 minutes, and moxibustion with moxi-cone applied. Once a day.

10. Effect

After 1 treatment, the pain was greatly relieved. Three treatments stopped the symptoms completely.

11. Essentials

Wen Tong Fa is one of the traditional methods for clearing obstruction of the channels, in which the needling sensation is urged and conducted to the affected area. Two techniques are used in it, one is to 'urge the sensation' and the other to 'connect it one point to the next'. By doing this, the channel Qi or needling sensation is led along the affected channel in order to remove obstruction and circulate Qi and Blood.

Urge the needling sensation along the channel to the diseased area includes four manipulations: Dragon swings the tail, Tiger shakes the head, Turtle drills the cave, and Phoenix flies up and down, namely the needle is manipulated swinging at the shallow level, shaking at the deep level, drilling around, and flying up and down. With the manipulation in this way, the Qi and Blood circulation is promoted to remove the obstruction of channels and collaterals. It is indicated in those syndromes of Qi stagnation and Blood stasis and for those patients for whom there is difficulty in having arrival of Qi due to the blockage of channel Qi by the joint.

Connect the needling sensation from one point to the next to the diseased area, like a relay race, the needling sensation is conducted from the point of the affected channel or a nearby point to where it is wanted. It is good in effect for treating hemiplegia, pains and Wei syndrome.

DRAGON SWINGS THE TAIL. TIGER SHAKES THE HEAD. TURTLE DRILLS THE CAVE. PHOENIX FLIES UP AND DOWN

Dragon swings the tail: The reinforcing method of acupuncture. In manipulation, the tip of the needle is directed toward the diseased area, when the needling sensation appears like being bitten, don't lift and don't thrust, swing the needle to both sides to strengthen the transmission of the needling sensation to urge and promote the Qi.

Tiger shakes the head: The reducing method of acupuncture. In manipulation, the left hand presses below the point to prevent the needling sensation going downward, while the right hand directs the needle tip toward the diseased area. When the needling sensation appears, bend the needle body a little, from down to up, make the needle move from the left side into a shape of a half circle, then from the same side, make the needle move from up to down to the original position with shaking and trembling to spread the needling sensation along the channel.

Turtle drills the cave: An even method of acupuncture. In manipulation, rotate the needle up and down and left and right while thrusting it deeper and deeper gradually, like a turtle drilling the Earth in all directions, to make the needling sensation appear repeatedly and transmit along the channel.

Phoenix flies up and down: An even method of acupuncture. In manipulation, thrust the needle to the Earth level first, wait for the Qi, then lift it to the heaven level, when the Qi comes under the needle with the tail shaking, thrust the needle again to the human level, lift and thrust and rotate it. After the needling sensation comes, the thumb and index finger of the right hand rotate the needle quickly up and down and left and right, rotate and release it repeatedly like a bird flying, to make the needling sensation transmit along the channel.

CASE III: LIU TAOXIN'S MEDICAL RECORD

1. General data

Mapuhko, male, 72, first visited on 1 Oct 1998.

2. Chief complaint

Pain on the medial aspect of the right thigh for about 2 years.

3. History of present illness

Pain on the medial aspect of the right thigh could last for hours and its severity varied from time to time. Pain was not fixed and became worse with movement or walking. Right leg movements were very much limited so that the patient needed a walking stick for assistance. He did not notice how the pain started and denied traumatic injury and occurrence of pain in relation either to weather change or to emotions. The pain annoyed him very much, anyway. He had a lot of treatment without effect. His left leg felt cold sometimes due to an injury during the Bosnia-Herzegovina War but never felt painful.

History of asthma characterized by difficult inspiration for 5–6 years. He experienced difficult breathing 6 days ago and felt good after taking tablets. He was allergic to dust especially in autumn. He often had yellowish sputum, shortness of breath and much spontaneous sweating and felt tired easily. His hands and body often felt hot.

No other complaints. Appetite good; sleep normal; defecation and urination normal.

4. Present symptoms

Severe pain on the medial aspect of the right thigh, limited movement. Reddish cheek; low voice and slight cough. Pain worse upon pressure but no obvious positive spots.

5. Tongue and pulse

Red to deep red tongue with white coating; right pulse wiry and Lung position weak, left pulse wiry and Kidney position weak.

6. Differentiation and analysis

Obstruction of meridians and collaterals resulting in pain.

His asthma was due to deficiency of Qi and Yin of the Lung and Kidneys. Lung Qi deficiency caused shortness of breath, fatigue, spontaneous sweating and production of Phlegm which obstructed the Qi passages making Lung Qi ascending and Kidney deficiency caused difficult inspiration. Yellowish sputum, feverish sensation in hands and body and red to deep red tongue all indicated internal Heat due to Yin deficiency. Weak left Kidney pulse was a sign of Kidney deficiency.

7. Diagnosis

TCM:

- Painful Bi syndrome (right thigh).

- Asthma.

Although the pain was not fixed, nor was it mobile so that meant it was diagnosed it as painful Bi.

Western medicine:

- Atypical femoral adductor muscle syndrome?
  Causes remained unknown and diagnosis unsure so that the only treatment of taking painkillers could not help much.

- Allergic asthma.

8. Treating principle

To open the meridians and activate the collaterals to stop pain. Also to regulate the function of the Lungs and Kidneys with reinforcing Qi and Yin method.

9. Prescription

- To puncture two spots in each of the three foot Yin meridians of the right thigh, one spot below the groin and the other above the knee to cover the whole painful area; applying even techniques.

- To puncture Taiyuan (L 9) and Taixi (K 3) gently.

Treatment to be given once every 2 days.

10. Effect

Second treatment: Pain reduced for only several hours after treatment. The same prescription plus Taichong (LR 3), Taibai (SP 3) and Sanyinjiao (SP 6).

Third treatment: Pain stopped for only half a day. Trying contra-lateral puncture by examining the medial aspect of the left upper arm and puncturing few positive spots found.

Fourth treatment: Effect lasted again only for several hours. Combining local points with Yuan-Source points and He-Sea points.

Fifth treatment: Pain stopped for a longer time but still came back. Adding ear point of medial aspect of thigh.

Sixth treatment: The same treatment.

Seventh treatment: Watching the patient dragging his right leg into the clinic the doctor thought with a sudden inspiration 'Qiao Meridian should be treated' and then punctured Zhaohai (KI 6), the Confluent point connecting with the Yinqiao Meridian. The pain disappeared immediately when the needle was inserted and when treatment was over, his leg movement was completely free.

One day a month later the patient came to the clinic telling the doctor that his pain stopped completely and he enjoyed travelling in Belgrade. He praised acupuncture as treatment with a miracle effect.

Doctor then offered the patient advice on diet to help prevent attacks of asthma.

11. Essentials

The doctor ignored Qiao meridians when treating pain of the lower limbs due to Bi syndrome having been present before, so he applied the methods of selecting points along the meridians, puncturing Ashi points and combining body acupuncture with ear acupuncture respectively. Ashi points, Yuan-Source points, He-Sea points were punctured but the effect could not keep long. Doctor's sudden inspiration of treating the Qiao Meridian for limitation of leg movement helped the patient by puncturing only one point to achieve a cure. This experience made the doctor examine and treat Qiao meridians for failure of treatment of leg pain and often got good results.

SECTION TWENTY-SEVEN • RE BI (FEBRILE BI)

CASE I: YANG YONGXUAN'S MEDICAL RECORD

1. General data

Anonymous female, 59.

2. Chief complaint

A burning pain in the left shoulder for 2 days.

3. History of present illness

Two days ago, she had a fever suddenly, restlessness, and burning pain in the left shoulder.

4. Present symptoms

Burning pain in the left shoulder with difficulty in lifting the arm, redness, swelling, and hotness of the shoulder, accompanied by thirst and constipation.

Examination: Body temperature: 39.6°C.

5. Tongue and pulse

Red tongue, peeled coating with cracks in the middle, rolling rapid pulse.

6. Differentiation and analysis

Heat Bi is usually manifested as abrupt onset of a burning pain in joints and accompanied by thirst and fullness in the chest. Red tongue, peeled coating with cracks in the middle, and rolling rapid pulse imply the damage of Yin by excessive Heat.

7. Diagnosis

TCM: Heat-febrile Bi (Yin consumed and Fire excessive).

Western medicine: Scapulohumeral periarthritis.

8. Treating principle

Clear Heat, remove obstruction of channels.

9. Prescription

Left side: Jianyu (LI 15), Jianliao (TE 14), Quchi (LI 11), Waiguan (TE 5), Hegu (LI 4).

The technique *Yang Zhong Yin Yin* was adopted at Jianyu (LI 15) and Jianliao (TE 14); the reducing method of lifting-thrusting adopted at Quchi (LI 11), Waiguan (TE 5) and Hegu (LI 4).

Herbal decoction, 1 dose, oral taking:

- Chuan Gui Zhi (川桂枝 *Ramulus Cinnamomi*) 3g

- Sheng Shi Gao (生石膏 *Gypsum Fibrosum*) 30g (decocted first)

- Zhi Mu (知母 *Rhizoma Anemarrhenae*) 9g

- Sheng Shan Zhi (生山栀 *Fructus Gardeniae*) 9g

- Chao Chi Shao (炒赤芍 *Radix Paeniae Rubra*) 9g

- Dan Zi Qin (淡子芩 *Radix Scutellariae*) 6g

- Ren Dong Teng (忍冬藤 *Caulis Lonicerae*) 9g

- Ren Dong Hua (忍冬花 *Flos Lonicerae*) 9g

- Zhi Da Huang (制大黄 *Radix et Rhizoma Rhei Preparata*) 6g

- Sheng Gao Cao (生甘草 *Radix Glycyrrhizae*) 3g.

10. Effect

On the following day, the herb Jin Hu (金斛 *Herba Dendrobii*) 9g was added.

On the third day, the body temperature was lowered to 36.9°C, pain in the shoulder was relieved, and the movement of the shoulder joint improved, red tongue becoming moist, thready rolling pulse. Acupuncture and herbs were continued. In total she was treated for 5 days, then her shoulder pain disappeared and the movement became normal.

11. Essentials

The patient is treated with both acupuncture and herbs. The formula is the modification of Baihu Jia Guizhi Tang (White Tiger Decoction with Cinnamon).

YANG ZHONG YIN YIN: REINFORCE FIRST AND THEN REDUCE
Manipulate the needle at shallow and deep levels in the following way:
The needle is inserted to the shallow level first and manipulated to reinforce with 9 times of quick thrusting and slow lifting, and then thrust to the deep level and manipulated to reduce with 6 times of quick lifting and slow thrusting. It is applied to treat the disease with Cold first and then Heat.

This is a technique opposite to **Yin Zhong Yin Yang** (see p.83). Both of these techniques are indicated in complicated syndromes with deficiency and excess at the same time.

CASE II: RECORD IN *ACUPUNCTURE-MOXIBUSTION FOR DIFFICULT DISEASES*

1. General data

Zhao, male, 32, visited on April 6, 1983.

2. Chief complaint

Swelling and pain of the right index finger joints for 1 month.

3. History of present illness

Swelling and pain of the right index finger joints occurred without clear reasons.

4. Present symptoms

The pain was with motor impairment. The erythrocyte sedimentation rate (ESR) was high.

5. Tongue and pulse

Red tongue, thin yellow coating, rapid pulse.

6. Differentiation and analysis

The patient is diagnosed with Heat-febrile Bi for he has redness, swelling and burning pain of joints. Red tongue, thin yellow coating, and rapid pulse indicate interior Heat.

7. Diagnosis

TCM: Heat-febrile Bi (pathogenic Heat obstructing in the channels and collaterals).

Western medicine: Arthritis.

8. Treating principle

Clear Heat, remove obstruction of channels and collaterals.

9. Prescription

Right side: Sanjian (LI 3).

The technique of *penetrating-heaven coolness* was applied. The needle was manipulated once every 5 minutes and retained for 30 minutes.

10. Effect

After withdrawal of the needle, the redness and swelling disappeared, and the finger could move freely. On the second visit, the pain basically stopped. One more treatment for consolidation was done and he was cured.

11. Essentials

The treatment focuses on the affected area with local points selected. According to the principle that Heat syndromes should be treated by clearing Heat, the reducing method is adopted to reduce the pathogenic Heat.

SUMMARY

Bi means obstruction. Bi syndrome refers to those diseases characterized by pain, swelling and heaviness of the muscles and joints caused by invasion of pathogenic Wind, Cold and Damp which obstruct the channels and collaterals. Of the pathogenic factors, if the Wind is predominant, the wandering Bi will take place; if the Cold is severe, painful Bi will be the outcome; if the Damp is more than the other two, there will be an onset of fixed Bi, and in a prolonged case, the Heat is transformed, and there will be Heat Bi.

Removing the pathogenic factors from the channels and collaterals is the principle for treatment of Bi syndrome. Acupuncture is mainly adopted for wandering Bi; moxibustion with acupuncture is applied for painful Bi, and intradermal needling therapy may be used in combination for those with serious pain; acupuncture and moxibustion are taken for fixed Bi, and for Heat Bi, the reducing method of acupuncture is what to do.

The points of Yang channels in the affected area are selected and with distal points along the affected channels in combination.

Main points: Houxi (SI 3), Shenmai (BL 62), Dabao (SP 21) and Geshu (BL 17) are chosen for pain all over the body; Yaoyangguan (GV 3) for pain in the lower back; Huantiao (GB 30), Juliao (GB 29) and Yanglingquan (GB 34) for iliac joint pain; Xiyan (EX-LE5) and Dubi (ST 35), Yinlinquan (SP 9), and Yanglingquan (GB 34) for knee joint pain; Chengshan (BL 57) and Feiyang (BL 58) for leg numbness and pain; Jiexi (ST 41), Qiuxu (GB 40) and Taixi (KI 3) for ankle pain; Jianyu (LI 15), Jianliao (TE 14), Jianneiling (Extra) and Quchi (LI 11) for shoulder joint pain; Quchi (LI 11), Shousanli (LI 10) and Tianjing (TE 10) for elbow joint pain; Yangchi (TE 4), Yangxi (LI 5), Wangu (SI 4), Houxi (SI 3) and Ashi points for wrist, palm and finger joint pain.

Use Dazhu (BL 11) in the case of deformity of joints; use Shenshu (BL 23) and Guanyuan (CV 4) if Cold is prevalent; use Geshu (BL 17) and Xuehai (SP 10) in cases where Wind is obvious; use Sanyinjiao (SP 6) and Yinlingquan (SP 9) for when Damp is serious; use Dazhui (GV 14) to treat fever.

SECTION TWENTY-EIGHT • NUMBNESS OF THE EXTREMITIES

CASE I: YANG JIEBIN'S MEDICAL RECORD

1. General data

Ye, female, 24.

2. Chief complaint

Numbness of the fingers of the left hand for half a year.

3. History of present illness

The patient had numbness of the thumb gradually without reason and half a month later the index, middle and ring fingers become numb too. The various physico-chemical examinations didn't show any abnormal findings. Muscular injection of vitamin B1 and B12 and herbal decoction didn't relieve her much. Recently in the last 2 months, the numbness was getting worse.

4. Present symptoms

Her left arm and fingers were not swelling, and the skin was a normal colour.

5. Tongue and pulse

Red tongue, thin white coating, thready pulse.

6. Differentiation and analysis

The numbness is caused by the obstruction of channels and collaterals. Yang Qi is stagnated and Blood circulation will be not smooth. The skin and muscles are de-prived of nourishment, resulting in numbness.

7. Diagnosis

TCM: Jin-Muscular Bi (arthralgia with muscles involved).

Western medicine: Numbness of extremities.

8. Treating principle

Remove obstruction to connect Qi, activate Blood, dissolve stasis.

9. Prescription

Shaoshang (LU 11), Shangyang (LI 1), Zhongchong (PC 9), Hegu (LI 4), Erjian (LI 2).

Affected side only. The Jing-Well points were pricked with a three-edged needle for bleeding; Hegu (LI 4) and Sanjian (LI 3) were reduced. Once every other day.

10. Effect

11. Essentials

The principle of treatment for numbness resulted from the poor nourishment of skin and muscles caused by the stagnated Qi and Blood is to remove the obstruction by activating Qi to circulate Blood. When the Blood is circulated well, the numbness will be stopped. Pricking the Jing-Well points for bleeding is to promote Blood circulation to remove obstruction so as to supply Blood to extremities. Thus numbness is stopped.

CASE II: YANG JIEBIN'S MEDICAL RECORD

1. General data

Bo, female, 50, came on October 28, 1978.

2. Chief complaint

Pain and numbness of both arms for 6 years.

3. History of present illness

The patient lived in a Damp place. She began to have pain and numbness of arms since November 1972, with formication in fingers and a cold pain in shoulder and neck. Four months ago her blood pressure was high. The treatment of Western medicine was not effective, so she came for acupuncture.

4. Present symptoms

She had the numbness and pain in both arms and formication in fingers, and a cold pain in shoulder and neck.

5. Tongue and pulse

6. Differentiation and analysis

Living in a Damp place, weak constitution, 50 years old. Pathogenic Wind Cold invades easily and blocks the channels and collaterals, making Qi and Blood stagnated, so pain and numbness occurs.

7. Diagnosis

TCM: Jin-Muscular Bi (Wind Cold Damp blocking the muscles).

Western medicine: Rheumatic numbness of the extremities.

8. Treating principle

Remove obstruction of channels and collaterals, dissolve Damp, stop pain.

9. Prescription

Zhongchong (PC 9), Shangyang (LI 1), Guanchong (TE 1) and Shaoshang (LU 11) were pricked to bleed 0.5–1ml; Jianwaishu (SI 14) and Fengmen (BL 12) pricked and cupped to bleed about 5ml.

10. Effect

With 10 treatments, she was basically cured.

11. Essentials

For such a prolonged case of obstruction of Qi and Blood, acupuncture can remove the pathogenic Cold Damp directly by bleeding the points. Once the obstruction is removed, the Qi and Blood circulation will be improved, the pain and numbness stopped.

SUMMARY

Mamu, numbness, known in ancient time as Buren, is a subjective symptom of the patient, manifested by anesthesia or hypoesthesia. Professor Yang Jiebin holds that pathological changes of Qi and Blood are the cause although there are also many other reasons believed in. For the treatment, the principle 'remove obstruction of channels and collaterals, regulate the circulation of Qi and Blood' should be followed. Based on his clinical experience of many years, Professor Yang pricks Jing-Well points for bleeding to connect channel Qi by activating Blood to dissolve stasis, and applies other proper therapeutics accordingly for symptomatic treatment. When the channels and collaterals are cleared of obstruction and Qi and Blood are freed from stagnation, the numbness of the extremities will be quickly relieved.

SECTION TWENTY-NINE • WEI SYNDROME

CASE I: CHENG XINNONG'S MEDICAL RECORD

1. General data

Hu, female, 21, first visited on July 23, 1992.

2. Chief complaint

Non-growth of breasts for 5–6 years.

3. History of present illness

Her breasts were as flat as that of a small girl. She had a gynaecological examination in a hospital and the result showed the normal indices of hormones, a slightly smaller uterus with retroversion, a mass 2×3.5cm in the right lower abdomen.

4. Present symptoms

The patient whose breasts were as flat as that of a small girl was introverted and pettish in character generally. Her menophania came when she was 15 and the menstruation was profuse in flow with clots, accompanied by pain in the lower abdomen and lumbosacral region. She had dizziness, fullness in the chest, irritability, dream-disturbed sleep, and poor appetite. She had a sallow complexion and a mass in the right lower abdomen with a dull pain or no pain.

5. Tongue and pulse

Purplish tongue, tip red, white coating, thready wiry pulse.

6. Differentiation and analysis

The breasts and lower abdomen are the distributing areas of the Liver Channel, dominated by the Liver, which is known as a General, needing to be soothed. The Liver Qi stagnation caused her slow development of breasts. Qi disease makes the Blood involved, thus there is a mass in the lower abdomen. Liver overacts on Spleen, the production of Qi and Blood is poor, thus there is poor appetite and dizziness. Qi stagnation transforms into Fire, disturbing the Mind stored in Heart, thus there is irritability and insomnia. With Qi stagnation and Blood stasis, Liver fails to store Blood and Spleen fails to control Blood, thus the menstruation flow was profuse and with clots, and there was pain in lower abdomen and lumbosacral region.

7. Diagnosis

TCM: Wei syndrome (Liver Qi stagnation).

Western medicine: Maldevelopment of breasts.

8. Treating principle

Soothe Liver, regulate Qi and Blood circulation.

9. Prescription

Shanzhong (CV 17), Yingchuang (ST 16), Tianchi (PC 1), Rugen (ST 18), Qimen (LR 14), Qihai (CV 6), Guilai (ST 29), Neiguan (PC 6), Hegu (LI 4), Zusanli (ST 36), Sanyinjiao (SP 6), Ququan (LR 8), Yanglingquan (GB 34), Taichong (LR 3).

Qihai (CV 6), Zusanli (ST 36) and Sanyinjiao (SP 6) were punctured with the reinforcing method, others with even method.

10. Effect

Eight treatments later, her breasts and mammary areola began to develop and the mass became smaller, appetite was improved, and body weight gradually increased. With 3 courses of treatment, all symptoms were greatly relieved, her breasts were bigger, with the mass appearing and disappearing. She didn't continue the treatment because she lived a long way away.

11. Essentials

This is a Wei syndrome of breasts, namely the non-development of breasts of young females. The breasts are dominated and supported by Jueyin Liver and Yangming Stomach channels, therefore the treating principle should be to soothe the Liver, circulate its Qi, and strengthen the Spleen and Stomach. The commonly used points are Rugen (ST 18), Tianchi (PC 1), Yingchuang (ST 16), Qimen (LR 14), Shanzhong (CV 17), Hegu (LI 4), Taichong (LR 3), Zusanli (ST 36), Sanyinjiao (SP 6), Shaoze (SI 1), Zhongwan (CV 12), Qihai (CV 6), etc.

CASE II: CHENG XINNONG'S MEDICAL RECORD

1. General data

Wu, male, 43, first visited on November 2, 1985.

2. Chief complaint

Muscular atrophy in the right leg for 20 years.

3. History of present illness

Twenty years ago, he began to have muscular atrophy in the right leg without any clear reasons, now the thigh also began to have muscular atrophy.

4. Present symptoms

The right leg was weak with muscular atrophy. The right side of the body felt cold, and sometimes with a migrating pain. The right teeth were weak in chewing. Walking was difficult. Appetite was normal, urine and stools normal.

Examination: Muscular atrophy in the right leg.

5. Tongue and pulse

Light red tongue, with cracks in the middle, toothprints on the borders, thin coating, wiry thready pulse.

6. Differentiation and analysis

This patient was constitutionally weak in Spleen and Stomach, and with the prolonged disease, his Qi of Middle Burner is injured further. The functions of Spleen and Stomach in receiving food, transporting and transforming were disordered, not enough Qi and Blood were produced, thus, the Zang Fu organs and tendons and bones lack nourishment, the joints are impaired in movements and muscles too weak to use. Cold in the right side of the body is because of Qi and Blood deficiency.

7. Diagnosis

TCM: Wei syndrome (Qi and Blood deficiency).

Western medicine: Muscular atrophy.

8. Treating principle

Remove obstruction of channels and collaterals, strengthen Spleen and Stomach, replenish Qi and Blood.

9. Prescription

Baihui (GV 20), Dazhui (GV 14). Right side: Jianyu (LI 15), Jianliao (TE 14), Quchi (LI 11), Waiguan (TE 5), Fengshi (GB 31), Yinlingquan (SP 9), Yanglingquan (GB 34), Zusanli (ST 36), Sanyinjiao (SP 6), Taichong (LR 3).

Sibai (ST 2) and Quanliao (SI 18) areas were tapped gently with the plum blossom needle and Foot-Yangming Channel of the leg tapped heavily.

10. Effect

The above treatment was given 10 times, and the symptoms were relieved. The tip of the tongue tenderly red, wiry pulse. The points Jiache (ST 6) (right), Hegu (LI 4) (right) and Houxi (SI 3) (right) were added.

With more than 40 treatments, the right side of his body was not feeling cold any more, the strength of his right arm was restored, but the right leg and ankle were still weak. The treatment continued for 15 more times. The weakness of the leg got better. His 20 years' intractable disease was obviously relieved with 60 treatments.

11.Essentials

The Ancient Medical Book says: 'The Yangming Channel is the sea of five Zang and six Fu organs, dominating moistening the tendons, which control the bones and move the joints.'

The plum blossom needle is used to tap heavily the Foot-Yangming Channel on the leg and tap gently the points Sibai (ST 2) and Quanliao (SI 18) in order to promote the circulation of Qi and Blood. In the Wei syndrome, the tendons and muscles are flaccid. The Yangming Channel is responsible for moistening the tendons. The Liver dominates the tendons, and is related externally–internally with the Gallbladder. Thus, the points of Yangming Channel, Jianyu (LI 15), Quchi (LI 11) and Zusanli (ST 36), the points of Shaoyang Channel, Jianliao (TE 14), Waiguan (TE 5), Fengshi (GB 31) and Yanglingquan (GB 34), the points of Liver Channel, Taichong (LR 3) are selected for treatment. Zusanli (ST 36), Sanyinjiao (SP 6) and Yinlingquan (SP 9) are used together to strengthen the acquired foundation. Yanglingquan (GB 34), an Influential point of the tendons, is used to regulate Qi of channels to replenish Qi and Blood to moisten and nourish tendons and bones. Baihui (GV 20) and Dazhui (GV 14) are points to regulate Yin and Yang to smooth Qi and Blood circulation. All the points in this group are functioning well in removing obstructions of the channels and collaterals, strengthening the Spleen and Stomach, and replenishing Qi and Blood.

CASE III: CHENG XINNONG'S MEDICAL RECORD

1. General data

Li, male, 14, first visited on February 25, 1987.

2. Chief complaint

Muscular atrophy of the left limbs, hemiplegia for 13 years.

3. History of present illness

He couldn't open his right eye since he was born. Half a year later, his left hand was found to be not able to hold things, and his left leg was weak. Xuanwu Hospital diagnosed him as having 'Congenital Infantile Paralysis'. Injection of galanthamine and vitamin together with acupuncture didn't make him better. His movement was impaired, and intelligence normal.

4. Present symptoms

Ptosis of right eyelid, muscular atrophy of left limbs.

5. Tongue and pulse

Red tongue, thin white coating, deep pulse.

6. Differentiation and analysis

This patient has congenital deficiency. In the case of Liver and Kidney Essence and Blood deficiency, the tendons, bones and muscles lack nourishment over a long period and as a result there is muscular atrophy.

7. Diagnosis

TCM: Wei syndrome (Liver and Kidney Essence and Blood deficiency).

Western medicine: Sequelae of poliomyelitis.

8. Treating principle

Replenish Essence and marrow, remove obstruction of channels, strengthen tendons.

9. Prescription

Baihui (GV 20), Dazhui (GV 14), Fengchi (GB 20), Hegu (LI 4), Zusanli (ST 36), Taichong (LR 3), Sanyinjiao (SP 6), Yanglingquan (GB 34).
　　Left side: Jianyu (LI 15), Shousanli (LI 10), Waiguan (TE 5), Houxi (SI 3), Yangxi (LI 5), Zhongquan (EX-UE3).
　　Right side: Yangbai (GB 14), Toulinqi (GB 15).
　　The Hand-Yangming Channel was tapped gently with a plum blossom needle.

10. Effect

On May 15, 1987, after 60 treatments, the functions of his left hand were greatly recovered, and the muscle of the upper arm was much improved. The swelling of the left wrist was relieved and the pain better. Baihui (GV 20), Dazhui (GV 14), Fengchi (GB 20), Hegu (LI 4), Taichong (LR 3), Sanyinjiao (SP 6), Yanglingquan (GB 34). Right side: Yangbai (GB 14), Toulinqi (GB 15), Sibai (ST 2), Zanzhu (BL 2). Left side: Jianyu (LI 15), Jianliao (TE 14), Pianli (LI 6), Shousanli (LI 10), Yangxi (LI 5), Zhongquan (EX-UE3). The Hand-Yangming Large Intestine Channel was tapped gently with a plum blossom needle.

　　On August 7, 1987, with 5 months' treatment, the movement of his left limbs, especially of the fingers and wrist, was improved, the muscle of the left upper arm was much improved. The ptosis of the right eyelid was better and the papebral fissure bigger. Because he needed to go home for school, he continued treatment later in the local hospital of his home town.

11. Essentials

Baihui (GV 20), a meeting point of Yang channels, regulate Yin and Yang, circulate Qi and Blood. Dazhui (GV 14) disperses Yang Qi. Hegu (LI 4) is a Yuan-Source point, pertaining to Yang, dominating Qi. Taichong (LR 3) is a Yuan-Source point, pertaining to Yin, dominating Blood. They are also known as Four Gates; when used together, Qi and Blood will be harmonized and Yin and Yang adjusted. Jianyu (LI 15) is a point of Yangming Channel, which is believed to be full of Qi and Blood. Waiguan (TE 5) is a Luo-Connecting point of Hand-Shaoyang Triple Burner Channel. Houxi (SI 3) is a point of Taiyang Channel, leading to Governor Vessel. The combination of this group is to clear obstruction of the channel Qi of the upper limbs. Zusanli (ST 36) is the Lower He-Sea point of Yangming Stomach Channel. Sanyinjiao (SP 6) is a meeting of Liver, Spleen and Kidneys. The combination of this group is to strengthen Spleen and Stomach, reinforce Liver and Kidneys, regulate Qi and Blood, and clear obstructed channels and collaterals. Yanglingquan (GB 34) is the Influential point of the tendons, so is used to strengthen tendons and soothe the Liver. Yangbai (GB 14) and Toulinqi (GB 15) circulate Qi and Blood in the local area.

ZHONGQUAN

Zhongquan (EX-UE3), located in the transverse crease on the dorsal carpus, in the depression on the radial side of the tendon of musculus extensor digitorum communi, is indicated by hotness of the palm, abdominal distention and pain, cough and asthma.

CASE IV: BO ZHIYUN'S MEDICAL RECORD

1. General data

Zhang, male, 11, first visited on January 16, 1992.

2. Chief complaint

Motor impairment of both hands, weakness of the right lower limb for 11 years.

3. History of present illness

He was born in a difficult labour and had an intracranial haemorrhage due to the usage of obstetric forceps, so he stayed in hospital for 52 days for treatment. Since birth, his thumbs flexed to the palm, unable to extend and although the other four fingers could do flexion and extension, he couldn't do anything with his hands.

4. Present symptoms

His thumbs were flexed, unable to extend. The other four fingers could do flexion and extension, but his hands were useless. He was unable to take care of himself in daily life. His right lower limb was weak, the right foot couldn't leave the ground when he walked, so he fell down very often.

5. Tongue and pulse

6. Differentiation and analysis

The child was injured when he was born. The Kidneys failed to produce marrow to nourish the bones. This caused Wei-flaccidity.

7. Diagnosis

TCM: Wei-flaccidity syndrome (Spleen and Kidney deficiency).

Western medicine: Sequelae of cerebral paralysis.

8. Treating principle

Reinforce Spleen and Kidneys, unobstruct channels.

9. Prescription

Abdominal Heaven–Earth acupuncture, Huaroumen (ST 24).

10. Effect

With 5 minutes of needling, his thumbs could stretch. Retaining needles for 30 minutes, his thumbs could hold a pencil, but were not free in movement. Two more treatments made his thumbs move much more freely and he could eat by himself. The right foot was stronger in walking. He was asked to do more exercises.

11. Essentials

Bo's Abdominal Acupuncture Therapy was applied to this patient. The Heaven–Earth points were Zhongwan (CV 12) and Guanyuan (CV 4), reinforcing Spleen and Kidneys. The Kidneys dominate bones and produce marrow. When it is deficient, the bones will be weak. The Spleen dominates the muscles and limbs. When it is deficient, the limbs and muscles will lack nourishment. Therefore, all the diseases related to Spleen and Kidney deficiency may be treated with the Abdominal Heaven–Earth acupuncture.

SUMMARY

Wei syndrome is characterized by flaccidity and atrophy of the limbs with motor impairment. The causative factors are attributed to invasion of the Lungs by virulent Heat pathogen, exhaustion of Blood and Body Fluid, affect of warm and Heat pathogen, depriving the tendons and muscles of nourishment. It is seen in acute myelitis, progressive myatrophy, myasthenia gravis, multiple neuritis, periodic paralysis, and so on.

The Ancient Medical Book says: 'The Yangming Channel is the sea of five Zang and six Fu organs, dominating moistening the tendons, which control the bones and move the joints.' 'Points along the Yangming channels are mostly selected in treating Wei syndrome.' So, tapping the Yangming course with a plum blossom needle is always adopted, and the symptomatic points are applied for needling as well.

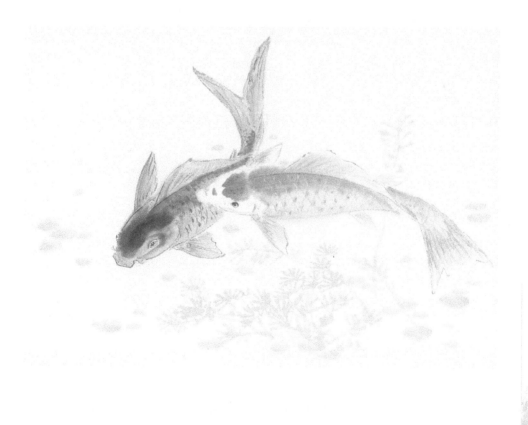

SECTION THIRTY • PTOSIS

CASE I: ZHENG KUISHAN'S MEDICAL RECORD

1. General data

Zeng, female, 7, first visited on October, 2003.

2. Chief complaint

Ptosis of right eye.

3. History of present illness

Without obvious reasons, she had ptosis of the right eye, and the dropped eyelid made the part of the eye above her pupil covered.

4. Present symptoms

She couldn't close her eye completely. The dropped eyelid made the part of the eye above her pupil covered. She was limited in blinking her eyes. She had lacrimation when it was Windy, increase of eye secretion, Dryness in the eye, and blurred vision.

5. Tongue and pulse

6. Differentiation and analysis

This is the ptosis falling into the category of Spleen Qi deficiency with the Windstroke in collaterals.

7. Diagnosis

TCM: Ptosis (Spleen Qi deficiency, Windstroke in collaterals).

Western medicine: Ptosis.

8. Treating principle

Dispel Wind, remove obstruction, strengthen Spleen, tonify Qi.

9. Prescription

Zanzhu (BL 2), Taiyang (EX-HN5), Yuyao (EX-HN4), Sibai (ST 2), Fengchi (GB 20), Zusanli (ST 36), Pishu (BL 20).

The warm-reinforcing method was adopted. Once a day, 10 times as 1 course.

10. Effect

With 2 months' treatment, the symptoms were obviously relieved. She could blink and close the eye. Looking straight forward, her eyes were basically symmetrical.

11. Essentials

Zusanli (ST 36) and Pishu (BL 20) are used to strengthen the Spleen and reinforce Qi and the other points for dispelling Wind to remove obstruction of the channels and collaterals. This is the treatment for both the symptoms and the root course.

WARM REINFORCING METHOD

This is the creation of Professor Zheng Kuishan. The stimulation severity is between Setting the Mountain on Fire and Inserting Fire for Reinforce. Clinically it is extensively used for the treatment of all deficiency Cold syndromes and the effect is good.

The manipulation: The left thumb or index finger presses the point, the right hand inserts the needle in, after the Qi arrives, the left hand presses hard while the right thumb rotates the needle forward continuously 3-5 times. After a heaviness and tightness come under the needle, press heavily and lift slowly for 3-5 times, the thumb rotates the needle forward for 3-5 times again, keep the needle tip at the place where the sensation is induced to keep the Qi there in order to continue the heaviness and tightness to produce a warm sensation. After retaining the needle, withdraw it slowly and press the point to close it quickly. Apply it once a day, 10 times as 1 course. Or it may be applied every other day accordingly.

CASE II: XIAO SHAOQING'S MEDICAL RECORD

1. General data

Cai, male, 27, first visited on November 19, 1988.

2. Chief complaint

Ptosis of both eyes for 10 years.

3. History of present illness

Ten years ago, he had ptosis of both eyes with no obvious reasons and accompanied by hoarseness, lassitude of the loins and legs, which were better in the morning when he got up or after taking a rest, and worse when tired. The provincial hospital diagnosed him with 'myasthenia gravis'. With medication of pyridostigmine, potassium chloride and prednisone for 8 days and 10 doses of herbal medicine, there was no improvement, so he came for acupuncture.

4. Present symptoms

Ptosis of both eyes, difficulty in opening the eyes, the pupils being covered. He had to raise his head, raise his eyebrow, and frown when he looked at things.

5. Tongue and pulse

Pale tongue, thin white coating, thready weak pulse.

6. Differentiation and analysis

The Spleen dominates the muscles. The upper eyelid pertains to the Spleen. In the case of Spleen Qi deficiency, clean Yang fails to ascend, or the Wind affects the collaterals with obstruction as the outcome, causing ptosis. In differentiation of syndromes, there is Spleen Qi deficiency and Wind affecting the collaterals.

The actual patient here has the condition of Spleen Qi deficiency and Kidney Yang deficiency.

7. Diagnosis

TCM: Ptosis (sinking of Qi of Middle Burner).

Western medicine: Myasthenia gravis.

8. Treating principle

Strengthen the Middle Burner, reinforce Spleen Qi, ascend the clean Yang, tonify Kidneys to consolidate the root, build up tendons and muscles, open the throat to treat hoarseness.

9. Prescription

Acupuncture and herbal decoction in combination.

Points:

- Shangming (EX-HN), Yangbai (GB 14) penetrating to Yuyao (EX-HN4), Tiantu (CV 22), Qihai (CV 6), Guanyuan (CV 4), Zusanli (ST 36), Xiangu (ST 43), Neiting (ST 44).

- Chengqi (ST 1), Sibai (ST 2), Fengchi (GB 20), Dazhui (GV 14), Yamen (GV 15), Lianquan (CV 23) penetrating to Haiquan (EX-HN11), Tongli (HT 5), Shenshu (BL 23) penetrating to Mingmen (GV 4).

The 2 groups of points were used in turn, once a day, with the needles retained for 30 minutes, 10 times as 1 course.

Herbal prescription: Modification of Bu Zhong Yi Qi Wan (中益气丸 Bolus for Reinforcing the Middle Burner and Replenishing Qi) plus You Gui Wan (右归丸

Bolus for Reinforcing the Kidney Yang). One dose each day. The herbs were decocted and the decoction taken 3 times a day. The ingredients were:

- Huang Qi (黄芪 *Radix Astragali*) 15g

- Dang Shen (党参 *Radix Codonopsis*) 9g

- Dang Gui (当归 *Radix Angelicae Sinensis*) 9g

- Zhi Gan Cao (炙甘草 *Radix Glycyrrhizae Preparata*) 5g

- Chen Pi (皮 *Pericarpium Citri Reticulatae*) 5g

- Sheng Ma (升麻 *Rhizoma Cimicifugae*) 6g

- Chai Hu (柴胡 *Radix Bupleuri*) 6g

- Baizhu (白术 *Rhizoma Atractylodis Macrocephalae*) 10g

- Shu Di (熟地 *Radix Rehmanniae Prepared*) 6g

- Chao Shan Yao (炒山 *parched Rhizoma Dioscoreae*) 15g

- Gou Qi Zi (枸杞子 *Fructus Lycii*) 6g

- Zi Dan Shen (紫丹参 *Radix Salviae Miltiorrhizae*) 15g

- Du Zhong (杜仲 *Cortex Eucommiae*) 8g

- Rou Gui (肉桂 *Cortex Cinnamomi*) 5g

- Zhi Fu Pian (制附片 *Radix Aconiti Preparata*) 5g

- Shan Zhu Yu (山茱萸 *Fructus Corni*) 6g

- Lu Jiao Jiao (鹿角胶 *Colla Cornus Cervi*) 15g

- Rou Cong Rong (肉 蓉 *Herba Cistanchis*) 6g

- Chao Yi Yi Ren (炒薏苡仁 *Semen Coicis*) 9g

- Po Gu Zhi (破故 *Fructus Psoraleae*) 6g

- Sha Ren (砂仁 *Fructus Amomi*) 3g (smashed).

10. Effect

After 1 course of treatment with acupuncture and herbs, his appetite was improved, the lifting of his eyelids was better, the hoarseness relieved, and his loins and legs felt warm and stronger. After 2 courses, the lifting of the eyelids became even stronger, speech clearer, and the loins and legs felt especially improved. In total, 30 times of acupuncture and 28 doses of herbs were applied, he was cured.

11. Essentials

For the patient with Spleen Qi deficiency and Kidney Yang deficiency, the principles for treatment are to strengthen the Middle Burner, reinforce Spleen Qi, ascend the clean Yang, tonify Kidneys to consolidate the root, build up tendons and muscles, and open throat to treat hoarseness. In acupuncture, the local and distal points are used in combination.

Locally, Zanzhu (BL 2), Sibai (ST 2), Yangbai (GB 14) penetrating to Yuyao (EX-HN4), Shangming (EX-HN) and Chengqi (ST 1) are reinforced to activate and regulate the Qi of Foot-Taiyang, Yangming and Shaoyang channels to promote the recovery of functions of muscles and tendons. Tiantu (CV 22), Yamen (GV 15), Lianquan (CV 23) penetrating to Haiquan (EX-HN11), and Tongli (HT 5) are punctured with even method to open throat to treat hoarseness. Qihai (CV 6), Guanyuan (CV 4), Zusanli (ST 36), Xiangu (ST 43), and Neiting (ST 44) are to strengthen the Middle Burner, reinforce Spleen Qi, and ascend the clean Yang. Fengchi (GB 20) and Dazhui (GV 14) are to send Yang to surface to eliminate internal and external Wind to treat diseases of eye and head. In addition, Shenshu (BL 23) and Mingmen (GV 4), penetrating is to reinforce, moxibustion is to warm, tonify the Kidneys to consolidate the root and strengthen the Mingmen Fire to reinforce the Spleen Yang.

As for the herbs, Bu Zhong Yi Qi Tang, aims at reinforcing the Middle Burner and replenishing Qi to ascend the clean Yang; You Gui Wan aims at reinforcing the Kidney Yang to replenish Essence and Blood and make strong the Mingmen Fire to promote Spleen Yang. In this way, the Spleen Qi is tonified, Qi and Blood produced, the function of eyelids in lifting will be restored, thus, the ptosis is cured.

SUMMARY

Ptosis is a disease manifested as a partial or complete drop of the upper eyelid due to the incompetence or descent of the levator muscle and Miller's smooth muscle. In a mild case, a part of the pupil, in a severe case, the whole pupil, is hidden from view, hindering the appearance and vision.

Congenital ptosis appears mostly to both sides or sometimes one side; being hereditary, an operation needs to be adopted for correction.

Acquired ptosis, owing to different causes, is divided into the following:

1. Oculomotor nerve paralytic ptosis.

2. Sympathetic nerve paralytic ptosis.

3. Muscular ptosis, often seen in those patients with myasthenia gravis, and is better in the morning, worse in the afternoon, becoming mild with rest while if not rested for days it would be aggravated immediately.

4. Mechanical ptosis, caused by the weight of the eyelid muscle, such as in severe trachoma, eyelid tumour or hyperplasia, etc.

5. Others, like traumatic ptosis, hysteric ptosis and so on.

Professor Zheng Kuishan says it is related with the Spleen and Kidneys in pathology, because the former is the production source of Qi and Blood, dominating muscles, while the latter is the congenital root, storing Essence and producing marrow, to nourish the eyes. For the treatment of ptosis, acupuncture functions to strengthen the Spleen and Kidneys, reinforce the Middle Burner to replenish Qi, and remove obstruction of the channels and collaterals, able to prevent the sequelae of operation, including incomplete closure of the eyelid, exposure keratitis, etc. For infantile cases, better to treat when they are 2–4 years old, because the intrapsychical self image will be established at the age of 3, with the appearance of ptosis, and their normal psychological development may be hindered.

Main points: Jingming (BL 1), Zanzhu (BL 2), Taiyang (EX-HN5), Yuyao (EX-HN4), Sibai (ST 2), Fengchi (GB 20).

Supplementary points: Mingmen (GV 4), Sanyinjiao (SP 6) and Taixi (KI 3) are added to warm and reinforce the Kidney Yang in the case of congenital Kidney Yang deficiency; Zusanli (ST 36), Pishu (BL 20) and Weishu (BL 21) are added to reinforce the Spleen Qi in the case of acquired Spleen and Stomach deficiency; Waiguan (TE 5) and Hegu (LI 4) are added to dispel Wind in cases where Wind strikes the collaterals of the eyelid.

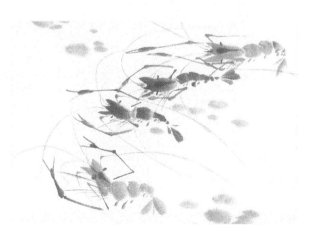

SECTION THIRTY-ONE • FACIAL SPASM

CASE I: CHENG XINNONG'S MEDICAL RECORD

1. General data

Xu, male, 62, first visited on August 3, 1992.

2. Chief complaint

Facial spasm on the right side for 10 years.

3. History of present illness

According to the patient, his facial spasm was caused by exposure to Wind after sweating and tiredness. Treated in many hospitals for years, he was not yet improved. The exposure to Wind, nervousness and tiredness would induce its onset.

4. Present symptoms

His facial spasm was frequent and as serious as contraction, causing the eyes and mouth to become deviated and cause salivation in sleep. He had sweating, aversion to wind, and aching of the shoulder and back. His complexion was dark.

5. Tongue and pulse

Pale tongue, tooth prints on borders, white coating, thready soft pulse.

6. Differentiation and analysis

His facial spasm is caused by invasion of Wind on the occasion of disharmony between Ying and Wei, making the defence weak. The Wind is characterized by constant movement and rapid change, upward and outward dispersion, invading the upper part of the body, and the face to cause the facial spasm. The patient is also constitutionally weak in Qi and Blood, and the muscles more seriously lack nourishment, therefore the spasms are so frequent and severe.

7. Diagnosis

TCM: Facial spasm (disharmony between Ying and Wei systems, muscles lack of nourishment).

Western medicine: Facial spasm.

8. Treating principle

Dispel Wind, harmonize Ying and Wei, replenish Qi and Blood.

9. Prescription

Dazhui (GV 14), Chengjiang (CV 24), Fengchi (GB 20), Sibai (ST 2), Quanliao (SI 18), Waiguan (TE 5), Hegu (LI 4), Zusanli (ST 36), Sanyinjiao (SP 6). Left side: Taiyang (EX-HN5), Juliao (ST 3), Dicang (ST 4), Jiache (ST 6).

The reinforcing method was adopted for the affected side, while the reducing method adopted for the healthy side.

10. Effect

With 8 treatments, the frequency of spasms was greatly reduced, the intensity of contraction lowered, and the dark complexion improved. The treatment was continued. The spasm occurred only occasionally. In total 3 courses were applied and this cured him. Three months later, the follow-up found no recurrence.

11. Essentials

Dazhui (GV 14), Fengchi (GB 20), Waiguan (TE 5), Hegu (LI 4) are selected to dispel pathological Wind; Neiguan (PC 6), Zusanli (ST 36), Sanyinjiao (SP 6) to harmonize Ying and Wei and replenish Qi and Blood; Sibai (ST 2), Quanliao (SI 18), Taiyang (EX-HN5), Juliao (ST 3), Dicang (ST 4), Jiache (ST 6), Chengjiang (CV 24) to treat locally.

CASE II: YANG YONGXUAN'S MEDICAL RECORD

1. General data

Hu, female, 38.

2. Chief complaint

Facial spasm on the left side for 7 years.

3. History of present illness

Her facial spasm was paroxysmal with irregular attacks for 7 years. She tried various kinds of treatment but without improvement.

4. Present symptoms

Facial spasm on the left side, paroxysmal, irregular.

5. Tongue and pulse

6. Differentiation and analysis

The facial region is a Yang area. Facial spasm will occur in cases where the Liver Wood is hyperactive, the Wind disturbs upward, making the Wood move frequently.

7. Diagnosis

TCM: Facial spasm.

Western medicine: Facial spasm.

8. Treating principle

Stop Wind.

9. Prescription

Left side: Fengchi (GB 20), Taiyang (EX-HN5), Quanliao (SI 18), Heliao (LI 19), Zanzhu (BL 2). Right side: Lieque (LU 7).

    The reinforcing-reducing of Nine-Six method was adopted. Lieque (LU 7) was reinforced while others reduced. The needles were retained for 20 minutes.

10. Effect

More than 20 acupuncture treatments gradually relieved and cured her facial spasm.

11. Essentials

The reducing method should be adopted for the points in the facial region to remove the pathogenic factors.

SUMMARY

Facial spasm is a disease manifested as irregular contracture of muscles on one side of the face. The causes are attributed to 'from Wind and involvement of Liver', and sometimes fright. Its characteristics are mostly endogenous Wind, less often exogenous Wind, mostly deficiency syndrome, in a few cases excess syndrome; slow onset but intractable. According to Professor Cheng, the healthy side should be treated together with the affected side, with fewer points on the affected side and the reinforcing method, and more points on the healthy side and the reducing method. The treating principle should be:

1. Replenishing Yin and Blood, soothing Liver to stop Wind.

2. Harmonizing Ying and Wei, dispelling Wind, activating collaterals.

3. Regulating Qi and Blood, resting the Heart to calm the Mind.

Main points: Baihui (GV 20), Fengchi (GB 20), Sibai (ST 2), Quanliao (SI 18), Dicang (ST 4), Jiache (ST 6), Waiguan (TE 5), Hegu (LI 4), Zusanli (ST 36), Sanyinjiao (SP 6).

To soothe the Liver, Sanyinjiao (SP 6), Taixi (KI 3) and Taichong (LR 3) should be added; to dispel Wind, Dazhui (GV 14), Quchi (LI 11) and Fengmen (BL 12) added; to harmonize Ying and Wei, Dazhui (GV 14) and Neiguan (PC 6) added; to rest the Heart and calm the Mind, Sishencong (EX-HN1) and Shenmen (HT 7) added.

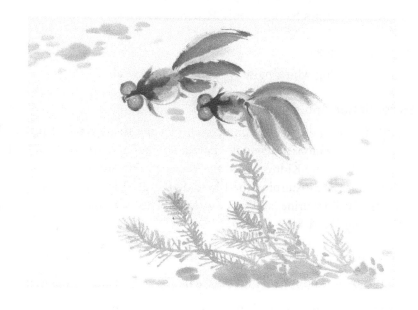

SECTION THIRTY-TWO • CHAN SYNDROME (TREMOR)

CASE I: CHENG XINNONG'S MEDICAL RECORD

1. General data

Li, male, 37, first visited on March 12, 1992.

2. Chief complaint

Tremor of hands and feet for 10 years and worse for 5 years.

3. History of present illness

He had treatment in a hospital, without clear diagnosis, so the result was ineffective.

4. Present symptoms

The tremor of hands and feet was obvious in the morning when got up and it became worse when he was in a hot temper. He was unable to write, work and use chopsticks, and this was accompanied by insomnia, restlessness, forgetfulness, yellow urine, and sometimes bloody stools. His complexion was dark.

5. Tongue and pulse

Tongue tip red, coating white, pulse wiry rolling, Chi weak.

6. Differentiation and analysis

From the symptoms and pulse, it can be seen that the tremor is due to Yin Blood deficiency, thus the tendons and muscles have not enough nourishment. The disharmony between Heart and Kidneys with the deficient Fire flaring up lead to restlessness and insomnia. Fire disturbing the Blood due to Yin Blood deficiency gives rise to forgetfulness, yellow urine, and bloody stools. This is a syndrome of Yin Blood deficiency causing Wind Yang stirring.

7. Diagnosis

TCM: Chan-tremor syndrome (yin Blood deficiency, Wind Yang stirring).

Western medicine: Tremor requiring further examination.

8. Treating principle

Replenish Yin to subdue Yang, moisten tendons and muscles.

9. Prescription

Fengchi (GB 20), Shousanli (LI 10), Hegu (LI 4), Neiguan (PC 6), Shenmen (HT 7), Yanglingquan (GB 34), Zusanli (ST 36), Sanyinjiao (SP 6), Xuanzhong (GB 39), Taixi (KI 3), Taichong (LR 3).

Fengchi (GB 20) and Taichong (LR 3) were reduced; Zusanli (ST 36), Sanyinjiao (SP 6) and Taixi (KI 3) reinforced; other points, even method.

10. Effect

One course of treatment relieved the accompanying symptoms and 5 courses made the tremor greatly better. The tremor was occasionally repeated only. The patient quit treatment.

11. Essentials

Replenishing Yin and Blood is the principle for treatment.

SUMMARY

Tremor of hands and feet, a common disease in old people, males more than females, is caused by the Liver and Kidney Yin and Blood deficiency with not enough nourishment for the tendons and muscles, and diseased Governor Vessel (manifested with brain symptoms), and Liver Qi stagnation, or even nervousness. 'Yin shows quietness, Yang shows movement.' Replenishing Yin and Blood is the basic principle for treatment. Zusanli (ST 36) and Shousanli (LI 10) are the main points, and the symptomatic points should be selected. Reinforcing and reducing should be adopted accordingly.

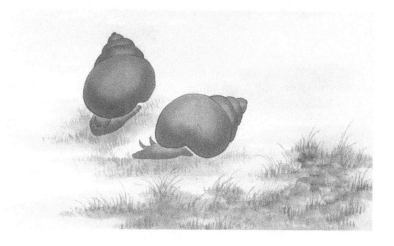

SECTION THIRTY-THREE • STIRRING OF THE LIVER WIND

CASE I: CHENG XINNONG'S MEDICAL RECORD

1. General data

An, male, 7, first visited on December 4, 1986.

2. Chief complaint

Restlessness and murmuring to himself for 3 years.

3. History of present illness

Three years ago, the boy began to be restless and began murmuring to himself. Before the onset, he had a fever followed by contractions. The Children's Hospital diagnosed him with 'intellectual disturbance' and medicated him with piracetam, but it was ineffective. He was term birth. His mother suffered from toxemia of pregnancy from the eighth month of pregnancy.

4. Present symptoms

The boy was restless, murmuring, irritable, unable to answer questions. His sleep and appetite were normal, urine and stools normal.

5. Tongue and pulse

Red tongue, thin coating, deep thready pulse.

6. Differentiation and analysis

In the episode of previous disease, the pathogens were not completely eliminated, and this consumed Liver Yin, and transformed into Wind disturbing the channels and collaterals, so the limbs are restless, disturbing the Mind stored in the Heart, so he murmurs.

7. Diagnosis

TCM: Stirring of the Liver Wind (Kidney deficiency, Liver hyperactivity).

Western medicine: Intellectual disturbance.

8. Treating principle

Remove pathogenic factors, clear obstruction of the channels and collaterals, rest the Heart, calm the Mind.

9. Prescription

Baihui (GV 20), Sishencong (EX-HN1), Fengfu (GV 16), Fengchi (GB 20), Dazhui (GV 14), Lianquan (CV 23), Neiguan (PC 6), Daling (PC 7), Shenmen (HT 7), Zusanli (ST 36), Sanyinjiao (SP 6), Waiguan (TE 5), Hegu (LI 4), Taichong (LR 3).
   Without retaining of needles.

10. Effect

More than 20 treatments, he was much improved.

11. Essentials

Baihui (GV 20) soothes the Liver to stop Wind waking up consciousness. Sishencong (EX-HN1) rests the Heart to calm the Mind to promote intelligence. Fengfu (GV 16), on Governor Vessel, at the place where the Wind stays, dispels Wind, opens the brain, and smooth the circulation of Qi. Fengchi (GB 20) dispels Wind to soothe the Liver. Dazhui (GV 14) rests the Heart to calm the Mind and to disperse Yang Qi. Lianquan (CV 23) clears the throat. Daling (PC 7), Neiguan (PC 6) and Shenmen (HT 7) rest the Heart and calm the Mind. Zusanli (ST 36) and Sanyinjiao (SP 6) strengthen the Spleen to promote intelligence and tonify the Liver and Kidneys. Waiguan (TE 5), Luo-Connecting point and Confluent point, clears Heat to unobstruct collaterals. Hegu (LI 4) and Taichong (LR 3), the Four Gates, tranquilize the patient to soothe the Liver to stop Wind.

TOXEMIA OF PREGNANCY

This refers to a critical condition that appears after 20 weeks of pregnancy, in which the manifestations are hypertension, oedema and albuminuria. If serious, there can be convulsions, coma, Heart failure, renal failure, even death of the mother and foetus. It is also harmful for the newly born baby, and there may be developmental retardation, apparent death, death, or a premature infant.

SUMMARY

Although acupuncture is effective for Liver Wind, the family, school, and society should be concerned about patients who are children and provide them with patient teaching and psychotherapy for their behaviour modification.

Main points: Baihui (GV 20), Dazhui (GV 14), Fengchi (GB 20), Hegu (LI 4), Taichong (LR 3).

Add Sishencong (EX-HN1) for intellectual disturbance; add Neiguan (PC 6), Daling (PC 7) and Shenmen (HT 7) for irritability; and add Zusanli (ST 36) and Sanyinjiao (SP 6) for improving the weak constitution.

SECTION THIRTY-FOUR • EPILEPSY

CASE I: YANG JIASAN'S MEDICAL RECORD

1. General data

Wei, female, 12, first visited on September 28, 1992.

2. Chief complaint

Epilepsy for 6 years.

3. History of present illness

She was hot tempered. She began to have epilepsy at the age of 6, once daily at least, sometimes 5–6 times.

Anamnesis: She was suffocated when she was born.

4. Present symptoms

During an attack, she stared with the consciousness lost for seconds and then woke up. In serious cases, the convulsions started from her mouth or fingers and quickly involved the limbs or half of the body. EEG showed a serious epilepsy wave. The diagnosis was epilepsy. Medication was not effective. She had poor appetite, grinding teeth in sleep, dry stools like sheep faeces and once every 3–4 days, urine normal. Dull expression in her eyes and on her face.

Examination: MRI showed an uneven distribution of grey matter on the left side of occipital parietal region.

5. Tongue and pulse

Red tongue, yellow sticky coating, wiry rolling pulse.

6. Differentiation and analysis

The epilepsy is mainly due to Wind, Phlegm, and reversed passage of Qi. Red tongue, yellow sticky coating, and wiry rolling pulse imply Phlegm Heat retention.

7. Diagnosis

TCM: Epilepsy (Wind Phlegm brought up by the reversed Qi).

Western medicine: Epilepsy.

8. Treating principle

Stop Wind, dissolve Phlegm, calm the Mind, promote resuscitation.

9. Prescription

Dazhui (GV 14), Fengchi (GB 20), Benshen (GB 13), Shenting (GV 24), Sishencong (EX-HN1), Tianshu (ST 25), Zhongwan (CV 12), Qihai (CV 6), Waiguan (TE 5), Zulinqi (GB 41).

Qihai (CV 6), even method. Others, the reducing method. Waiguan (TE 5) penetrating to Neiguan (PC 6). Fengchi (GB 20), toward the tip of nose, 0.5–0.9 cun, no retaining of needle. Dazhui (GV 14), perpendicularly 0.8–1.2 cun, no re-taining of needle. Benshen (GB 13), Shenting (GV 24) and Sishencong (EX-HN1), obliquely 0.3 cun to the subcutaneous level.

The above-mentioned treatment was applied once every other day, retaining the needles for 30 minutes.

10. Effect

She didn't have an attack until October 9, 1992, on which day, her convulsions suddenly started from the mouth to the limbs when waiting for treatment in wait-ing-room. She was carried to the bed quickly and pressed at Renzhong (GV 26), Hegu (LI 4), Taichong (LR 3), Houxi (SI 3) and Shenmai (BL 62). Ten minutes later, she woke up. After a short rest, she was treated again with the previous method. During lunch that day, she had another attack. Thereafter, without attack, her spir-itual condition improved, she was Fire-eyed, not hot tempered as before, becoming stronger with better appetite and sleep and normal urine and stools.

EEG examination on January 7, 1993, compared with EEG taken on September 25, 1992, showed a great improvement. Acupuncture was continued to reduce the dosage of medicine and stop the medication.

11. Essentials

During an attack of epilepsy, Renzhong (GV 26), Yongquan (KI 1), Baihui (GV 20), Hegu (LI 4) and Taichong (LR 3) should be selected. Add Houxi (SI 3) and Shenmai (BL 62) to promote resuscitation to stop convulsions. In the relieved period, stop Wind, dissolve Phlegm, pacify Heart and calm the Mind are the principles to be adopted to treat the root cause, i.e. Wind and Phlegm.

Waiguan (TE 5), Luo-Connecting point of Hand-Shaoyang Triple Burner Channel which is indicated in those diseases with disordered Qi, is to regulate Qi and dissolve Phlegm, penetrating to Neiguan (PC 6), indicated in mental disorders. Zulinqi (GB 41) soothes Liver, stops Wind, and dissolves Phlegm. They are paired Confluent points, helping each other in soothing Liver, stopping Wind, regulating Qi, and dissolving Phlegm, selected as the main points for epilepsy. Fengchi (GB 20) is a point where Wind enters the brain, important for stopping Wind. Dazhui (GV 14), a point of the Governor Vessel which goes into the brain directly, is able to calm the Mind and promote resuscitation. Wind is Yang pathogenic factor, transforming into Heat easily, and Dazhui (GV 14) clears Heat too.

Shenting (GV 24), a meeting point of Foot-Taiyang with Governor Vessel, Benshen (GB 13), a meeting point of Foot-Shaoyang with Yangwei Vessel, are reduced to treat the Wind, Fire and Phlegm of epilepsy with foam on lips. Sishencong (EX-HN1) is the established point for calming the Mind and promoting resuscitation. The Spleen is said to be the source of Phlegm, so Zhongwan (CV 12), Front-Mu of the Stomach, is to dissolve Phlegm. Tianshu (ST 25), Front-Mu of the Large Intestine, is to clear obstructed intestines for treating the Stomach. Qihai (CV 6), Sea of Qi, is to regulate Qi for dissolving Phlegm. These four points are called Four Gates, and are good at regulating Qi, dissolving Phlegm, strengthening Spleen and harmonizing Stomach.

CASE II: CHENG XINNONG'S MEDICAL RECORD

1. General data

Yu, male, 35, first visited on November 7, 1986.

2. Chief complaint

Intermittent disturbance of consciousness for 16 years.

3. History of present illness

Sixteen years ago, when he worked in the countryside, he used to be frightened suddenly, and got intermittent unconsciousness, lasting for 5–10 minutes each time. In Friend Hospital, the EEG showed the epilepsy wave. Now he was taking luminal and diazepam every day. He had 6–7 attacks each month.

Anamnesis: He was born in a difficult labour with a history of neonatal asphyxia.

4. Present symptoms

When the attack was about to start, his complexion became yellowish blue, limbs weak, or he had a cough and red face. During the attack, he was pale, with purple lips, staring eyes, unconsciousness, sometimes foam on lips, stiffness of the right limbs and involuntary movement, or urinary incontinence. He was generally hot tempered with irritability. He had a cough with profuse Phlegm which was difficult to spit, retarded movement, poor appetite, poor sleep, belching, abdominal distension, dry mouth with preference for hot drinks, dry stools, and yellow urine.

5. Tongue and pulse

Swollen pale tongue, thin coating, slightly sticky, deep thready wiry pulse.

6. Differentiation and analysis

His epilepsy started from the fright, which makes Qi disordered in circulation, and as a result, the Body Fluid cannot be transported in the normal passages, so Qi stagnates, Phlegm is retained, and these elements are always ready to be induced to block channels and collaterals. Failure of Qi and Blood to nourish causes pale complexion and purple lips. The staring of the eyes and unconsciousness are due to poor nourishment of the brain. Prolonged disease results in deficiency of Qi and Blood, so there is a pale complexion, pale tongue, deep thready pulse. The Liver stagnation, failing to keep free flow of Qi, affects the Spleen Earth, there exists belching, abdominal distention, and poor appetite. This is an example of a syndrome of Qi and Blood deficiency with Qi stagnation and Phlegm retention.

7. Diagnosis

TCM: Epilepsy (Qi stagnation, Phlegm retention).

Western medicine: Epilepsy.

8. Treating principle

Regulate Qi, dissolve Phlegm, replenish Qi and Blood.

9. Prescription

Baihui (GV 20), Sishencong (EX-HN1), Fengchi (GB 20), Guanyuan (CV 4), Houxi (SI 3), Shenmen (HT 7), Zusanli (ST 36), Fenglong (ST 40), Shenmai (BL 62), Sanyinjiao (SP 6), Taichong (LR 3), Taixi (KI 3).
   Even method.

10. Effect

With 30 acupuncture treatments, his pathological condition was greatly relieved.

11. Essentials

Shenmen (HT 7) is good for mental disorders and epilepsy. Baihui (GV 20) and Sishencong (EX-HN1) are good to strengthen the brain for resuscitation. Guanyuan (CV 4) and Zusanli (ST 36) are good to improve the functions of Spleen and Stomach to produce Blood. Taichong (LR 3) is good to promote Qi circulation. Fenglong (ST 40) is good for dissolving Phlegm.

SUMMARY

Epilepsy occurs in seizures, known as Yang Xian Feng, including grand mal, petit mal, focal and psychomotor seizures, etc. Grand mal epilepsy is manifested by falling down in a fit, loss of consciousness, or screaming with eyes staring upward, and convulsions. After some minutes, consciousness returns, and the condition becomes normal. Petit mal epilepsy is manifested only with a momentary loss of attention with eyes staring directly forward, but no convulsions. The principle for treatment is to promote resuscitation, dissolve Phlegm, pacify Liver, and stop Wind.

During seizure: Baihui (GV 20), Renzhong (GV 26), Hegu (LI 4) penetrating to Laogong (PC 8).

After seizure: Baihui (GV 20), Fengchi (GB 20), Dazhui (GV 14), Jinsuo (GV 8), Jiangshi (PC 5), Yaoqi (EX-B9).

Grand mal epilepsy: Daytime seizure: add Shenmai (BL 62); night seizure: add Zhaohai (KI 6).

Petit mal epilepsy: Add Shenmen (HT 7), Neiguan (PC 6), Yintang (EX-HN3).

Focal seizure: Add Hegu (LI 4), Taichong (LR 3), Yanglingquan (GB 34).

Yaoqi (EX-B9) is 2 cun directly above the tip of the coccyx, in the depression between the sacral horns. In combination with Dazhui (GV 14) and Baihui (GV 20), it is indicated in epilepsy. The insertion of needle is subcutaneously upward along the Governor Vessel 2–3 cun.

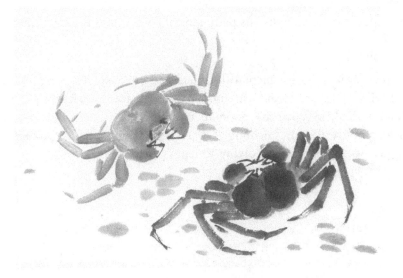

SECTION THIRTY-FIVE • HYSTERIA

CASE I: RECORD IN *ACUPUNCTURE-MOXIBUSTION FOR DIFFICULT DISEASES*

1. General data

Fang, female, 27, first visited on June 9, 1986.

2. Chief complaint

Capricious in laughing and crying, irregular convulsions of four limbs for 4 years.

3. History of present illness

She was capricious in laughing and crying, had irregular convulsions of all four limbs for 4 years, and decline of memory year by year. The symptoms were aggravated, for the previous treatment, including Western medicine and Chinese medicine, was not effective.

4. Present symptoms

Her laughing and crying and the convulsions of the four limbs became more and more frequent. She had attacks more than 10 times during the day and it was worse at night.

5. Tongue and pulse

Pale tongue, thin coating, thready pulse.

6. Differentiation and analysis

This is hysteria with epileptic seizure.

7. Diagnosis

TCM: Hysteria.

Western medicine: Hysteria.

8. Treating principle

9. Prescription

Shenting (GV 24).

   Chou Qi Fa (lifting method) was applied. The needle was lifted with a strong break-out force in quick frequency, and retained for 48 hours. The patient was asked to relax by thought-breathing exercises with concentration on the Dantian while thoracic breathing.

10. Effect

After needling, the symptoms stopped. For the duration of the time the needles were retained and for 1 day after, in total 72 hours, she had only 2 occurences of laughing and crying.

11. Essentials

Shenting (GV 24), a point of Governor Vessel, functions to treat headache, epilepsy, and rhinorrhoea with turbid discharge. To use it in the treatment for different diseases, different methods of manipulation should be adopted and supplemented with different thought-breathing exercises.

CHOU TIAN FA AND TOU ZHEN DAO YIN FA

Chou Tian Fa, including Chou Qi Fa and Tian Qi Fa, is a compound technique of lifting-thrusting for reinforcing and reducing.

Chou Qi Fa (lifting method) is reducing, while Tian Qi Fa reinforcing. The needle is retained for 2-24 hours, even as long as 24-48 hours. For the duration, the needle is manipulated 1-2 times. Chou Qi Fa in the scalp acupuncture is done in this way: after routine disinfection, a filiform needle, #30 or 32, 1.5 cun, is inserted quickly through the skin with a 15° angle to the lower level of galea aponeurotica, thrust slowly horizontally about one cun, and then lifted 3 times with a strong break-out force. The needle body is not moved or only 0.1 cun moved, and thrust slowly about 1 cun again. Repeat the lifting and thrusting until De Qi. **Tian Qi Fa** (thrusting method) is done with the manipulation of needle in the opposite way.

Tou Zhen Dao Yin Fa (scalp acupuncture plus thought-breathing exercises) includes active and passive exercises. In the active exercise, the doctor and the patient both do Yinian-thought and body movement. Yinian-thought is to treat Shen-spirit. While he manipulates the needle, the doctor asks the patient to do Yinian-thought with the concentration on the affected area. Yinian-thought brings the affected limb to move. Yinian-thought and the body movement should be co-ordinated with each other. Yinian-thought has two functions. One is to activate and conduct channel Qi to the affected area, the other is to lead the pathogen out. The passive exercise is adopted for those who are unable to move, the person's healthy limbs, or other people should help the affected side to move. For instance, for the patient with urine retention, during manipulation and retention of the needle, when the patient does abdominal breathing and urinating, the doctor or a family member presses his lower abdomen toward the urethra; for the patient with hemiplegia, the doctor helps him to sit up repeatedly, and to walk. Those who are unable to sit should do flexing of knees, stretching of legs, flexing of elbows, and stretching of arms in bed.

CASE II: CHENG XINNONG'S MEDICAL RECORD

1. General data

Xi, male, 18, first visited on November 16, 1987.

2. Chief complaint

Unable to speak for 1 day.

3. History of present illness

Yesterday at about 11 o'clock, he was suddenly unable to speak for no reasons, and lost his way home when he was out and then was brought back. He had tetany and aphasia when he was 7. Treated by Professor Cheng, he was relieved and could do physical labour. For more than 10 years, he had no recurrence.

4. Present symptoms

Apart from being unable to speak, his sleep and appetite were good and urine and stools normal.

Examination: Dull eyes.

5. Tongue and pulse

Red tongue, thin white coating, thready rapid pulse.

6. Differentiation and analysis

The delicate child had tetany due to Xu-Wind disturbance. Now his Yin and Blood were exhausted, which deprived the channels of nourishment, and blocked the mouth, so he was unable to speak. Shen-Mind lacks nourishment, so he has dull eyes.

7. Diagnosis

TCM: Hysteria (Heart and Spleen deficiency).

Western medicine: Hysteric aphasia.

8. Treating principle

Regulate Qi and Blood, open mouth, promote resuscitation.

9. Prescription

Baihui (GV 20), Dazhui (GV 14), Lianquan (CV 23), Hegu (LI 4), Sanyinjiao (SP 6), Lieque (LU 7), Zhaohai (KI 6), Taichong (LR 3).

Lianquan (CV 23), no retention of needle. Other points, even method.

10. Effect

He could speak in the afternoon after needling. Another 4 acupuncture treatments were done to consolidate, with Baihui (GV 20), Lianquan (CV 23) (no retaining), Hegu (LI 4), Lieque (LU 7), Zhaohai (KI 6), Taichong (LR 3).

11. Essentials

Baihui (GV 20) promotes resuscitation in order to open the mouth. Dazhui (GV 14) calms the Mind and disperses Yang Qi. Lianquan (CV 23) is the local point for aphasia. Lieque (LU 7), of the Lung Channel, leads to the Conception Vessel ascending to the throat; Zhaohai (KI 6), of the Kidney Channel, leads to the Yinqiao Vessel ascending to throat. The combination of the two opens the throat to speak. TCM holds that the Kidneys are the root of speech and the Lungs the door of the voice. These two points are effective in treating aphasia and hoarseness. Hegu (LI 4), Sanyinjiao (SP 6) and Taichong (LR 3) regulate Qi and Blood. The combination of the group of points functions well in regulating Qi and Blood, improving the state of the brain and opening the mouth.

CASE III: LIU JIAYING'S MEDICAL RECORD

1. General data

Su, female, 25 years old, waiting for employment.

2. Chief complaint

Sudden loss of consciousness for 2 hours.

3. History of present illness

The patient had a quarrel with her boyfriend and later with her mother, so she was unhappy. Subsequently she lost consciousness with a locked jaw, stiff neck and closed eyes. She was sent to the emergency room and was found to have no abnormalities in the nervous system. Diagnosed as hysteria, the girl was referred to acupuncture for treatment.

4. Present symptoms

Unconsciousness, closed eyes, locked jaw, stiff neck.

5. Tongue and pulse

Her tongue could not be seen because of the locked jaw. Her pulse was thready and string-taut.

6. Differentiation and analysis

The spiritual stimulation caused the mental depression, disordered Qi activities, and upward disturbance of Liver Qi. The Phlegm and Qi stagnation in combination disturbed the brain, resulting in unconsciousness and trismus and closed eyes.

7. Diagnosis

TCM: Syncope.

Western medicine: Hysteria.

8. Treating principle

Smooth Qi circulation, wake up the brain, promote resuscitation.

9. Prescription

Renzhong (GV 26), Neiguan (PC 6), Taichong (LR 3). Medium stimulation, even method, continuous manipulation of needles, retaining for 25 minutes.

10. Effect

After continuous manipulation of the needles for 5 minutes, the patient gave a long sigh and 'en...en...' Ten minutes' continuous manipulation of needles past, she burst out with a cry suddenly and became clear minded and spoke normally.

11. Essentials

This patient is a young girl. The emotional stimulation causes her mental depression and the Liver Qi stagnation. The brain is disturbed and she lost consciousness. With clear diagnosis, Renzhong (GV 26), the Emergency point, is used to wake up the brain and smooth the Qi circulation. Neiguan (PC 6) is used for smoothing Qi and calming the Mind. Taichong (LR 3) is a point used for soothing the Liver Meridian to subdue the upward disturbance of Liver Qi. The patient is restored from unconsciousness through this correct differentiation and proper stimulation in acupuncture.

SUMMARY

Hysteria is a kind of neurosis. TCM holds that it is usually caused by emotional depression and over thinking. The patient has a sudden onset of mental disorder with violent behaviour and laughing and crying, or sleeping all the time, or dysphonia, or limb paralysis, or trembling and spasm like epilepsy, or sudden loss of hearing and vision, but without organic pathological changes found in examination. Acupuncture may be applied together with suggestion therapy.

Main points: Renzhong (GV 26), Neiguan (PC 6), Shenmen (HT 7).

Hegu (LI 4) and Taichong (LR 3) are added for epileptic cases; Yamen (GV 15), Huantiao (GB 30) and Yanglingquan (GB 34) are added for paralysis; Daling (PC 7) and Yongquan (KI 1) added for sleeping all the time; Tiantu (CV 22) added for globus hestericus; Jingming (BL 1) added for loss of vision; Tinggong (SI 19) and Yifeng (TE 17) added for loss of hearing; Lianquan (CV 23) and Tongli (HT 5) added for inability to speak.

SECTION THIRTY-SIX • DEPRESSION

CASE I: CHENG XINNONG'S MEDICAL RECORD

1. General data

Zhang, female, 21, first visited on September 27, 1984.

2. Chief complaint

The sensation of a foreign body in the throat for 1 year.

3. History of present illness

One year ago, she began to feel blocked in the throat and uncomfortable in the chest due to unhappiness at work. Diagnosed pharyngeal neurosis, she was medicated but not relieved.

4. Present symptoms

Blocked sensation in the throat, menstruation scanty in volume and dark in colour.

5. Tongue and pulse

Pale tongue, thready rapid pulse.

6. Differentiation and analysis

Mei He Qi (globus hysterics), mostly seen in females, is a subjective sensation as if a plum pit is stuck in the throat or the throat is compressed, caused by the Liver Qi stagnation bringing Phlegm up owing to emotional injuries.

7. Diagnosis

TCM: Mei He Qi (globus hysterics) (Qi stagnation, Phlegm retention).

Western medicine: Pharyngeal neurosis.

8. Treating principle

Regulate Liver, dissolve Phlegm.

9. Prescription

Tiantu (CV 22), Shanzhong (CV 17), Taichong (LR 3), Hegu (LI 4), Zusanli (ST 36), Neiguan (PC 6), Fenglong (ST 40), Lieque (LU 7).

Fenglong (ST 40) was reduced. Other points, even method.

10. Effect

Five treatments of acupuncture relieved the symptoms greatly.

11. Essentials

For globus hysterics, regulate Liver Qi and dissolve Phlegm are the principles for treatment.

Taichong (LR 3), Yuan-Source of Liver Channel, pertaining to Yin, dominating Blood, can regulate Liver Qi; Hegu (LI 4), Yuan-Source of the Large Intestine Channel, pertaining to Yang, dominating Qi, can ascend and disperse to treat depressions. These are the Four Gates, used to harmonize Qi and Blood and regulate Yin and Yang.

Shanzhong (CV 17), Influential point of Qi, which acts on the Qi circulation of the whole body, together with Tiantu (CV 22), is used to circulate the stagnated Qi. 'Strengthen the Spleen first to prevent it from being involved when the Liver is diseased'. Zusanli (ST 36), He-Sea of Stomach, is selected to strengthen the Spleen and Stomach beforehand, and Fenglong (ST 40) to strengthen Spleen to dissolve Phlegm.

CASE II: CHENG XINNONG'S MEDICAL RECORD

1. General data

Geng, female, 17, first visited on July 14, 1980.

2. Chief complaint

Insanity for 2 weeks.

3. History of present illness

Because she had to take an examination to enter university, she was nervous and worked too hard, and it happened to be the time when her period was coming; then she became mentally disordered, being unclear minded, scared and restless. Taking diazepam and herbal medicine was not very effective.

4. Present symptoms

She was mentally disordered, and had no desire for food. Her stools were normal.

5. Tongue and pulse

Red tongue, thick yellowish coating, wiry rapid pulse.

6. Differentiation and analysis

This patient reached her depressive mental disorder due to over thinking and emotional depression, when the Liver Qi fails to circulate well, the Spleen fails to carry out its function of transportation and transformation well, thus the fluid is retained into Phlegm, which disturbs the brain and the Mind. In pathology, Hand-Shaoyin Heart, Foot-Jueyin Liver, Foot-Taiyin Spleen channels are involved.

7. Diagnosis

TCM: Hysteria (accumulation of Phlegm with Heat).

Western medicine: Hysteria.

8. Treating principle

Regulate Qi, remove depression, dissolve Phlegm, promote resuscitation.

9. Prescription

Baihui (GV 20), Sishencong (EX-HN1), Renzhong (GV 26), Shanzhong (CV 17), Neiguan (PC 6), Shenmen (HT 7), Daling (PC 7), Sanyinjiao (SP 6), Taichong (LR 3).

In addition An Gong Niu Huang Wan (Cow-bezoar Bolus for Resurrection) was administered, 1 bolus each day.

10. Effect

On her second visit, Fenglong (ST 40) and Zanzhu (BL 2) were added. On her seventh visit, she was in a recovered state. Renzhong (GV 26) was omitted, Houxi (SI 3) added. On her thirteenth visit, Baihui (GV 20), Sishencong (EX-HN1), Shanzhong (CV 17), Neiguan (PC 6), Shenmen (HT 7), Sanyinjiao (SP 6), Taichong (LR 3) were used. Three more treatments resulted in her basic recovery.

11. Essentials

For this complicated case with Hand-Shaoyin Heart, Foot-Jueyin Liver, Foot-Taiyin Spleen channels involved, the points from multiple channels should be selected to regulate Yin and Yang: Baihui (GV 20), Sishencong (EX-HN1) and Renzhong (GV 26) for promoting resuscitation and waking up the Spleen; Shanzhong (CV 17), Neiguan (PC 6), Daling (PC 7) and Shenmen (HT 7) for regulating Qi circulation in the chest to calm the Mind; Sanyinjiao (SP 6) for strengthening Spleen Qi; Fenglong (ST 40) for dissolving Phlegm; Taichong (LR 3) for soothing the Liver; and Houxi (SI 3), leading to the Governor Vessel, for dispersing Yang Qi, resting the Heart, and calming the Mind.

The good therapeutic outcome is achieved by using the group of points mentioned above for the purpose of dissolving Phlegm and promoting the brain to relieve depression.

CASE III: JI XIAOPING'S MEDICAL RECORD

1. General data

Yan, female, 43 years old, came on September 19, 2002 for the first visit.

2. Chief complaint

Melancholy, anxiety, irritability, and sadness for 1 year and 3 months.

3. History of present illness

Because her work was not smooth and she had interpersonal relationship disagreements, she became melancholy, anxious, worried, and irritable, she had dream-disturbed sleep, and sometimes she cried without reasons. In June 2001 Beijing Medical University diagnosed her with depression, and prescribed her anti-melancholy medicines Deanxit (Flupentixol-melitracen) 2 tablets daily, Fluoxetine 1 tablet daily, and Rola 2 tablets daily taken orally. During medication she was relieved of the symptoms, but since stopping taking medicines in January 2002, her symptoms were again as before. Therefore she came for acupuncture treatment.

4. Present symptoms

She was melancholy, anxious, worried, irritable, crying without reason, having suicidal intentions, distention in chest and hypochondrium, poor appetite, and dream-disturbed sleep.

5. Tongue and pulse

Red tongue tip and borders, white sticky coating; string-taut and rapid pulse (120/min).

6. Differentiation and analysis

The cause of her pathological condition is depression damaging the Liver. The Liver Qi stagnation causes her distention in the chest and hypochondrium. Prolonged Liver Qi stagnation turns into Fire, thus red tongue tip and borders and string-taut rapid pulse. Liver is the Wood and Spleen the Earth. Strong Wood overacts on Earth. The Spleen is related to worries, so she has anxiety, poor appetite, and white sticky tongue-coating. Liver Wood is the mother of Heart Fire, the mother disease involves the child, Liver Fire causes Heart Fire, so there appears irritability, palpitations, dream-disturbed sleep, and red tip of tongue. Generally Lung Metal acts on Liver Wood, but here the Liver Wood is too strong, counter-acting on Lung Metal, which is related to sadness, which is why she often has unreasonable crying.

In short, this is Liver Qi stagnation, Heart and Liver Fire preponderance, Lung Qi obstruction producing Heat, and Spleen Qi deficiency.

7. Diagnosis

TCM: Yuzheng-melancholia.
Western medicine: Depression.

8. Treating principle

Smooth the Liver for relieving Liver Qi stagnation, clear Heart Fire and Liver Fire, remove Lung Heat, strengthen Spleen and Stomach, replenish Kidney Yin to subdue Heart and Liver Fire.

9. Prescription

Taichong (LR 3), Guangming (GB 37), Xingjian (LR 2), Xiaxi (GB 43), Neiguan (PC 6), Shenmen (HT 7), Yuji (LU 10), Zusanli (ST 36), Sanyinjiao (SP 6), Taixi (KI 3).

The reinforcing method for Zusanli (ST 36), Sanyinjiao (SP 6), Taixi (KI 3). The reducing method for the rest points. Retain the needles for 30 minutes. Three times a week.

10. Effect

After 5 treatments, she was relieved in terms of melancholy, anxiety, worries, and irritability, her heart rate became 100/min. Altogether she was treated 28 times; her symptoms all disappeared and heart rate changed to 80/min. Five-year follow-up found her with no relapse.

11. Essentials

TCM holds that emotional activity is closely related with the five Zang organs, which are thus named the five Shen-emotional organs. Emotions may injure the Zang organs and dysfunctions of the Zang organs may cause abnormal emotions. At the beginning in this case, anger damaged the Liver. Liver Qi stagnation disorders the functions of Heart, Liver, and Lungs, so the patient was anxious, irritable, and crying without reason.

In the differentiation, the relation of the Five Elements in producing, acting, overacting, and counteracting are applied to get the conclusion, dysfunctions of Liver, Heart, Spleen and Lungs.

The points were selected according to the correct differentiation and treating principle, at the same time, the specific functions of five Shu points were made full use of in treatment.

Taichong (LR 3), the Yuan-Source point of the Liver Meridian, Guangming (GB 37), the Luo-Connecting point of the Gallbladder Meridian, are the combination of Yuan-Luo for smoothing the Liver to regulate Liver Qi. They are important points for depression. Xingjian (LR 2), Ying-Spring point of the Liver Meridian, is used to clear the Liver Fire, whilst Xiaxi (GB 43), the Ying-Spring point of the Gallbladder Meridian, is to clear the Gallbladder. Shenmen (HT 7), the Yuan-Source point of the Heart Meridian, is for clearing the Heart Fire, and Neiguan (PC 6), the Luo-Connecting point of the Pericardium Meridian, is for treating irritability and palpitations. Yuji (LU 10) is the Ying-Spring point of Lung Meridian, removing the Lung Heat. Zusanli (ST 36) and Sanyinjiao (SP 6) strengthen Spleen and Stomach to subdue Liver Wood. Taixi (KI 3) reinforces Kidney Yin to reduce Heart and Liver Fire.

The prescription of points selected to smooth the Liver to relieve Liver Qi stagnation, clear Heart Fire and Liver Gallbladder Fire, remove Lung Heat, strengthen Spleen and Stomach, and replenish Kidney Yin, functions well to lead to a positive result.

SUMMARY

Depression is caused by emotional injury and Qi stagnation, manifested as being mentally depressed, restless and irritable, crying, and feeling as if there is a plum pit lodged in the throat, etc. The principle for treatment is to regulate Shen-Mind, circulate Qi, soothe Liver, and remove depression.

Main points: Renzhong (GV 26), Neiguan (PC 6), Shenmen (HT 7), Taichong (LR 3).

SECTION THIRTY-SEVEN • IMPOTENCE

CASE I: LU SHOUYAN'S MEDICAL RECORD

1. General data

Wang, male, 48, first visited on August 17, 1965.

2. Chief complaint

Impotence, incontinence of urine.

3. History of present illness

He took part in the war of liberation in 1947, slept in cold damp places for a long time. From 1959, he suffered from impotence and incontinence of urine.

4. Present symptoms

He suffered from impotence and incontinence of urine. He felt soreness and pain in the lower back, and weakness of the four limbs. His urine was sometimes white colour and with white clumps in it, and he had painful urination. He had headache and dizziness.

5. Tongue and pulse

Pale tongue, soft pulse.

6. Differentiation and analysis

This is impotence caused by invasion of Cold Damp, making the Kidney Yang exhausted and the Essence deficient and Cold.

7. Diagnosis

TCM: Impotence (invasion of Cold Damp, Kidney Yang deficiency).

Western medicine: Impotence.

8. Treating principle

Dispel Cold, warm Yang, reinforce Kidney Yin.

9. Prescription

- Guanyuan (CV 4), Zhongji (CV 3).
- Mingmen (GV 4), Yaoshu (GV 2).
- Shenshu (BL 23).

The 3 groups of points were used in turn. Moxibustion with 7 grain-sized cones was done at each point.

10. Effect

After 6 times of moxibustion, his impotence was cured and he became energetic again.

11. Essentials

Professor Lu selected Guanyuan (CV 4) and Zhongji (CV 3) which are in the location of the Dantian, the place where the male Essence is stored. Treating with moxibustion here is to dispel the Cold of the Essence. Moxibustion at Mingmen (GV 4) is to reinforce the genuine Fire. Moxibustion at Yaoshu (GV 2) is to warm Yufang (jade house) which is between Baihuanshu (BL 30), a point also named Yufangshu and its Qi connecting with Yufang. The ancient alchemists said to 'store Essence in the jade house'. The Back-Shu points are rooted in the Taiyang Channel and correspond to the Governor Vessel. Thus, moxibustion at Yaoshu (GV 2) can also warm up Yufang. Moxibustion at these two points functions to dispel Cold Damp of the Governor Vessel. Moxibustion at Shenshu (BL 23) reinforces the Kidney Yang to produce the genuine Yin. In this way, the 6 moxibustion treatments cured the patient and made her energetic again.

CASE II: CHENG XINNONG'S MEDICAL RECORD

1. General data

Tao, male, 55, first visited on October 15, 1985.

2. Chief complaint

Impotence for half a month.

3. History of present illness

Half a month ago, he became impotent and got testis redux because he and his wife had a quarrel during intercourse. Since then, he had been emotionally depressed.

4. Present symptoms

Impotence and testis redux, accompanied by emotional depression, fullness in the chest, shortness of breath, dizziness, soreness in the lower back, dry mouth but no desire to drink, poor appetite, and poor sleep with only 2–3 hours sleep each night.

5. Tongue and pulse

Red tip and borders of tongue, wiry and a little rapid pulse, Chi weak.

6. Differentiation and analysis

This patient became impotent from emotional depression, which injures the Liver, so the Yang Qi of Liver and Kidneys cannot be dispersed. Red tip and borders of tongue, wiry and a little rapid pulse, and Chi weak are the manifestations of failure of the Yang Qi of the Liver and Kidneys in dispersing.

7. Diagnosis

TCM: Impotence (Liver stagnation, Kidney deficiency).

Western medicine: Impotence.

8. Treating principle

Soothe Liver to relieve stagnation, tonify Kidney Yang.

9. Prescription

Baihui (GV 20), Guanyuan (CV 4), Neiguan (PC 6), Sanyinjiao (SP 6), Taichong (LR 3).

10. Effect

On his first visit, psychotherapy was also applied by explaining to him that his problem was only temporary. On the following day, he said after the first time of acupuncture he could do intercourse already. The above-mentioned treatment was continued and he was cured after 4 treatments.

11. Essentials

Complete Works of Zhang Jingyue (*Impotence*) says: 'Impotence is mostly caused by the decline of Mingmen Fire, the deficiency of Essence and Qi, or emotional injuries, damaging the production of Yang Qi.' *Miraculous Pivot* (*Jing Jin*) says: 'The Muscle Region of Foot-Jueyin, is diseased…the penis fails to act, when caused by endogenous factor it cannot erect.'

For the patients with disease caused by emotional damage, an effective result can be achieved by relieving his worries and fears. Guanyuan (CV 4) is selected to strengthen the Kidney Yang. Sanyinjiao (SP 6) is to regulate the three Yin channels for tonifying Yang. Baihui (GV 20) is to lift Yang Qi. Taichong (LR 3) is to smooth the Qi of the Jueyin Channel. Neiguan (PC 6) is to rest the Heart to calm the Mind.

SUMMARY

Impotence is generally due to indulgence in sexual activities, which makes Mingmen Fire decline and exhausts the Kidney Essence. It may also be due to worry, which damages the Heart and Spleen. Or fear and fright injure the Kidneys. Or Damp Heat driving downward makes the penis unable to erect.

Main points: Mingmen (GV 4), Shenshu (BL 23), Guanyuan (CV 4), Sanyinjiao (SP 6).

Shenshu (BL 23) is used to reinforce the Kidneys, Mingmen (GV 4) and Guanyuan (CV 4) to replenish the genuine Fire of the Lower Burner, Sanyinjiao (SP 6), the meeting point of the three Yin channels of foot, all of which distribute to the lower abdomen and knot at the external genitals, to reinforce the three Yin organs.

Add Xinshu (BL 15), Shenmen (HT 7), Zusanli (ST 36) for Qi deficiency of Heart and Spleen, add Xingjian (LR 2) and Taichong (LR 3) for mental depression, and add Yinlingquan (SP 9) for Damp Heat driving downward.

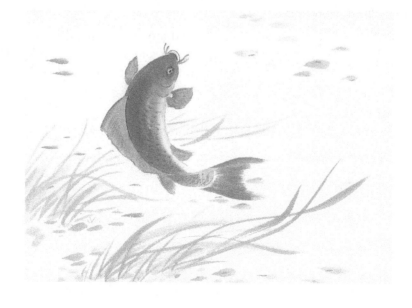

SECTION THIRTY-EIGHT • HERNIA

CASE I: RECORD IN *ACUPUNCTURE-MOXIBUSTION FOR DIFFICULT DISEASES*

1. General data

Gao, male, 51, first visited on June 3, 1994.

2. Chief complaint

Paroxysmal abdominal pain for 2 days.

3. History of present illness

Two days ago, he began to have a paroxysmal abdominal pain and a swelling and pain of the scrotum on the left side.

4. Present symptoms

Paroxysmal abdominal pain, swelling and pain of the scrotum on the left side. Vomiting. Without bowel movements for 2 days.

Examination: His abdomen was a little bulged with the intestines visible, soft, no tenderness and rebound tenderness, but a strengthened bowel sound.

5. Tongue and pulse

Red tongue, thin coating, wiry rapid pulse.

6. Differentiation and analysis

Foot-Jueyin Liver Channel distributes to and around the genitals. The Liver Qi is stagnated and goes in the opposite direction, as a result a hernia appears. The stagnated Liver Qi attacks the Spleen Earth, so that there is vomiting.

7. Diagnosis

TCM: Hernia (Qi of Liver and Spleen channels going adversely).

Western medicine: Hernia.

8. Treating principle

Soothe Liver and circulate Qi, regulate Liver and Spleen.

9. Prescription

Yinbai (SP 1), Dadun (LR 1).

　　Moxibustion was done for 40 minutes each time after needling Yinbai (SP 1), once a day.

10. Effect

With moxibustion, he felt a burning pain in the local area. After 7 treatments, his swelling and pain disappeared. There was no recurrence.

11. Essentials

Wai Tai Mi Yao (*The Medical Secrets of an Official*) says: 'For hernia of the scrotum… do moxibustion at the medial side of the great toe, at the junction of the red and white muscle (Yinbai, SP 1)…' *Miraculous Pivot* (*Jing Mai*) says: 'Foot-Jueyin…when its Qi reverses upward, the testicle is diseased hernia, in excess, it is stiff, in deficiency, it is itching. Dadun (LR 1) is selected for treatment.'

Following the principle given by the Classics, Dadun (LR 1) and Yinbai (SP 1) are selected, and moxibustion is applied to enhance the effect. The Qi of the Liver and Spleen channels is circulated, the pain is stopped since the obstruction is removed.

CASE II: CHENG XINNONG'S MEDICAL RECORD

1. General data

Li, male, 50, first visited on January 27, 1992.

2. Chief complaint

Testicle pain for nearly 40 years, aggravated for 1 month.

3. History of present illness

He said he got this pain when he played football when he was young.

4. Present symptoms

His testicles were swollen and painful, especially worse when tired and attacked by Wind. He couldn't sleep well because of the pain.

5. Tongue and pulse

Tongue tip was red, coating white, pulse wiry and rolling.

6. Differentiation and analysis

From his pulse and symptoms, with Yin Qi accumulated in the interior and Cold Damp invasion, his Conception Vessel and Liver Channel were blocked, leading to the testicles' swelling and pain.

7. Diagnosis

TCM: Hernia (Cold Damp retention).

Western medicine: Hernia.

8. Treating principle

Soothe Liver and regulate Qi, warm and dissolve Cold Damp.

9. Prescription

Baihui (GV 20), Guanyuan (CV 4), Guilai (ST 29), Ququan (LR 8), Zhongfeng (LR 4), Taichong (LR 3), Dadun (LR 1), Sanyinjiao (SP 6), Ganshu (BL 18), Shenshu (BL 23).

Moxibustion was applied to Guanyuan (CV 4). Ganshu (BL 18) and Shenshu (BL 23), without retaining the needles. Other points were punctured with even method.

10. Effect

With 5 courses of treatment given intermittently, the swelling disappeared, only a mild pain appeared occasionally. He was basically cured.

11. Essentials

To warm the channels and collaterals and dissolve the Damp, moxibustion is done at Guanyuan (CV 4) to dispel Cold. To soothe the Liver and regulate Qi, Taichong (LR 3), Dadun (LR 1), Ganshu (BL 18), and Shenshu (BL 23) are used in combination to treat the Liver and Kidneys simultaneously.

SUMMARY

Hernia is a disease characterized by protrusion of the contents from the body cavity, manifested as swelling and pain of testicles and scrotum. The causative factors are said to be the invasion of Cold, Heat and Damp, leading to the obstruction of Qi and Blood in the Conception Vessel and Liver Channel. Although there are different types of hernia, pain in the lower abdomen is the common manifestation. The points are mainly selected from the Conception Vessel and Liver Channel. Moxibustion with ginger or direct moxibustion is applied for its treatment.

Main points: Guanyuan (CV 4), Dadun (LR 1), Sanyinjiao (SP 6).

SECTION THIRTY-NINE • PROLAPSE OF RECTUM

CASE I: SHAO JINGMING'S MEDICAL RECORD

1. General data

Zhao, female, 56, first visited on August 18, 1977.

2. Chief complaint

Prolapse of rectum for 3 years.

3. History of present illness

At the beginning, she only felt a bearing-down in the anus after bowel movements, as if something had prolapsed, and when she stood up the prolapsed rectum restored itself. With the development of the condition, it became worse, so she came for treatment.

4. Present symptoms

The prolapse of the rectum became worse, more than 4cm, and it couldn't restore itself automatically. Even in coughing or walking, the rectum could prolapse. The frequency of bowel movements was increased. She had a sallow complexion and listlessness.

5. Tongue and pulse

Pale tongue with white coating. Soft weak pulse.

6. Differentiation and analysis

This patient has hypofunction of Spleen and Stomach, so the sinking of Qi of the Middle Burner causes the weakness of Qi in lifting and looseness of the anus in astringing the rectum.

7. Diagnosis

TCM: Prolapse of rectum (sinking of Qi of Middle Burner).

Western medicine: Prolapse of rectum.

8. Treating principle

Lift and reinforce Yang Qi.

9. Prescription

Baihui (GV 20), Changqiang (GV 1), Huangang (Empirical point for prolapse of rectum).

Acupuncture and moxibustion were applied to Baihui (GV 20). The patient should be in a lateral recumbent position when Changqiang (GV 1) and Huangang (Extra) are punctured. The 3 cun filiform needle was used with 2.5 cun inserted. For the duration of retaining the needles for 20–30 minutes, the needle was manipulated twice to strengthen the needling sensation, during which the patient would feel a contraction in the anus.

10. Effect

After the first time of moxibustion, she didn't have prolapse of rectum when she had a bowel movement. Only a bearing-down sensation appeared when walking and tired. One week later, the same moxibustion treatment was given again and the bearing-down sensation disappeared. Another treatment was applied just to consolidate the effect.

11. Essentials

Acupuncture and moxibustion at Baihui (GV 20) promote Yang Qi to lift the rectum. Changqiang (GV 1) and Huangang (Extra) are in the local area of the anus, deep insertion can strengthen the controlling and astringing of the anus and regulate the Governor Vessel to lift the Qi of the Middle Burner.

> **HUANGANG**
>
> Huangang (Extra) is located in the local area of the anus, at 3 o'clock and 9 o'clock. It is the empirical point for prolapse of the rectum.

CASE II: XIAO SHAOQING'S MEDICAL RECORD

1. General data

Zhu, male, 12, first visited on May 12, 1956.

2. Chief complaint

Prolapse of the rectum for 3 years.

3. History of present illness

Three years ago, his rectum started to prolapse after a bout of chronic enteritis. Later, the diarrhoea was cured, but the prolapse of the rectum continued, without effective treatment.

4. Present symptoms

Prolapse of the rectum, sallow complexion, emaciation, accompanied with dizziness and poor appetite.

5. Tongue and pulse

Thin white tongue-coating, thready weak pulse.

6. Differentiation and analysis

The patient is weak in constitution owing to the chronic diarrhoea. Sinking of Qi of the Middle Burner causes the failure of contraction of the anus, thus there is prolapse of the rectum.

7. Diagnosis

TCM: Prolapse of the rectum (sinking of Qi of the Middle Burner).

Western medicine: Prolapse of the rectum.

8. Treating principle

Reinforce the Qi of the Middle Burner, lift Qi to raise the rectum.

9. Prescription

Baihui (GV 20), Changqiang (GV 1), Qihai (CV 6), Tianshu (ST 25), Dachangshu (BL 25).

The reinforcing-reducing achieved by rapid and slow insertion and withdrawal of the needle was used and the needles were retained for 20 minutes. After needling, moxibustion was done. Once every other day.

10. Effect

With 2 treatments, the anus was able to contract, but prolapsed again when passing stools. Six treatments made the prolapse stop, even when carrying heavy loads there was no prolapse. Three more treatments were given to consolidate the good effect.

11. Essentials

Qihai (CV 6) and Guanyuan (CV 4) are selected to reinforce the Qi of the Middle Burner. Moxibustion at Baihui (GV 20) is to activate Yang Qi to lift the prolapsed rectum. Changqiang (GV 1) is to strengthen the contraction of the anus. Tianshu (ST 25) combined with Dachangshu (BL 25) is to regulate the Qi of the Large Intestines to promote the recovery of their normal functions.

SUMMARY

Prolapse of the rectum is mostly caused by prolonged diarrhoea or dysentery owing to the sinking of the Qi of the Middle Burner. In a mild case, the rectum can be restored after bowel movements, but in severe cases, it prolapses even with coughing and carrying heavy loads.

Main points: Baihui (GV 20), Changqiang (GV 1).

Qihai (CV 6), Zusanli (ST 36), Pishu (BL 20) and Shenshu (BL 23) are added for those who have a weak constitution, and moxibustion is applied for the cases of Yang deficiency.

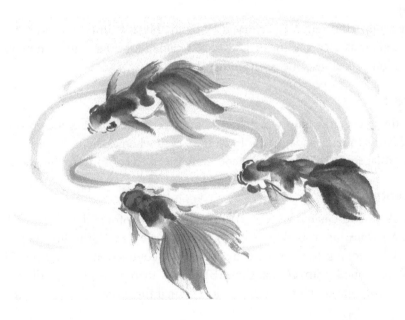

SECTION FORTY • HIGH FEVER

CASE I: WU ZHONGCHAO'S MEDICAL RECORD

1. General data

Li, female, 53 years old.

2. Chief complaint

High fever and unconsciousness for 1 week.

3. History of present illness

One week ago, the patient had a high fever suddenly, 41–42°C, without a clear cause. She was admitted into a big Western medicine hospital. All kinds of examinations failed to find the cause, and the treatment was not effective in relieving the fever, so she left the hospital. In the past she had a history of Sjogren syndrome.

4. Present symptoms

High fever, unconsciousness, restlessness of hands and feet, the whole body a dark purple colour.

5. Tongue and pulse

Thorny tongue in dark purple colour, dry coating; surging rapid pulse.

6. Differentiation and analysis

The patient had a history of Sjogren syndrome, although the pathological condition was stable at present, the evil Heat stagnated inside her body. It was induced suddenly without clear reasons. Her whole body was a dark purple colour, like pig's Liver. 'Heat enters the Ying Blood...macule and papule'. It was thought to be the macule and papule covering the skin. The dark purple tongue with thorns on it, and the surging rapid pulse showed the signs of strong Heat damaging the collaterals and Blood stasis. And the Mind stored in the Heart was disturbed by the evil Heat, therefore the patient was unconscious with restlessness of hands and feet. This pathological condition was differentiated as the Heat entering the Blood system causing high fever (strong Heat).

7. Diagnosis

TCM: High fever (strong Heat), (Heat entering the Blood system).

Western medicine: High fever requiring further examination.

8. Treating principle

Clear Heat, treat exterior syndrome, cool the Blood, activate Blood circulation.

9. Prescription

Dazhui (GV 14), Weizhong (BL 40), Quchi (LI 11), Hegu (LI 4), Fengchi (GB 20), Xuehai (SP 10), Neiguan (PC 6).

Bloodletting was applied at Dazhui (GV 14) and Weizhong (BL 40) alternately with an interval of half an hour. Quchi (LI 11), Hegu (LI 4), Fengchi (GB 20), and Xuehai (SP 10) were punctured with the reducing method, and Neiguan (PC 6) with the reinforcing method.

10. Effect

With the bloodletting at Dazhui (GV 14) and Weizhong (BL 40) alternately, the dark purple colour of the whole body became lighter quickly and the restlessness greatly relieved. Together with acupuncture at other points, her high fever was stopped. At dawn, her body temperature became normal, the dark colour of the body changed to normal, her restlessness disappeared, and consciousness was restored. Xijiao Dihuang Tang (Decoction of Rhinoceros Horns and Rehmannia) and Qingying Tang (Decoction for Clearing Heat in the Ying System) were administered for recuperation.

Dazhui (GV 14) is an important point to reduce Heat. Weizhong (BL 40), known as a Blood cleft, is a quick point for treating the acute case of Heat in Blood. Bloodletting at these two points can clear the evil Heat from the Blood directly, resulting in 'removing Blood stasis'. Quchi (LI 11) and Hegu (LI 4), good at circulating Qi and Blood to remove obstruction of the meridians and collaterals, are reduced to reduce the excessive Yangming Heat. Fengchi (GB 20) is a crossing point of Foot-Shaoyang and Yang-Link Vessel, effective in dispelling Wind, activating Blood, treating head and eyes, and regulating Qi and Blood. The Heart is dominating the Blood and vessels and stores the Mind. Neiguan (PC 6), the Luo-Connecting point of Pericardium Meridian, circulates Qi and Blood, and calms the Mind. Xuehai (SP 10) is reduced to cool the Blood to activate Blood and remove Blood stasis.

11. Essentials

Treatment based on syndrome differentiation is the most important characteristic of TCM. In this specific case, the whole body of the patient which was a dark purple colour like pig's Liver is differentiated as the sudden onset of macules and papules due to Heat entering the Blood system, which is the key point of the pathological condition. The tongue and pulse show the signs of strong Heat, and unconsciousness indicates the disturbance of the Mind stored in the Heart. The diagnosis is clearly confirmed as high fever (strong Heat) resulted from Heat entering the Blood system. Following the principle given by Ye Tianshi that 'Heat entering Blood will cause exhaustion of Blood and accelerate the Blood. To cool the Blood and remove Blood stasis is the treating principle for the treatment.', bloodletting is used to cool the Blood and clear the Heat in the Blood system and remove Blood stasis. The reducing method at other points is for the purpose of clearing evil Heat, cooling the Blood, activating Blood, removing stasis and calming the Mind. The treatment is so effective that the high fever stopped and consciousness was restored.

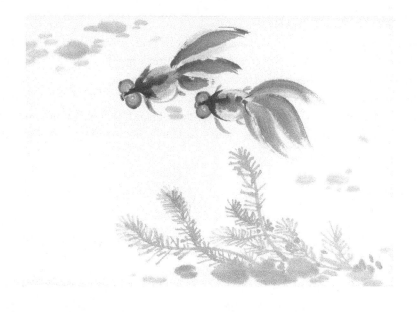

SECTION FORTY-ONE • BLOOD SYNDROME

CASE I: WU ZHONGCAO'S MEDICAL RECORD

1. General data

Zhao, male, 60 years old.

2. Chief complaint

Haematemesis and haematochezia accompanied with a decrease in blood pressure for 6 hours.

3. History of present illness

Two weeks ago, the patient suddenly had cerebral thrombosis. With anticoagulation and dilatancy treatment his condition became stable and he was discharged from the hospital. From yesterday, he had sudden retention of urine and in catheterization he was found to have haematuria; the haemostatics was not effective in stopping bleeding, and during the operation it was discovered that his Bladder had hyperaemia. And later he had haematemesis and haematochezia, and all treatments to stop bleeding were of no use for him.

4. Present symptoms

Cold extremities, unconscious, blood pressure too low to detect.

5. Tongue and pulse

Red tongue, thin coating; thready weak pulse.

6. Differentiation and analysis

The patient had ischaemic Windstroke with the Blood stasis in the meridians and collaterals of the brain. With the treatment of Western medicine in the principle of activating Blood and dissolving stasis, his pathological condition became worse. And the transmission of his disease was quick, manifested as haematemesis, haematochezia, and haematuria, indicating that Qi deficiency failed to control the Blood. Now his cold extremities and unconsciousness were the critical signs of Qi collapse resulting from Blood loss.

7. Diagnosis

TCM:

- Blood syndrome (haematemesis, haematochezia, haematuria). Qi and Blood deficiency, failure of Qi in controlling Blood.
- Ischaemic Windstroke (recovery stage). Qi deficiency and Blood stasis.

Western medicine:

- Generalized stress ulcer.

- Cerebral embolism.

8. Treating principle

Reinforce Yuan-Primary Qi, produce Blood.

9. Prescription

Baihui (GV 20), Shenque (CV 8). Moxibustion for 30 minutes.

The Governor Vessel, 'the sea of Yang meridians', governs the Yang Qi of the whole body and is indicated in mental disorders. Baihui (GV 20) is located on the top of the head, at the place where the meridians meet with each other, therefore it functions to regulate the meridians, increase Yuan-Primary Qi, and restore consciousness. The Conception Vessel is 'the sea of Yin meridians'; it reinforces all Yin meridians. Shenque (CV 8) is the place of Yuan-Primary Qi, therefore it functions to restore Yang to treat collapse. The combination of the two is not only to reinforce Qi to produce Blood, but also to regulate Yin and Yang and harmonize Qi and Blood. Moxibustion is used to warm and reinforce Yang for treating collapse. The points and moxibustion used in this way result in a good effect to reinforce Yuan-Primary Qi to stop bleeding.

10. Effect

This is an acute case. When the acute symptom is relieved, the treatment can be stopped. Thirty minutes of moxibustion made the patient's extremities begin to get warm, and blood pressure began to increase. Haematemesis still existed, but was greatly relieved. Then with Shihui San (Carbonized ten herbs) and Dushen Tang (Ginseng Decoction) prescribed to reinforce Qi and stop bleeding, his blood pressure was restored and all symptoms greatly relieved.

11. Essentials

Moxibustion is always thought of as a method for keeping fit, seldom used to treat acute diseases. In this case, it was just the moxibustion that saved the patient. Bianque's Experiencial Therapy (Bianque Xinshu): 'Genuine Qi deficiency causes people to become diseased, genuine Qi collapse causes people to die. To save life, moxibustion is the first choice.' It can be seen that moxibustion is a good treatment for the critical condition of collapse of Yang Qi.

The application of moxibustion is a simple but effective way to save the patient in the critical stage and gives time to prepare the herbal decoction, laying the foundation for the later treatment.

There are only two points used, one from the Governor Vessel and the other from the Conception Vessel. These two promote mutual production of Yin and Yang to treat collapse, and the other advantage is, that it is convenient for the doctor to do moxibustion, making the effect realized quickly.

GYNAECOLOGICAL AND PAEDIATRIC DISEASES

SECTION ONE • DYSMENORRHOEA

CASE I: SHAO JINGMING'S MEDICAL RECORD

1. General data

Li, female, 22.

2. Chief complaint

Dysmenorrhoea for 8 years.

3. History of present illness

She had the menarche with pain when she was 14, but she didn't have treatment because the pain was not serious at that time. Four years ago, she was caught by the rain while she was having a period and the pain became worse. With medication the pain stopped but she had a serious abdominal pain whenever she menstruated since then.

4. Present symptoms

She was having a period now, and she had a serious abdominal cold pain in the lower abdomen, and the pain was worse on pressure. The menstrual flow was small in quantity, dark in colour and with clots. She was slim with cold limbs, suffering complexion, and sweating.

5. Tongue and pulse

The tongue was slightly dark, the coating thin, the pulse wiry.

6. Differentiation and analysis

TCM holds that dysmenorrhoea is caused by obstruction of Qi and Blood. The pathogenic factors leading to the obstruction of Qi and Blood are Cold Damp retention, Liver Qi stagnation, Qi and Blood deficiency and so on. This patient's dysmenorrhoea is due to Cold obstructed in the uterus.

7. Diagnosis

TCM: Dysmenorrhoea (Cold stagnated in the uterus).

Western medicine: Dysmenorrhoea.

8. Treating principle

Warm the channels to dispel Cold, circulate Qi to activate Blood.

9. Prescription

Guanyuan (CV 4), Sanyinjiao (SP 6), Ciliao (BL 32).

The reinforcing and reducing achieved by lifting and thrusting and rotating the needle was used. Moxibustion was applied as well.

Guanyuan (CV 4) was inserted 1.5 cun, leading the needling sensation to the perineum. Sanyinjiao (SP 6) was inserted perpendicularly 1–1.5 cun along the posterior border of the tibia, leading the needling sensation to the sole of the foot. Ciliao (BL 32) was inserted 1.5–2 cun into the posterior sacral foramen, leading the needling sensation to the lower abdomen and perineum.

10. Effect

Her pain was immediately relieved after the arrival of Qi and disappeared 10 minutes later. The needle was retained for 30 minutes and manipulated twice in the duration. Later, she was treated regularly 3–5 days before the menstruation until it started, in succession for 3 periods, and she was cured. The follow-up for 2 years found no recurrence.

11. Essentials

For dysmenorrhoea due to Cold obstructed in the uterus, Guanyuan (CV 4) is used to reinforce the Kidney Yang to dispel Cold, circulate Qi and regulate her menstruation; Sanyinjiao (SP 6) is used to strengthen the Spleen to circulate Qi and activate the Blood; and Ciliao (BL 32) is to regulate the Lower Burner and adjust Chong and Ren.

SUMMARY

Dysmenorrhoea refers to the pain appearing in the lower abdomen and lower back before, after or during menstruation. Acupuncture-moxibustion is effective for its treatment, not only to stop the pain immediately, but also to have a good long-term result. The pain before or during menstruation is mostly excess syndrome of Cold retention and/or Qi stagnation; while pain after menstrual flow is usually deficiency syndrome. The excess syndrome should be treated through warming the channels to dispel Cold and regulating Qi to remove stasis. The deficiency syndrome should be treated through regulating and reinforcing the Liver and Kidneys and replenishing Qi and Blood. Acupuncture-moxibustion is applied 3–5 days before menstruation, once a day, until the flow comes. For severe and prolonged cases, acupuncture-moxibustion should be given for 3–4 cycles at least.

Main points: Guanyuan (CV 4), Sanyinjiao (SP 6), Taichong (LR 3).

Zhongji (CV 3), Ciliao (BL 32) and Diji (SP 8) are added for the cases of abdominal pain worsened by pressure; Neiguan (PC 6), Yanglingquan (GB 34) and Qihai (CV 6) are added for cases of pain with hypochondrium and breasts involved; and Shenshu (BL 23) and Zusanli (ST 36) added for cases of abdominal pain with soreness in the lower back.

SECTION TWO • AMENORRHOEA

CASE I: RECORD IN *ACUPUNCTURE-MOXIBUSTION FOR DIFFICULT DISEASES*

1. General data

Yan, female, 43, first visited on October 12, 1980.

2. Chief complaint

Her menstruation stopped for half a year.

3. History of present illness

Her menstruation was usually normal in cycles, colour, quantity and quality. Half a year ago, on day when she was having a period, she waded in cold water. Since then her menstruation stopped.

4. Present symptoms

Amenorrhoea, soreness in lower back, tiredness of limbs, aversion to wind, headache, cold sensation in lower abdomen. Her profuse leucorrhoea was without abnormal colour and smell.

5. Tongue and pulse

Pale tongue, thin white coating, deep and a bit slow pulse.

6. Differentiation and analysis

Synopsis of Prescriptions of the Golden Chamber (*Women's Miscellaneous Diseases*) (金 要 略) says: 'In women's diseases, due to deficiency, accumulation of Cold, and stagnation of Qi, menstruation stops.'

Aversion to Wind, headache, cold sensation in lower abdomen, profuse leucorrhoea, pale tongue, thin white coating, deep and a bit slow pulse were the symptoms of pathogenic Cold stagnated in the uterus.

7. Diagnosis

TCM: Amenorrhoea (Cold retention, Blood stasis).

Western medicine: Amenorrhoea.

8. Treating principle

Warm the channels to dispel Cold.

9. Prescription

Guanyuan (CV 4).

Moxibustion was applied with a medicinal cake as isolation. The medicinal cake was made with the powder of Hu Jiao (胡椒 *Fructus Piperis Nigri*), Ding Xiang (丁香 *Flos Caryophylli*) and Rou Gui (肉桂 *Cortex Cinnamomi*). Moxibustion with 6 cones was done.

10. Effect

On the following day, she said her menstruation started again.

11. Essentials

Guanyuan (CV 4) is a meeting point of Ren with three foot Yin channels and a place from where the Qi of the Triple Burner originates, being one of the tonifying points for the whole body. Hu Jiao (胡椒), Dingxiang (丁香) and Rou Gui (肉桂) are pungent and warm materials, warming channels and dispelling Cold to stop pain. They can strengthen Kidney Yang, dispel Cold, unobstruct channels and regulate Ren for smoothing menstrual flow.

CASE II: CHENG XINNONG'S MEDICAL RECORD

1. General data

Hu, female, 40, first visited on January 3, 1992.

2. Chief complaint

Her menstruation stopped for 2 years.

3. History of present illness

Two years ago, she had a quarrel with somebody. It was during her menstruation which was not coming regularly later due to her mental depression.

4. Present symptoms

Amenorrhoea, accompanied with distention in lower abdomen, cold pain in loin radiating to back, fullness in chest, sighs, irritability, numbness of limbs, loose stools 2–3 times a day. Her cheeks and lips were dark purple.

5. Tongue and pulse

Tongue purplish, coating thin yellow, pulse wiry, Chi weak.

6. Differentiation and analysis

In emotional factors, anger damages Liver, the Liver Qi stagnates, Blood stasis is formed, so the menstruation stops. Qi and Blood circulation is blocked, so she has pain in her back and loins and numbness of limbs. Prolonged stagnation produces Heat, so she has irritability and yellow tongue-coating.

7. Diagnosis

TCM: Amenorrhoea (Qi stagnation with Blood stasis).

Western medicine: Amenorrhoea.

8. Treating principle

Regulate Qi, remove stasis.

9. Prescription

Shanzhong (CV 17), Qihai (CV 6), Zhongji (CV 3), Hegu (LI 4), Xuehai (SP 10), Sanyinjiao (SP 6), Taichong (LR 3), Xingjian (LR 2).
    Zhongji (CV 3) was treated with moxibustion, other points, even method.

10. Effect

She insisted on treatment for 7 courses of treatment, although not regularly. Her menstruation started again with regular cycles and other symptoms disappeared.

11. Essentials

Taichong (LR 3) and Xingjian (LR 2) are especially good for soothing the Liver and circulating its Qi, and clearing the Liver Fire.

SUMMARY

Amenorrhoea, if due to exhaustion of Blood caused by loss of Blood, indulgence in sexual activities, many deliveries or prolonged disease, is known as exhaustive amenorrhoea; if due to emotional anger and invasion of Cold, is known as stasis amenorrhoea.

Main points: Guanyuan (CV 4), Sanyinjiao (SP 6), Xuehai (SP 10).

Pishu (BL 20), Shenshu (BL 23), Qihai (CV 6) and Zusanli (ST 36) are added for exhaustive amenorrhoea to reinforce Kidney Qi, strengthen Spleen and Stomach and replenish Yin and Blood.

Zhongji (CV 3), Hegu (LI 4) and Xingjian (LR 2) are added for stasis amenorrhoea to reduce Heat and remove stasis to produce new Blood. Moxibustion is used for those Cold cases.

SECTION THREE • BENG LOU (UTERINE BLEEDING)

CASE I: CHENG XINNONG'S MEDICAL RECORD

1. General data

A 31-year-old female, named Liu, visited on May 13, 1992.

2. Chief complaint

Menstrual leaking for 14 days.

3. History of present illness

Fourteen days ago, her menstrual flow started, light colour, accompanied with soreness in the lumbar region. Medication was not effective. She had the menarche when she was 14. The cycle, colour and quantity of her menstruation were all normal. She got married at the age of 27, and had an abortion twice within 2 years after marriage.

4. Present symptoms

Menstrual flowing for 14 days without stopping. She was always tired, afraid of cold, and inactive in talking. She had a pale complexion.

5. Tongue and pulse

Pale tongue, thin coating, deep thready pulse.

6. Differentiation and analysis

Two abortions causes her Chong and Ren deficiency. Lack of taking care of herself causes Qi and Blood deficiency, so Chong and Ren non-consolidation, Liver and Spleen lose their controlling and storing functions, so Beng Lou (uterine bleeding).

7. Diagnosis

TCM: Beng Lou (Chong and Ren deficiency, Kidney Qi deficiency).

Western medicine: Dysfunctional uterine bleeding.

8. Treating principle

Regulate and reinforce Chong and Ren, reinforce Qi to control Blood.

9. Prescription

Baihui (GV 20), Guanyuan (CV 4), Zusanli (ST 36), Sanyinjiao (SP 6), Yangchi (TE 4), Yinbai (SP 1).

Yinbai (SP 1) was treated with moxibustion; other points, the reinforcing method.

10. Effect

With 5 treatments, the uterine bleeding was reduced and she felt better in spirit and physical strength. After 7 treatments, the bleeding stopped. Another 7 treatments to consolidate the improvement made all her symptoms disappear.

11. Essentials

Baihui (GV 20) is used to lift Qi of the Middle Burner; Guanyuan (CV 4) to reinforce Yuan-Source Qi to regulate Chong and Ren; Zusanli (ST 36), Sanyinjiao (SP 6), Yinbai (SP 1) to harmonize Liver and Spleen to restore their functions in controlling and storing Blood and replenishing Qi and Blood; Yangchi (TE 4) is the Yuan-Source point of the Triple Burner Channel, functioning to regulate Chong and Ren and reinforce Qi to control Blood.

CASE II: XIAO SHAOQING'S MEDICAL RECORD

1. General data

A 24-year-old female, named Huang, visited on May 19, 1998.

2. Chief complaint

Irregular menstruation accompanied by uterine bleeding for 7 years.

3. History of present illness

She had the menarche when she was 15. The cycle, colour and quantity of her menstruation were all normal. Since 1992, the cycle became disordered, only once every 2 or 3 months or even once in 6 months, the flow was still profuse after 7 days and with big clots. Hundred doses of herbal medicine, many treatments with oestrogen-progesterone cyclic therapy, and three treatments of uterine curettage failed to cure her. She came for acupuncture treatment.

4. Present symptoms

Postdated menstruation lasting more than 7 days, small quantity, dark colour, distending pain in lower abdomen, big clots in flow, and accompanied with dizziness, headache, and palpitations. Sallow complexion.

5. Tongue and pulse

Yellow and slight sticky tongue-coating, thready and rapid pulse.

6. Differentiation and analysis

This patient suffers from irregular menstruation accompanied by Beng Lou for 7 years. She is inward looking and depressed. Thus for a long time, the Liver is disordered in keeping the free flow of Qi and Chong and Ren are disordered in storing and releasing the Blood. Because of the Liver's disorder, her menstruation is delayed.

7. Diagnosis

TCM: Beng Lou (Liver Qi stagnation, failure of Spleen in transportation and transformation).

Western medicine: Dysfunctional uterine bleeding.

8. Treating principle

Soothe the Liver and regulate Qi, strengthen the Spleen and replenish the Blood, regulate Chong and Ren.

9. Prescription

Acupuncture, moxibustion and herbal medicine were used in combination.

Points:

- Baihui (GV 20), Neiguan (PC 6), Zhongwan (CV 12), Tianshu (ST 25), Qihai (CV 6) penetrating to Guanyuan (CV 4), Qichong (ST 30), Xuehai (SP 10), Diji (SP 8), Sanyinjiao (SP 6), Taichong (LR 3).

- Shangxing (GV 23), Hegu (LI 4), Shenque (CV 8), Guanyuan (CV 4), Zusanli (ST 36), Gongsun (SP 4), Yinbai (SP 1), Taixi (KI 3), Shuidao (ST 28), Guilai (ST 29), Qimen (LR 14).

The above two groups of points were used by turn. The filiform needle was used, even method, retained for 30 minutes, in the duration, the Phoenix Flying technique was applied to manipulate the needles once every 10 minutes. At the same time, Zhongwan (CV 12), Shenque (CV 8), Tianshu (ST 25), Qihai (CV 6) and Guanyuan (CV 4) were treated with cupping for 5–10 minutes. Once a day, 1 month as 1 course.

Herbal medicine:

- Dan Zhi Xiaoyao Wan (丹栀逍 丸 Ease Bolus of Moutan Bark and Cape Jasmine Fruit), twice a day, 4g each time.

- Guipi Wan (归脾丸 Bolus for Invigorating the Spleen and Nourishing the Heart), twice a day, 4g each time.

These two medicines used together for the purpose to strengthen the Spleen for controlling Blood.

10. Effect

Seven courses, 210 times of treatment all together, treated her menstruation so that it became regular at about 40 days, the quantity, colour and quality were all improved, and the flow lasted 5–8 days, medium quantity, fresh red colour, small dark clots, without Beng Lou anymore.

11. Essentials

As *Recovery of Various Diseases* (*Wan Bing Hui Chun*) says: 'Menstruation comes late, dark and with clots, due to Qi stagnation and Blood stasis.' The treating principle is to soothe the Liver, regulate Qi and activate Blood for regulating menstruation. *Various Diseases in Verse* says: 'If menstrual cycles are not regular, Diji (SP 8) and Xuehai (SP 10) are the points for treatment.'

Diji (SP 8) is a Xi-Cleft point of Foot-Taiyin Spleen Channel, used together with Xuehai (SP 10), to activate Blood, regulate menstruation, and circulate Qi to stop pain. Qimen (LR 14), Taichong (LR 3), Shuidao (ST 28), Guilai (ST 29) are reduced to soothe the Liver and regulate Qi, and activate Blood to smooth menstrual flow. In this way, the Liver is regulated and the Stomach harmonized, and menstruation comes regularly. The Chong Vessel is the sea of Blood, Ren Vessel is responsible for fostering the foetus. In cases where they are disordered, the sea of Blood will be disordered in storing Blood, thus causing Beng Lou (uterine bleeding). Zhongwan (CV 12), Shenque (CV 8), Qihai (CV 6), Guanyuan (CV 4), Qichong (ST 30), Zusanli (ST 36), Sanyinjiao (SP 6) and Yinbai (SP 1) are selected for treatment. Acupuncture together with moxibustion functions to regulate Chong and Ren, reinforce the Qi of the Middle Burner, and strengthen the Spleen in controlling Blood. Because she has had Beng Lou for a long time, Qi and Blood are deficient, Heart and brain lack nourishment, manifested as dizziness, headache and palpitations. The head is the meeting place of all the Yang channels, the face is the distribution area of the Yangming Channel. Baihui (GV 20) of Governor Vessel is used together with the Yuan-Source and He-Sea point of Hand-Yangming Large Intestine Channel, reinforced, to ascend clean Yang to dispel Wind and stop pain. Neiguan (PC 6) leads to Yinwei Vessel, Gongsun (SP 4) leads to Chong Vessel, reinforced, to treat palpitations with the Mind stored in the Heart disordered. Taixi (KI 3) is the Yuan-Source point of Foot-Shaoyin Kidney Channel, reinforced, and is used to reinforce Kidney Yin to subdue the deficient Fire. Shangxing (GV 23) of the Governor Vessel is reinforced to activate Yang Qi of the Governor Vessel to help Baihui (GV 20) in dispelling Wind and stopping pain. The combination of acupuncture with herbal treatment functions to soothe the Liver and regulate Qi, strengthen the Spleen and replenish the Blood, reinforce Qi of the Middle Burner, and regulate Chong and Ren. In this way her stubborn disease of menstruation is cured.

SUMMARY

Beng Lou (uterine bleeding) is caused by worry, Blood stasis, or invasion of Cold or Heat, causing the failure of Chong and Ren in consolidating and Liver and Spleen in storing and controlling Blood. The basic treating principle is to reinforce Chong and Ren, regulate the Liver and Spleen, and replenish Qi to control Blood.

Main points: Baihui (GV 20), Guanyuan (CV 4), Ganshu (BL 18), Pishu (BL 20), Sanyinjiao (SP 6), Yinbai (SP 1), Yangchi (TE 4).

Add Mingmen (GV 4) and Qihai (CV 6) for Cold syndrome to promote Qi to dispel Cold. Add Xuehai (SP 10) and Shuiquan (KI 5) for Heat syndrome to clear Heat from Blood. Add Zhongji (CV 3) and Taichong (LR 3) for Blood stasis syndrome to remove stasis to produce new Blood.

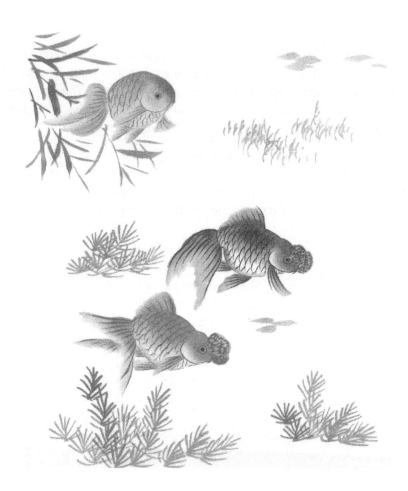

SECTION FOUR • RU PI (NODULES IN THE BREAST)

CASE I: GUO CHENGJIE'S MEDICAL RECORD

1. General data

A female aged 40, visited on May 6, 1980.

2. Chief complaint

Pain in her breasts with nodules for 6 years.

3. History of present illness

Six years ago, she had induced an abortion, and then her menstruation began to be postdated, the breast became hyperplasic with pain. By taking herbal medicine, the pain could be relieved. But it would start again when medication stopped. In the last 3 years, every month 15 days before menstrual flow, she had pain in the breasts, and nodules could be felt. So she came for acupuncture.

4. Present symptoms

She had pain and nodules in the breasts. Usually she was hot tempered, her menstruation was postdated, small quantity, pale colour, her pain in the breasts became worse before menstruation and when getting angry and tired. The accompanying symptoms were frontal headache, difficulty in falling asleep, dream-disturbed sleep, distending pain in the hypochondrium, bitter taste, and dry throat.

Examination: She was emaciated with pale complexion. Her breasts were normal in appearance, with no exudation from nipples. Patch-like, movable and smooth masses, 4.5cm × 3.5cm, with medium hardness, clear margins, obvious tenderness, were felt in the laterosuperior parts of the breasts. The cervical and subaxillary lymphnodes were enlarged.

5. Tongue and pulse

Red tongue, not moistened, thin white coating, wiry thready pulse.

6. Differentiation and analysis

The prolonged Liver Qi stagnation transforms into Fire that condenses the fluid into Phlegm staying in the breasts where the Liver Channel passes through, forming the nodules, so cause pain. Distending pain in hypochondrium, bitter taste, and dry throat are the symptoms of Liver Fire affecting upward. Liver and Kidney are of the same origin. In the prolonged case of Liver Fire, there appears Yin deficiency of Kidney, therefore the patient has blurred vision, tinnitus, soreness and weakness of lumbus and knees, difficulty in falling asleep, and dream-disturbed sleep. Red tongue, not moistened, thin white coating, wiry thready pulse are the manifestations of Yin deficiency of Liver and Kidneys.

7. Diagnosis

TCM: Ru Pi (Liver Kidney Yin deficiency).

Western medicine: Hyperplasia of mammary glands.

8. Treating principle

Reinforce Liver and Kidney, regulate Chong and Ren.

9. Prescription

- Tianzong (SI 11), Jianjing (GB 21), Ganshu (BL 18), Shenshu (BL 23).
- Wuyi (ST 15), Shanzhong (CV 17), Sanyinjiao (SP 6), Taixi (KI 3).

The 2 groups were used in turn, once a day, 10 times as 1 course, with a 4-day rest before the next course.

10. Effect

After 5 courses of treatment, the pain in the breasts before menstruation disappeared, and the masses decreased to 0.5cm × 0.5cm, no tenderness. She had no abnormal taste in the mouth during menstruation, no more irritability, no spitting of Blood, but still had a dry throat, difficulty in falling asleep, soreness and weakness in lumbar region. Two more courses of treatment cured all her symptoms. Three years later, the follow-up found no recurrence.

11. Essentials

In differentiation, this is a syndrome of Liver and Kidney Yin deficiency and Chong and Ren dysfunction. Wuyi (ST 15) lateral to the breast and Shanzhong (CV 17) were selected to regulate the channels of the breast to activate Blood; Ganshu (BL 18) to soothe Liver Qi; Jianjing (GB 21) to smooth Gallbladder Qi in order to smooth Liver Qi because they were externally–internally related; Tianzong (SI 11) was effective in removing obstructions of the channels and collaterals, good for breast diseases; Shenshu (BL 23) and Taixi (KI 3) to replenish Kidney Water for supplementing Kidney Yin; Sanyinjiao (SP 6) to strengthen Spleen and Stomach, reinforce Liver and Kidneys, regulate Qi and Blood, and remove obstructions of the channels and collaterals. The combination of these points functions to achieve the purpose of subduing swelling, dissolving masses and stopping pain.

CASE II: GUO CHENGJIE'S MEDICAL RECORD

1. General data

A female aged 25, visited on March 17, 1999.

2. Chief complaint

Distending pain in the breasts for 8 months.

3. History of present illness

Eight months ago, she began to have a distending pain in the breasts owing to being angry with somebody. Later the pain appeared repeatedly and got worse before menstruation.

4. Present symptoms

Distending pain and nodules in breasts, getting worse before menstrual flow. Recently, her menstruation was postdated and with distending pain in the abdomen.

Examination: A patch-like mass 3.5cm × 3.5cm felt in the laterosuperior part of the right breast, a mass 2.5cm × 2.5cm felt in the laterosuperior part of the left breast, movable and smooth, with tenderness, medium quality. The subaxillary lymphnodes were not felt. Infrared scanning showed hyperplasia of mammary glands.

5. Tongue and pulse

Light red tongue, wiry pulse.

6. Differentiation and analysis

Anger can cause Liver Qi stagnation. The breasts are the distributing areas of the Liver Channel. Qi stagnation with Phlegm retention produces the nodules in the breasts. Her wiry pulse is the sign of Liver stagnation.

7. Diagnosis

TCM: Ru Pi (Liver Qi stagnation).

Western medicine: Hyperplasia of mammary glands.

8. Treating principle

Soothe Liver and regulate Qi, soften and dissolve masses.

9. Prescription

Wuyi (ST 15), Rugen (ST 18), Hegu (LI 4), Yanglingquan (GB 34).
    Electric stimulation was applied for 30 minutes.

10. Effect

After the first treatment, she felt much relieved and she was very happy about it. With 3 treatments, the masses became considerably smaller and softened. Six treatments cured her completely.

11. Essentials

This is a syndrome of Liver Qi stagnation.

CASE III: GUO CHENGJIE'S MEDICAL RECORD

1. General data

A female aged 42, visited on March 30, 1999.

2. Chief complaint

A dull pain and masses in the breasts for 1 month.

3. History of present illness

She had a 10-year history of hyperplasia of mammary glands which was controlled by acupuncture-moxibustion and herb treatment. Recently, the pain started again due to tiredness.

4. Present symptoms

The patch-like, movable and smooth masses, 5cm × 4cm, with medium quality, clear margins, tenderness, felt in the laterosuperior parts of breasts. The cervical and subaxillary lymphnodes were not felt. She was tired all over the body, with soreness and weakness in her lumbus and knees, dizziness, blurred vision, and poor appetite. Her complexion was sallow.

5. Tongue and pulse

Pale tongue, deep thready pulse.

6. Differentiation and analysis

Her tiredness, sallow complexion, and the soreness and weakness in her lumbus and knees, dizziness, blurred vision, poor appetite, and pale tongue, deep thready pulse are all the symptoms of Qi and Blood deficiency. Obstruction and deficiency of Qi and Blood result in pain and masses in her breasts.

7. Diagnosis

TCM: Ru Pi (Qi and Blood deficiency).

Western medicine: Hyperplasia of mammary glands.

8. Treating principle

Replenish Qi and Blood, circulate Qi and activate Blood.

9. Prescription

- Wuyi (ST 15), Rugen (ST 18), Zusanli (ST 36).

- Jianjing (GB 21), Tianzong (SI 11), Pishu (BL 20).

Zusanli (ST 36) and Pishu (BL 20) were reinforced; for the other points, even method was used. The needles were retained for 30 minutes. Two groups of points were used in turn, once a day. Herbal medicine, the modified Sheng Yu Tang (圣愈汤 Decoction for Healing Wounds) was prescribed.

10. Effect

After 5 treatments, the pain was relieved and the masses began to be soft and smaller, but the symptoms of Qi deficiency still existed. The same treatment was continued for another 7 times and the pain and masses disappeared. Because she lived far from here, she didn't have more acupuncture treatments apart from taking 10 more doses of herb medicine to take at home. The follow-up next month found her cured.

11. Essentials

This is a syndrome of Qi and Blood deficiency.

CASE IV: GUO CHENGJIE'S MEDICAL RECORD

1. General data

A girl aged 12, visited on June 10, 1980.

2. Chief complaint

Pain and masses in breasts for 3 months.

3. History of present illness

Pain and masses in her breasts for 3 months with obvious tenderness. She couldn't touch the desk when having lessons in school. The painkiller was not helpful.

4. Present symptoms

Tenderness in breasts with the masses felt.

Examination: The body development was normal, the complexion was a little sallow but moistened. The colour of breasts was normal, but the hard nodules, movable, 2cm in size, felt below nipples, with obvious tenderness and clear margins.

5. Tongue and pulse

Tongue slightly red, pulse normal.

6. Differentiation and analysis

Qi and Blood are not flowing well. Phlegm in combination with stagnated Qi forms the masses in breasts.

7. Diagnosis

TCM: Ru Pi (Phlegm and Qi in stagnation).

Western medicine: Central type of mammary development problem of young girls.

8. Treating principle

Circulate Qi, activate Blood, disperse masses, stop pain.

9. Prescription

Shanzhong (CV 17), Wuyi (ST 15), Hegu (LI 4).

Even method was applied. Needles were retained for 15 minutes. Once every other day.

10. Effect

After 6 treatments, she felt the pain much reduced and the masses became soft. Four more treatments cured her completely. Six months later, the follow-up found no recurrence.

11. Essentials

This is a young girl's Ru Pi (mammary development problem).

CASE V: GUO CHENGJIE'S MEDICAL RECORD

1. General data

A 57-year-old male, visited on January 8, 1999.

2. Chief complaint

His left breast was painful with a mass in it for 5 months.

3. History of present illness

Initially, he just felt pain in his left breast, and the pain became gradually worse, and taking a painkiller was no use. One month later, the left breast began to be enlarged and a mass could be felt.

4. Present symptoms

Pain and mass were present in his left breast. He was generally in a hot temper.

Examination: The left breast was obviously enlarged, its nipple and colour were normal, but a flat mass, 2cm × 0.8cm in size, was felt under the mammary areola. The mass was medium hard quality, movable, smooth, with obvious tenderness. The cervical and subaxillary lymphnodes were not enlarged.

5. Tongue and pulse

Slightly dark tongue, thin white coating, wiry and a bit slow pulse.

6. Differentiation and analysis

Liver Qi stagnation for a long time causes Blood circulation to stagnate, producing mass in the breast.

7. Diagnosis

TCM: Ru Pi (Liver Qi stagnation).

Western medicine: Mammary development problem of males.

8. Treating principle

Soothe the Liver and regulate Qi, stop pain, disperse mass.

9. Prescription

Shanzhong (CV 17), Wuyi (ST 15), Hegu (LI 4), Ganshu (BL 18). The reducing method.

10. Effect

After 7 acupuncture treatments, the pain was stopped and the mass became soft. Fifteen times later, the mass was reduced to 0.5cm × 0.5cm. After 2 months, the follow-up found no recurrence of pain and the mass disappeared.

11. Essentials

This is a male Ru Pi (nodules in the breast) due to Liver Qi stagnation, causing Blood stasis, thus formed the mass in breast.

SUMMARY

Ru Pi (nodules in the breast), or hyperplasia of the mammary glands, with the pain aggravated before menstruation, or when becoming angry or being tired, and its mass becoming enlarged and hard, is, according to Professor Guo Chengjie, due to Liver Qi stagnation and obstruction of Qi of the Foot-Yangming Channel. The Liver keeps the free flow of Qi and stores Blood, its channel distributes to the chest and connects with the breasts. The Foot-Yangming Stomach Channel passes through the breasts. In cases where the Spleen is damaged by worry, causing a failure in transportation and transformation, the Liver is damaged by anger, causing Liver Qi to be stagnated, the Qi and Blood circulation of Liver and Stomach are obstructed, and Chong and Ren disordered, and what will take place is that, Ru Pi, the nodule, is formed due to the obstruction of Qi and Blood in the breasts. The treatment is started from circulating Qi, treating the Liver and Stomach, and regulating Chong and Ren. Based on the individual conditions of patients in clinic, Professor Guo divides it into the 4 syndromes below.

Liver Qi stagnation: Distending pain and masses in the breasts getting worse before menstruation and when getting angry, and radiating to the subaxillary region and shoulder and back, there is fullness in the chest, abdominal distention, poor appetite, irregular menstruation, tongue not red, pulse wiry.

Liver Fire: Distending pain with a burning sensation in breasts and hypochondrium, made worse by pressure, irritability, quick to get angry, bitter taste in mouth, dry throat, predated menstruation, yellow urine, yellow tongue-coating, wiry rapid pulse.

Liver and Kidney Yin deficiency: Mass and pain in breasts, sometimes better and sometimes worse, dizziness, blurred vision, dry mouth, hot sensation in the Five Centres, red tongue, little coating, thready wiry rapid pulse.

Qi and Blood deficiency: Nodules in breasts, dull pain, worse when tired, fatigue, poor appetite, dizziness, blurred vision, palpitations, pale complexion, pale tongue, deep thready pulse.

Main points: On chest: Wuyi (ST 15), Shanzhong (CV 17), Hegu (LI 4); on back: Jianjing (GB 21), Tianzong (SI 11), Ganshu (BL 18).

Add Taichong (LR 3) for Liver Fire syndrome, omit Hegu (LI 4), add Taixi (KI 3) for Yin deficiency syndrome, omit Hegu (LI 4), add Zusanli (ST 36) and Pishu (BL 20) for Qi and Blood deficiency syndrome, add Sanyinjiao (SP 6) for irregular menstruation cases.

Two groups of points used in turn, once a day, reinforcing and reducing achieved by lifting and thrusting and rotating the needle applied, reinforcing deficiency, reducing excess, 20–30 minutes for retaining of needles, 10 times as one course, 3–4 days for rest before the next course, no acupuncture during menstruation.

Wuyi (ST 15), on breast, and Shanzhong (CV 17), lateral to breast, can clear obstructed channel Qi to activate Blood of the breast; Ganshu (BL 18) can circulate Liver Qi; Jianjing (GB 21) can circulate Gallbladder Qi to regulate Liver Qi owing to their exterior–interior relation; Hegu (LI 4), Yuan-Source of Hand-Yangming, Zusanli (ST 36), He-Sea of Foot-Yangming – these two points can conduct the channel Qi of Hand and Foot-Yangming, and nourish the Stomach and strengthen the Spleen, the acquired foundation of the human body, to enhance the resistance to disease and prevent Liver Fire affecting the Stomach; Tianzong (SI 11) is effective for diseases of the breasts owing to its function in removing obstructions in channels and collaterals by soothing the Liver and regulating the Qi of Yangming; Taichong (LR 3) can reduce Liver Fire; Pishu (BL 20) can strengthen the Spleen so that Qi and Blood flourish; Taixi (KI 3) can replenish Kidney Water to make Liver Yin ample; Sanyinjiao (SP 6) can enhance the Spleen and Stomach, benefit the Liver and Kidneys, regulate Qi and Blood, and remove obstructions of the channels and collaterals.

From clinical observation, Professor Guo treats Ru Pi (nodules of breast) with a satisfactory result in both the short-term and long-term; the curative rate of the short-term effect is 63%, and the total effective rate is 97%.

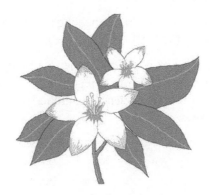

SECTION FIVE • LOU RU (ABNORMAL LACTATION)

CASE I: HE PUREN'S MEDICAL RECORD

1. General data

A 30-year-old female, named Chen, visited on May 29, 2002.

2. Chief complaint

Lou Ru (abnormal lactation) for 2 years.

3. History of present illness

Two years ago, she began to have Lou Ru (milk flowing) not in breast feeding period. When the breasts were pressed, white milk flowed out. In the recent 2 years, her body weight gained nearly 10kg. She went to the Gynaecological Department of Peking Union Medical College Hospital for treatment. The examination showed that her prolactin was normal; infrared scanning showed mild hyperplasia of the mammary glands; MRI of the head showed that everything was normal. It was thought to be an endocrine dyscrasia, so no particular medicine was administered for her.

Anamnesis: A history of hypertension for 2 years.

4. Present symptoms

There was milk white in colour flowing out when her breasts were pressed, and her breasts were not red in colour, were without swelling and pain, and without masses either. Her menstruation was less in quantity, pale in colour, lasting only 2 days each time.

Examination: The breasts were normal in appearance without redness and swelling and hard nodules.

5. Tongue and pulse

Pale tongue, white coating, deep thready pulse.

6. Differentiation and analysis

Lou Ru refers to an abnormal lactation without infantile sucking. Its pathogenesis is that of Qi and Blood deficiency, Yangming Qi non-consolidation, or the Liver Channel blocked by accumulated Heat, failure to keep free flow of Qi, so the milk is forced out. This patient has hypertension, her mental depression for a long time makes the Liver disordered in keeping the Qi free flowing, caused this abnormal lactation.

7. Diagnosis

TCM: Lou Ru (Liver stagnation, Spleen deficiency).

Western medicine: Abnormal lactation requiring further examination.

8. Treating principle

Soothe the Liver, strengthen the Spleen, replenish Qi and Blood, regulate Chong and Ren.

9. Prescription

Zulinqi (GB 41).

Acupuncture with 1 cun filiform needle, which was retained for 30 minutes. Twice a week.

10. Effect

After the first time of acupuncture, her abnormal lactation was greatly reduced. A total of 5 treatments cured her. The follow-up after 1 year found no recurrence.

11. Essentials

Zulinqi (GB 41) is selected to smooth Liver Qi because of the exterior–interior relation between Liver and Gallbladder. When Liver is normal in keeping the free flow of Qi, the milk secretion will be controlled. And Zulinqi (GB 41) is one of the Eight Confluent Points, leading to the Dai Vessel. Menstruation, pregnancy, delivery, and lactation are closely related with the Chong, Ren and Du vessels, with which the Dai Vessel is importantly connected. Therefore Zulinqi (GB 41) is punctured to regulate the functions of Chong, Ren and Dai Vessels to strengthen Qi and Blood to control milk secretion. Professor He uses Zulinqi (GB 41), the single point, to soothe the Liver, strengthen the Spleen, and strengthen Qi and Blood to treat Lou Ru with a remarkable effect. If bloody secretion is seen, the corresponding examinations should be done to find out the reasons, to see if it is mammary cancer.

SECTION SIX • RU NÜ (NIPPLE BLEEDING)

CASE I: GUO CHENGJIE'S MEDICAL RECORD

1. General data

A 45-year-old female, named Zhang, visited on March 2, 1982.

2. Chief complaint

Bleeding of the right nipple for 3 months.

3. History of present illness

Bleeding of the right nipple was gradually worse, but without pain. One month ago, she was diagnosed with 'tumour in the mammary duct' in a hospital. Unwilling to have an operation, she came for acupuncture-moxibustion treatment.

4. Present symptoms

The breasts were symmetrical, the nipple and mammary areola of normal colour, profuse pink fluid coming out from the right nipple and being ejected when the breast was pressed. No nodules were found. Mentally she was dejected. Her menstruation was small in quantity and irregular in cycle. She had irritability and insomnia.

5. Tongue and pulse

Dark tongue, yellowish coating, wiry pulse.

6. Differentiation and analysis

In differentiation, this is a syndrome due to mental depression, Liver Qi stagnation, which is transformed into Fire, Liver overacting on Spleen, which fails to control Blood, and the Heat forces Blood to extravasate from the breast.

7. Diagnosis

TCM: Ru Nü (nipple bleeding) (Liver stagnation transformed into Fire).

Western medicine: Tumour in the mammary duct.

8. Treating principle

Soothe Liver and regulate Qi, strengthen Spleen to control Blood.

9. Prescription

- Wuyi (ST 15), Rugen (ST 18), Hegu (LI 4), Zusanli (ST 36).
- Ganshu (BL 18), Geshu (BL 17), Pishu (BL 20).

Geshu (BL 17), Pishu (BL 20), Zusanli (ST 36) were reinforced; other points reduced. The two groups of points were used once a day on alternate days.

10. Effect

With 10 times of acupuncture, although the quantity of nipple bleeding was not reduced, the colour changed to become light, and the quality became clear. Another 10 times of treatment made the bleeding less, and without ejecting when the breast was pressed. The treatment was continued and the herbal decoction, modified Dan Zhi Xiaoyao San (丹栀逍 散 Ease Powder of Moutan Bark and Cape Jasmine Fruit), used in combination, 1 dose every day. In total, she had 3 courses of acupuncture-moxibustion and 8 doses of herb medicine, and then there was no more bleeding when the breast was pressed. It was cured in the short-term. Three months later, the follow-up found no recurrence.

11. Essentials

This is a case of mammary cancer.

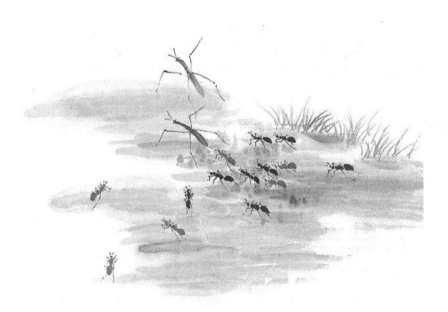

SECTION SEVEN • MACROMASTIA

CASE I: GUO CHENGJIE'S MEDICAL RECORD

1. General data

A 28-year-old female, named Wang, visited on August 3, 1980.

2. Chief complaint

Breasts quickly enlarged in 2 months.

3. History of present illness

She had breast-fed for 1 year after her first delivery, and had ceased lactation 6 months ago. Her menstruation was normal, but the breasts grew enormously, bigger than during the breast-feeding stage. She felt heavy with a bearing-down sensation, but without pain.

4. Present symptoms

Her body figure was normal. The breasts enlarged to the hypochondrium with the nipples coming down to the middle part of the abdomen. The mammary glands were rich and soft, with irregular nodules in them, no tenderness, no abnormal colour of nipples, mammary areola and breasts. The subaxillary lymphnodes were not felt. She had irritability, hot temper, and poor sleep.

5. Tongue and pulse

Light red tongue, thready and a rather slow pulse.

6. Differentiation and analysis

In differentiation, this is a case of enlarged breasts due to Liver Qi stagnation, unsmooth going of Qi and Blood of Liver and Stomach, making Blood obstructed, dysfunction of Chong and Ren, causing the leaking of Qi and Blood and disordered nourishment in breasts.

7. Diagnosis

TCM: Macromastia (disharmony between Liver and Stomach, Qi and Blood leaking, disordered nourishment in breasts).

Western medicine: Macromastia.

8. Treating principle

Soothe the Liver, circulate Qi, regulate Chong and Ren.

9. Prescription

- Wuyi (ST 15), Shanzhong (CV 17), Hegu (LI 4), Sanyinjiao (SP 6).

- Jianjing (GB 21), Tianzong (SI 11), Ganshu (BL 18).

Even method. The two groups were used once a day on alternate days, with the needles retained for 30 minutes.

10. Effect

With 5 treatments, the distention and bearing-down sensation was relieved. After 1 course, the breasts began to retract. After 4 courses, the breasts retracted to the lateral border of the chest and the nipples to the 6th rib, returning to the size of during breast-feeding, the glands were rich and soft, and no nodules felt.

11. Essentials

Qi and Blood leaking causing the disordered nourishment in breasts as a result of Liver Qi stagnation.

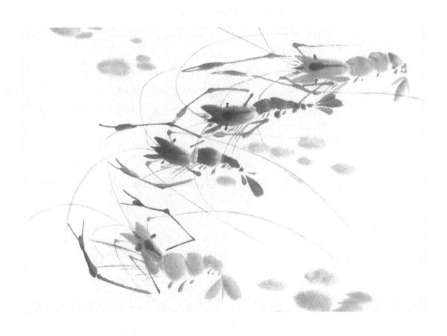

SECTION EIGHT • YIN TING (PROLAPSE OF UTERUS)

CASE I: RECORD IN *ACUPUNCTURE-MOXIBUSTION FOR DIFFICULT DISEASES*

1. General data
A 50-year-old female, named Gao, visited on June 15, 1986.

2. Chief complaint
Prolapse of uterus for many years.

3. History of present illness
A bearing-down sensation in lower abdomen aggravated by tiredness. Gynaecological examination: Prolapse of uterus in degree I.

4. Present symptoms
Bearing-down sensation in lower abdomen aggravated by tiredness and standing for a long time, listlessness, palpitations, shortness of breath, soreness in lumbus, frequency of urination, morbid leucorrhoea.

5. Tongue and pulse

6. Differentiation and analysis
Ptosis of the internal organs is the result of sinking of the Qi of the Middle Burner. This patient has a bearing-down sensation in the lower abdomen which is aggravated by tiredness and standing for a long time, listlessness, palpitations, shortness of breath, soreness in the lumbus, frequency of urination, and morbid leucorrhoea. All of these are the manifestations of sinking of the Qi of the Middle Burner.

7. Diagnosis
TCM: Prolapse of uterus (Qi deficiency, sinking of Qi).

Western medicine: Prolapse of uterus.

8. Treating principle
Lift Yang to raise the prolapse.

9. Prescription
Baihui (GV 20), Qihai (CV 6), Weidao (GB 28), Tianshu (ST 25), Guilai (ST 29).
    Tianshu (ST 25) penetrating to Guilai (ST 29). Once a day, 12 times as 1 course.

10. Effect

After 3 courses of treatment, she felt relieved in the bearing-down sensation. After another 3 courses, the uterus was restored to its normal position.

11. Essentials

Baihui (GV 20), is on the top of the head, selected for the lower disease and lifting the prolapse. Qihai (CV 6) reinforces Qi to restore the prolapsed uterus. Weidao (GB 28), a meeting point of the Foot-Shaoyang with the Dai Vessel, acts to astringe the uterus. Tianshu (ST 25) penetrating to Guilai (ST 29), acts to strengthen the lower abdominal muscles for astringe the uterus.

SUMMARY

Yin Ting, namely prolapse of uterus, refers to descent of the uterus into the vagina, or descent of the front wall of the vagina with the uterus. Usually it is the result of Liver stagnation, sinking of Qi due to Spleen deficiency. Mostly, deficiency syndromes are present, but sometimes Damp Heat flowing to the Liver Channel is seen, which is accompanied with hesitant urination, and irritability with internal Heat.

Main points: Baihui (GV 20), Weidao (GB 28), Guanyuan (CV 4), Sanyinjiao (SP 6).

Add Qihai (CV 6) and Zusanli (ST 36) for Qi and Blood deficiency.

Weidao (GB 28) is inserted with the tip of needle obliquely to a medial inferior direction, as deep as 2–3 cun, with a medium or strong stimulation. Once every day or every other day, 7 times as 1 course.

SECTION NINE • STERILITY

CASE I: LIU JIAYING'S MEDICAL RECORD

1. General data

Wang, female, 34 years old, free professional.

2. Chief complaint

Married for 3 years without pregnancy.

3. History of present illness

Because she was caught in the rain during her menstrual period, the menstrual flow became less in quantity and dark in colour in the late stage for about 10 days, accompanied with soreness in the lumbar region, cold feeling in the lower abdomen, and hyposexuality. She and her husband had had examinations but the result showed no abnormality of their reproductive system. She took Wuji Baifeng Wan (White Phoenix Bolus of Black-Bone Chicken) but the effect was not successful. She came for acupuncture on June 5, 2006.

4. Present symptoms

Forty days had passed since her last period. She was restless and anxious and this was accompanied by insomnia, cold pain in the lower abdomen, and cold extremities.

5. Tongue and pulse

Dark tongue, thin white coating; deep thready and a slightly slow pulse.

6. Differentiation and analysis

Catching cold during the menstrual period and the retention of cold in the body resulted in Blood stasis, and Chong and Ren were blocked by the Cold, which affected the uterus, thus menstruation was not coming on time (abnormality in ovulation), causing sterility.

7. Diagnosis

TCM: Sterility.

Western medicine: Primary sterility.

8. Treating principle

Remove obstruction of meridians and collaterals, dispel Cold, regulate Chong and Ren.

9. Prescription

Xuehai (SP 10), Guilai (ST 29), Qihai (CV 6). Acupuncture, medium stimulation, the reducing method. Moxibustion with a box at the lower abdomen for 20 minutes.

Zusanli (ST 36), Sanyinjiao (SP 6). Acupuncture, medium stimulation, the reinforcing method.

The needles were retained for 30 minutes. Once every other day, 10 times as 1 course.

10. Effect

She had 7 treatments and stopped for 2 weeks because she travelled abroad. The treatment was continued after she came back. Although her menstruation was not yet coming, her emotional state was good and the abdominal cold pain had stopped. Considering that two months ago she had had the last menstruation, she should have had the immunologic pregnancy test first. The result of the test was positive. The re-examination by the Obstetrical and Gynaecological Hospital confirmed that she was pregnant.

11. Essentials

The patient had invasion of Cold during menstruation. The pathogenic Cold stayed in the uterus, causing the dark menstrual flow and small quantity of Blood. The reducing method in acupuncture at Xuehai (SP 10), Guilai (ST 29), and Qihai (CV 6) to promote the Qi circulation and activate Blood is applied. Moxibustion at lower abdomen is to warm the uterus to dispel Cold. Reinforcing Zusanli (ST 36) is to strengthen the Spleen and Stomach to produce Qi and Blood. Reinforcing Sanyinjiao (SP 6) is for the purpose of tonifying the Liver and Spleen to produce more Essence. The restoring of meridian Qi and regulation of menstruation give the result of increase of conception rate. The successful treatment gets successful result.

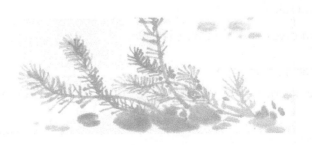

SECTION TEN • ENURESIS

CASE I: CHENG XINNONG'S MEDICAL RECORD

1. General data

A 15-year-old boy, named Du, visited on July 1, 1987.

2. Chief complaint

Enuresis for 6 years.

3. History of present illness

Six years ago, he began to have enuresis. The pathological condition was better in summer and worse in winter.

4. Present symptoms

He had enuresis at midnight every day. During the daytime, his urine was not large in quantity, and was white in colour. He had no lower back pain and soreness in lumbar region. His appetite, sleep, intelligence, memory, and bowel movement were normal. He was emaciated and sallow in complexion.

5. Tongue and pulse

Pale tongue with toothmarks on borders, thin yellow coating, thready weak pulse.

6. Differentiation and analysis

Systematic Classic of Acupuncture-Moxibustion says: 'Deficiency causes enuresis.' The Kidney dominates storage and controls Qi activities; the Bladder is the organ to store and discharge urine, depending on the warmth and nourishment of Kidney Yang. In case the Kidney Qi is deficient, the Bladder will be deficient and Cold, failing to control the Water passage, thus enuresis occurs. In cases where the Spleen is deficient, it will fail to produce Qi and Blood, the muscles and skin lack nourishment, and thus there is emaciation and sallow complexion. Yang is deficient, thus the tongue is pale with toothmarks and there is aversion to cold and thready weak pulse.

7. Diagnosis

TCM: Enuresis (Spleen Kidney Yang deficiency).

Western medicine: Enuresis.

8. Treating principle

Warm and reinforce Spleen and Kidney Yang, strengthen Qi to hold urine.

9. Prescription

Baihui (GV 20), Qihai (CV 6), Guanyuan (CV 4), Zusanli (ST 36), Sanyinjiao (SP 6), Shenshu (BL 23), Pishu (BL 20).

Moxibustion was applied at Guanyuan (CV 4); needles were not retained at Pishu (BL 20) and Shenshu (BL 23); other points were reinforced.

10. Effect

After 4 treatments, he could wake up to pass urine. In order to consolidate the good effect, the treatment was continued for 12 more times and he was cured.

11. Essentials

Baihui (GV 20) is a meeting point of Hand and Foot Yang channels with the Governor Vessel, ascending the clean to raise the sinking, and promote resuscitation to benefit the brain; Guanyuan (CV 4) and Qihai (CV 6) warm and reinforce Kidney Yang to control the Bladder; Sanyinjiao (SP 6) is a meeting point of three foot Yin channels, able to regulate and reinforce the Spleen and Kidneys. Shenshu (BL 23) and Pishu (BL 20) reinforce the Spleen and Kidneys.

CASE II: YANG YONGXUAN'S MEDICAL RECORD

1. General data

A 16-year-old boy, named Jin.

2. Chief complaint

Enuresis since he was small.

3. History of present illness

He had enuresis ever since he was small.

4. Present symptoms

Enuresis, 2–3 times each night, and in summer as well.

5. Tongue and pulse

Moistened tongue, a bit slow but forceful pulse.

6. Differentiation and analysis

The Kidneys dominate urination and defecation. The Kidney Qi is deficient, being unable to control urine, enuresis occurs as a result. This is mostly the congenital deficiency.

7. Diagnosis

TCM: Enuresis (Kidney Qi non-consolidation).

Western medicine: Enuresis.

8. Treating principle

Remove obstruction and reinforce Qi at the same time.

9. Prescription

Guanyuan (CV 4), Sanyinjiao (SP 6).

Rotating method in manipulation. Guanyuan (CV 4) was reinforced while Sanyinjiao (SP 6) reduced. Once every other day.

10. Effect

After 10 treatments, he could get up to pass urine but he still occasionally had enuresis. Since his Lower Burner was deficient, he couldn't control his urine. Warming and reinforcing the Spleen and Kidneys was applied. Sanyinjiao (SP 6) was reinforced now. Four treatments, once every other day, basically cured him. The follow-up found no recurrence.

11. Essentials

The causative factors of enuresis are complicated and it is an intractable disease. As people say, asthma is so suffering, enuresis is so hateful. Acupuncture is an effective treatment for it with a remarkable effective rate of more than 95%. In fact, all patients can be cured if they are not too tired in daytime and do not drink too much water before going to bed in evening, and are called to pass water regularly at night.

CASE III: MENG HONG'S MEDICAL RECORD

1. General data

Wang, male, 5 and half years old.

2. Chief complaint

Enuresis 2–4 times each night.

3. History of present illness

Every night, the child had enuresis at least twice, and when he was tired or drank more water, his enuresis could occur 3 or 4 times every night. The urine was clear and in increased volume.

4. Present symptoms

Pale complexion, cold limbs, especially in cold weather, weakness in legs when walking, easily tired.

5. Tongue and pulse

Pale tongue, white coating, deep slow weak pulse.

6. Differentiation and analysis

Kidney Yang deficiency.

Enuresis is related to the Kidneys and Bladder. The Kidneys dominate storage of Essence and Qi activities in urine discharge, while the Bladder dominates the storage and discharge of urine. The Kidneys are deficient, the Lower Burner will be deficient and Cold, causing the failure of the Bladder to control urine, so enuresis occurs.

7. Diagnosis

TCM: Infant enuresis (Kidney Yang deficiency).

Western medicine: Infant enuresis.

8. Treating principle

Reinforce the Kidneys to strengthen Yang.

9. Prescription

Baihui (GV 20), Zhongji (CV 3), Zusanli (ST 36), Sanyinjiao (SP 6), Shenshu (BL 23), Qihai (CV 6), Guanyuan (CV 4).

Acupuncture with medium stimulation, without retaining the needles, once a day or every other day. Moxibustion at Shenshu (BL 23), Qihai (CV 6), and Guanyuan (CV 4), once every other day, 15 minutes each time. Ten treatments as 1 course.

10. Effect

Two to 3 courses will achieve successful results. The premise is to treat the organic disease first.

11. Essentials

Infant is always characterized by Kidney Yang deficiency. The treating principle is to reinforce the Kidney Yang and good life habits should be built up. Before going to bed in the evening, don't drink too much water. The parent should not accuse, instead, should encourage the child so as to set up self-confidence.

SUMMARY

Enuresis refers to urination at night without self-awareness. As it is said in *Systematic Classic of Acupuncture-Moxibustion* 'Deficiency causes enuresis'. The deficiency is of Qi. For treatment, the principle is to regulate and reinforce Kidney Qi to strengthen the Qi activity of the Bladder.

Main points: Guanyuan (CV 4), Sanyinjiao (SP 6).

Add Shenmen (HT 7) for those who are not very clear minded before urinating; add Baihui (GV 20) for those who have frequent urination; add Shenshu (BL 23) and Pangguangshu (BL 28) for those who are weak in constitution due to prolonged disease.

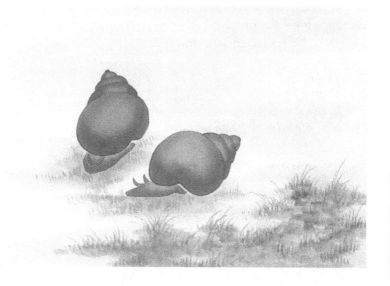

SECTION ELEVEN • ZHA SAI (MUMPS)

CASE I: CHENG XINNONG'S MEDICAL RECORD

1. General data

A 46-year-old female, named Shi, visited on April 7, 1980.

2. Chief complaint

The left parotid region was painful and swollen for 5 days.

3. History of present illness

Five days ago, she noticed a pain and swelling in the left mandible region and it diffused to the whole mandible region 3 days ago. Her body temperature was 37.8°C at that time. She used to have vomiting due to taking of acheomycin tablets. So she came for acupuncture.

4. Present symptoms

The left parotid region was swollen and painful, involving the left side of her head in paroxysmal pain. In the afternoon, she had a fever too. She had a cough, but mild. Her appetite was normal.

5. Tongue and pulse

Light red tongue, white dry coating, thready rolling pulse.

6. Differentiation and analysis

The invasion of exogenous epidemic pathogenic Heat blocks the Shaoyang Channel, making the Qi of this channel obstructed, thus there is onset of pain. The epidemic pathogen is usually of the evil Heat in nature, so it causes redness, swelling, hotness, and pain of the affected area, and fever.

7. Diagnosis

TCM: Mumps (invasion of epidemic pathogenic Heat).

Western medicine: Acute parotitis.

8. Treating principle

Regulate Shaoyang Channel, dissolve the accumulation, stop pain.

9. Prescription

Dazhui (GV 14), Waiguan (TE 5), Hegu (LI 4). Left side: Yifeng (TE 17), Jiache (ST 6), Tianrong (SI 17).

Even method.

10. Effect

After the first time of acupuncture, her pain was relieved. With 5 treatments, her mumps were cured.

11. Essentials

For the treatment of this patient, the points are mainly selected from the local area and the affected Shaoyang Channel to regulate its Qi circulation and remove obstruction to stop pain.

SUMMARY

Mumps, also known as Ha Ma Wen, is an acute infectious disease caused by exogenous epidemic pathogenic Heat, manifested as fever and swelling pain in the parotid region. It is mostly seen in children but sometimes adults. In modern medicine, it is epidemic parotitis. In some children, lower abdominal pain and testicle pain also occur.

Main points: Yifeng (TE 17), Jiache (ST 6), Hegu (LI 4).

Add Quchi (LI 11) for fever and Waiguan (TE 5).

Add Shaoshang (LU 11) and Shangyang (LI 1) for serious swelling pain, pricking to bleed.

Add Zhongji (CV 3), Sanyinjiao (SP 6) and Taichong (LR 3) for the accompanied testitis.

DISEASES OF THE EYES, EARS, NOSE AND THROAT

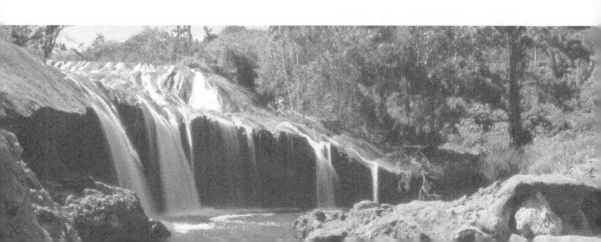

SECTION ONE • TINNITUS AND DEAFNESS

CASE I: CHENG XINNONG'S MEDICAL RECORD

1. General data

A 62-year-old male, named Shi, visited on February 25, 1982.

2. Chief complaint

Decline of hearing of the left ear for 3 months.

3. History of present illness

Three months ago, he had a common cold, then the hearing of his left ear became worse and this was accompanied by tinnitus. He went to Beijing Tongren Hospital, the examination showed 'a sunken drum membrane of the left ear' and he was diagnosed with sudden deafness of the left ear.

Examination: BP150/90mmHg.

4. Present symptoms

Hearing of left ear declined, accompanied with tinnitus, dry mouth, and dream-disturbed sleep.

5. Tongue and pulse

Pale flabby tongue with toothmarks, wiry rolling pulse.

6. Differentiation and analysis

The Gallbladde Channel runs 'to the forehead at the corner of hairline and down to the back of ear', 'from the back of ear it enters into the ear'. The Phlegm Damp is brought upward by the Liver and Gallbladder Fire to attack the ear, causing the sudden deafness.

7. Diagnosis

TCM: Sudden deafness (Phlegm Fire disturbing upward).

Western medicine: Sudden deafness.

8. Treating principle

Remove obstruction of ear, clear Fire, dissolve Phlegm.

9. Prescription

Baihui (GV 20), Fengchi (GB 20), Waiguan (TE 5), Hegu (LI 4), Zhongzhu (TE 3), Yanglingquan (GB 34), Sanyinjiao (SP 6), Taichong (LR 3). Left side: Yifeng (TE 17), Tinggong (SI 19).

Even method.

10. Effect

On March 1, 1982 he came again. Zhongwan (CV 12) and Zusanli (ST 36) were added for treatment. The hearing of his left ear was greatly improved.

11. Essentials

Baihui (GV 20) is selected to regulate Yin and Yang and Qi and Blood. Fengchi (GB 20), Tinggong (SI 19) and Yifeng (TE 17) remove obstruction of the ear. Waiguan (TE 5) and Zhongzhu (TE 3) circulate Qi of the Shaoyang Channel. Taichong (LR 3) and Hegu (LI 4) circulate Qi and activate Blood to remove obstruction. Zusanli (ST 36), Sanyinjiao (SP 6) and Zhongwan (CV 12) strengthen the Spleen and harmonize the Stomach, dissolve Phlegm and Damp. Yanglingquan (GB 34) soothe the Wood to strengthen the Earth.

CASE II: XIAO SHAOQING'S MEDICAL RECORD

1. General data

A 60-year-old male, named Fan, visited on October 25, 1994.

2. Chief complaint

Loss of hearing of the right ear for 2 years.

3. History of present illness

Two years ago, his wife died and he was very depressed and got a sudden dizziness accompanied by tinnitus and decline of hearing and then loss of hearing. Gulou Hospital diagnosed him with sudden deafness. Medication was not helpful.

4. Present symptoms

The hearing of his right ear was lost completely, he felt obstructed in the ear, especially on rainy days. He was irritable. His sleep, appetite, urination and defecation were normal.

5. Tongue and pulse

Light red tongue, white sticky coating, wiry rolling pulse.

6. Differentiation and analysis

This patient is mentally depressed and worried because of the death of his wife. Mental depression damages the Liver and worries damage the Spleen. The Liver Qi is stagnated and the Phlegm formed due to failure of Spleen in transportation and transformation. The Liver Qi brings the Phlegm upward to disturb the ear, causing deafness.

7. Diagnosis

TCM: Deafness (Liver Qi bringing the Phlegm upward to disturb the ear).

Western medicine: Sudden deafness.

8. Treating principle

Soothe Liver and regulate Qi, strengthen Spleen and dissolve Phlegm, remove obstruction of ear, restore hearing.

9. Prescription

Hegu (LI 4), Zusanli (ST 36), Sanyinjiao (SP 6), Taichong (LR 3). Right side: Tinghui (GB 2), Yifeng (TE 17), Zhongzhu (TE 3).

Even method. Retaining the needles for 20 minutes and manipulating once every 10 minutes. After removing the needles, indirect moxibustion with ginger was applied at Tinghui (GB 2); 5 cones were used until the skin became reddish. Once a day.

10. Effect

After 2 treatments, he felt the tinnitus and obstruction were relieved. Professor Xiao thought it was a sign that the auditory nerve was beginning to recover, so he changed the even method to the reducing method to excite the auditory nerve and taught the patient to do Self-Blow of Qi. With 11 treatments, the patient could distinguish the sound of music and speaking. One month's treatment made him hear clearly.

11. Essentials

Tinghui (GB 2) and Yifeng (TE 17) are local points for deafness. *Treatment of Diseases in Verse (Bai Zheng Fu)* says: 'For distention and obstruction in the ear, Tinghui (GB 2) and Yifeng (TE 17) are the points to treat.' These two points can regulate the Qi of Triple Burner and Shaoyang. Hegu (LI 4) and Taichong (LR 3) are the Four Gates, circulating Qi and activating Blood, to soothe the Liver and relieve depression. Zusanli (ST 36) and Sanyinjiao (SP 6) can strengthen the Spleen and Stomach to dissolve Phlegm for restoring hearing. As to the techniques of needling, according to Professor Xiao, the local points should be inserted deeply, otherwise they are useless. So Yifeng (TE 17) and Tinghui (GB 2) are inserted as deep as 1.5 cun. Indirect moxibustion with ginger at the local area can warm and remove obstruction of channels, and this is good for prolonged cases and deficiency syndromes.

> ## SELF-BLOW OF QI
> When getting up in the morning, after washing, the patient does deep respiration for more then 10 times, takes a break for 1-2 minutes, takes one deep inhalation, closes the mouth, pinches the nostrils with the right thumb and index finger, and blows the Qi from the Eustachian tube into the ear until the drum membrane gurgles.
>
> It is used to balance the pressure inside and outside the ear to treat the sunken drum.

CASE III: HAN BIN'S MEDICAL RECORD

1. General data

Wang, female, 27 years old.

2. Chief complaint

Sudden deafness and tinnitus of the right ear for 10 days.

3. History of present illness

Ten days ago after a strenuous exercise she began to have a sudden hearing decline, accompanied by tinnitus and dizziness. She had to be helped to stand. All the symptoms were tending to become aggravated. In hospital, the examination found her right ear hearing loss 60–90dB, so diagnosed her with sudden deafness. Treatment of Chinese and Western medicine didn't relieve her much. She came for acupuncture treatment.

4. Present symptoms

Deafness, tinnitus with a sound in the ear like waves in the sea, distending pain in the right ear, dizziness, blurred vision, nausea, red face, dry throat, bitter taste in mouth in the morning, irritability, hot temper, sometimes hypochondriac pain.

5. Tongue and pulse

Red tongue, thin yellow coating; string-taut forceful pulse.

6. Differentiation and analysis

Liver and Gallbladder Fire, Qi stagnation and Blood stasis.

The Fire of Liver and Gallbladder goes up along the Liver and Gallbladder meridians, the Shaoyang Meridian Qi is blocked, thus there is loss of hearing, tinnitus and distention in the ear. The Liver Fire together with Wind disturbs the head, causing dizziness, blurred vision, and nausea. Red face, dry throat, bitter taste, irritability, hot temper, hypochondriac pain, red tongue, yellow coating and string-taut forceful pulse are all the manifestations of Liver and Gallbladder Fire. Upward disturbing of Liver and Gallbladder Fire is the cause of Qi stagnation and Blood stasis in the collaterals around/in the ear, thus there is hearing loss.

7. Diagnosis

TCM: Sudden loss of hearing.

Western medicine: Sudden deafness.

8. Treating principle

Clear Fire of the Liver and Gallbladder, activate Blood circulation, remove obstruction of meridians and collaterals.

Select the points of Hand and Foot-Shaoyang and Foot-Jueyin meridians. The reducing method.

9. Prescription

Right side Yifeng (TE 17), right side Tinghui (GB 2), right side Shuaigu (GB 8), Fengchi (GB 20), right side Zhongzhu (TE 3), Yanglingquan (GB 34), Taichong (LR 3), right side Zulinqi (GB 41). Retain the needles for 20 minutes, 3 times a week, 10 times as 1 course.

10. Effect

After 1 course of treatment, most of her hearing was restored, only 8000Hz hearing still 20dB lost. Other symptoms disappeared. Three months' follow-up found no relapse. She was clinically cured.

11. Essentials

- Local point in combination with distal points of affected meridians: Yifeng (TE 17), Tinghui (GB 2), and Shuaigu (GB 8) of the affected side are selected to promote the Blood circulation in the local area. The distal points of Shaoyang meridians are to remove obstruction of the meridians and collaterals. Yifeng (TE 17) is the Crossing point of Hand and Foot Shaoyang meridians, in anatomy, the great auricular nerve is distributed here, and deeper, is the site where the facial nerve perforates out of the stylomastoid foramen.

- Yanglingquan (GB 34) and Taichong (LR 3) are used for clearing the Liver and Gallbladder Fire.

SUMMARY

Tinnitus and deafness are of excess and deficiency nature in differentiation. The excess syndrome is caused by the Liver and Gallbladder Fire or Phlegm Fire upward disturbing, or by Wind and Heat invasion, blocking the Qi of the channel in the ear. The deficiency syndrome is caused by Kidney Qi deficiency, in which the essential Qi is not ample enough to nourish the ear, or by sinking of the Qi of the Middle Burner, as a result of which the ear lacks nourishment. In the case of deafness due to traumatic injury, the tongue-coating and pulse can be normal, it is regarded as an excess syndrome and treated accordingly.

Main points: Yifeng (TE 17), Zhongzhu (TE 3), Tinggong (SI 19). (Erment (TE 21), Tinggong (SI 19) and Tinghui (GB 2) can be used by turns.)

Add Fengchi (GB 20) and Xingjian (LR 2) for Liver and Gallbladder Fire; add Fenglong (ST 40) for Phlegm Fire upward disturbing, add Shenshu (BL 23), Taixi (KI 3) and Qihai (CV 6) for Kidney Yin deficiency, add Baihui (GV 20) for sinking of the Qi of the Middle Burner; and add Dazhui (GV 14) and Hegu (LI 4) for invasion of exogenous pathogenic factors.

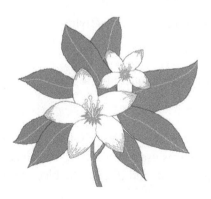

SECTION TWO • CONGESTION, SWELLING AND PAIN OF THE EYE

CASE I: SHAO JINGMING'S MEDICAL RECORD

1. General data

A 40-year-old female, named Wang, visited on May 20, 1992.

2. Chief complaint

Congestion, swelling and pain of two eyes for 4 days.

3. History of present illness

Her eyes were congested, swollen and painful, difficult to open because of photophobia and lacrimation. She had had blurred vision for 4 days already. Gentamycin intramuscular injection and chloromycetin eye drops didn't help her much.

4. Present symptoms

Swelling of eyelids, seriously congestive palpebral conjunctiva, big patches of bleeding at the bulbar conjunctiva at the temporal side of eyeballs, a large amount of sticky discharge.

5. Tongue and pulse

Red tongue, wiry rapid pulse.

6. Differentiation and analysis

Invasion of epidemic pathogenic Heat affects upward to the eyes along the Liver and Gallbladder channels, causing the swelling and pain of her eyes.

7. Diagnosis

TCM: Congestion, swelling and pain of eyes (hyperactivity of pathogenic Heat).

Western medicine: Acute blepharoconjunctivitis.

8. Treating principle

Clear Heat, remove toxins, relieve swelling, stop pain.

9. Prescription

Taiyang (EX-HN5), Zanzhu (BL 2), Erjian (EX-HN6). Ear points: Eye, Liver.

The three-edged needle was used for pricking for bleeding. Taiyang (EX-HN5) was pricked for bleeding 2–3 ml, and in case the bleeding is not enough, cupping with a small cup could be done to draw more Blood out. Zanzhu (BL 2) and Erjian (EX-HN6) were pricked to squeeze about 1ml of Blood out. The ear points Eye and Liver were pricked to squeeze 2–3 drops of blood out.

10. Effect

After 1 bleeding treatment, the patient's pain was relieved. On the following day, the swelling and pain disappeared and the congestion relieved. Two more times of bleeding at Taiyang (EX-HN5), Zanzhu (BL 2) and Erjian (EX-HN6) were done and she was cured.

11. Essentials

Pricking to cause bleeding is very effective in treating eye diseases, such as acute conjunctivitis, keratitis, stye, corneal opacity, trachoma, and electric ophthalmia, etc. Using the three-edged needle to prick Taiyang (EX-HN5) for bleeding can improve the Blood circulation of the eye tissues to dispel Wind, activate Blood, clear Heat and promote vision. Just as *Jade Dragon Songs* (Yu Long Ge) says: 'For congestion and swelling and pain of eyes with aversion to light, puncturing Jingming (BL 1) and pricking Taiyang (EX-HN5) for bleeding will result in a cure.'

Zanzhu (BL 2) has the function of smoothing the channel Qi to dispel Wind, clear Heat, remove obstruction of channels, and stop pain. Erjian (EX-HN6) functions to reduce fever, treat inflammation, calm the Mind and stop pain. The ear points Eye and Liver function to clear Fire of the Liver, cool Blood and promote vision. This group of points is effective to clear Heat, remove toxins, relieve swelling, and stop pain, so the therapeutic result is satisfactory.

CASE II: WEI LIXIN'S MEDICAL RECORD

1. General data

Zhang, female, 48 years old.

2. Chief complaint

Dry feeling in the eyes for 2 years.

3. History of present illness

In the recent 2 years, she felt dry in her eyes, and when it was serious, it was accompanied with pain, hotness and blurred vision. Lacrimal secretion (Schirmer's test) was 1mm and 2mm respectively. Western medicine diagnosed her Xerophthalmia and treated with artificial tears. Her symptoms were not relieved. Her lacrimal secretion became 0mm.

4. Present symptoms

Dry and painful eyes, irritability, insomnia, sudden hotness in the body, soreness and weakness in the lumbus and knees, appetite normal, constipation.

5. Tongue and pulse

Dark red and thin tongue, little coating; string-taut thready pulse, a little rapid.

6. Differentiation and analysis

The Liver opens into the eyes. Eye diseases are always related to the Liver. Dryness of the eyes is owing to the failure of Liver Blood in nourishing the eyes. The patient is 48 years old, her Kidney functions are declining. The Kidneys are the organ storing Essence which moisten and nourish the eyes. When the Kidneys are deficient, they fail to do this. The Kidney deficiency further causes the Liver Yin deficiency. Thus Yin deficiency of both Liver and Kidneys is the original reason for hotness in the body, irritability, and insomnia. Kidney deficiency results in soreness and weakness in the lumbus and knees. The Kidneys dominate urination and defecation. Kidney Yin deficiency, failing to moisten the Large Intestine, leads to constipation. Dark red and thin tongue, little coating, and string-taut thready rapid pulse are also the signs of Liver and Kidney Yin deficiency.

7. Diagnosis

TCM: Dry eyes (Liver and Kidney Yin deficiency).

Western medicine: Xerophthalmia.

8. Treating principle

Nourish the Liver and Kidneys.

9. Prescription

Acupuncture on Jingming (BL 1), Zanzhu (BL 2), Taiyang (EX-HN5), Sibai (ST 2), Baihui (GV 20), Shenting (GV 24), Fengchi (GB 20), Quchi (LI 11), Hegu (LI 4), Tianshu (ST 25), Zusanli (ST 36), Sanyinjiao (SP 6), Taixi (KI 3), Taichong (LR 3), Ganshu (BL 18), Shenshu (BL 23), Xinshu (BL 15).

10. Effect

Alleviation of dry and painful eyes was realized after 5 treatments. Sleep got better and bowel movement became normal. Ten treatments resulted in increase of lacrimal secretion to 2mm, alleviation of irritability and hotness in the body, and good sleep.

11. Essentials

The age of the patient is quite important in differentiation. Females between the ages of 45 and 52 years old always have menopausal symptoms, such as irritability and sudden hotness in the body. The menopause symptoms are mainly related with the Kidneys, which decline around this age. Regardless of whatever symptoms she has, reinforcing the Kidneys is a must, so Sanyinjiao (SP 6), Taixi (KI 3), and Shenshu (BL 23) are selected. Moreover, calming the Mind, using Baihui (GV 20) and Shenting (GV 24), should not be neglected.

SUMMARY

Congestion, swelling and pain of eyes is involved in acute conjunctivitis, mostly seen in spring and autumn, accompanied by photophobia and lacrimation and sticky discharge. In cases caused by invasion of Wind Heat, the accompanying symptoms will be headache, fever, and superficial rapid pulse; in cases caused by Liver and Gallbladder Fire, the accompanying symptoms will be bitter taste in mouth, irritability, and wiry pulse.

Main points: Jingming (BL 1), Fengchi (GB 20), Hegu (LI 4), Taiyang (EX-HN5).

Taiyang (EX-HN5) is pricked for bleeding. Add Shaoshang (LU 11), Erjian (LI 2) and Zanzhu (BL 2) for the Wind Heat syndrome; add Taichong (LR 3) and Taiyang (EX-HN5) penetrating to Shuaigu (GB 8) for the Liver and Gallbladder Fire syndrome.

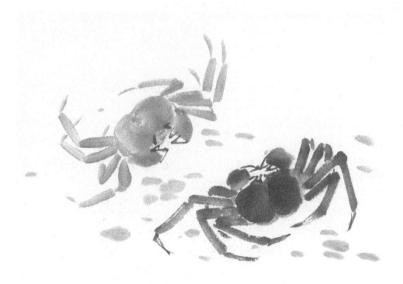

SECTION THREE • BLURRED VISION

CASE I: CHENG XINNONG'S MEDICAL RECORD

1. General data

A 73-year-old male, named Xu, visited on May 16, 1992.

2. Chief complaint

Decline of vision of both eyes for 4 years.

3. History of present illness

In 1988, he was diagnosed with Optic Atrophy. He came for acupuncture treatment.

4. Present symptoms

He had blurred vision with a corrected vision 0.2. When he was tired, his blood pressure would be higher. His spirits and complexion were normal.

5. Tongue and pulse

Sticky yellow coating, the left pulse thready and wiry, Chi pulse of both sides weak.

6. Differentiation and analysis

The Liver opens into eyes, the Kidneys store Essence and dominate the pupils. The patient is old in age, his Liver Blood and Kidney Yin are deficient, not able to nourish the eyes, so he has blurred and declining vision.

7. Diagnosis

TCM: Blurred vision (Liver and Kidney deficiency).

Western medicine: Optic atrophy.

8. Treating principle

Reinforce Liver and Kidneys, replenish Blood, promote vision.

9. Prescription

Baihui (GV 20), Sibai (ST 2), Tongziliao (GB 1), Yanglao (SI 6), Neiguan (PC 6), Hegu (LI 4), Guangming (GB 37), Sanyinjiao (SP 6), Taixi (KI 3), Taichong (LR 3), Geshu (BL 17), Ganshu (BL 18), Shenshu (BL 23).

Sanyinjiao (SP 6), Taixi (KI 3), Geshu (BL 17), Ganshu (BL 18) and Shenshu (BL 23) were reinforced, and other points, even method.

10. Effect

With 4 courses of treatment, the patient felt that his eyes did not get tired easily and the blurred vision was relieved. Two more courses were given for consolidation, he could then see clearly and he stopped treatment.

11. Essentials

The treatment here is based on 'replenishing the Kidney Water and Liver Yin, and clearing the Liver Fire to improve the vision', that is, reinforcing anti-pathogenic Qi and reducing pathogenic Qi at the same time, thus, the effect is good.

SUMMARY

Blurred vision, a common condition in old people, is caused by deficiency of Yin and Blood and hypofunction of the Liver and Kidneys. The essential substances of the five Zang and six Fu organs pour upward to nourish the eyes, which have an especially close relationship with the Liver and Kidneys. With enough nourishment of Blood, the eyes can see clearly, without enough Blood for nourishment, there will be blurred vision. Therefore the basic principles for treatment are reinforce the Liver and Kidneys and replenish Blood to promote vision.

Main points: Jingming (BL 1), Sibai (ST 2), Yanglao (SI 6), Guangming (GB 37), Taichong (LR 3), Geshu (BL 17), Ganshu (BL 18), Shenshu (BL 23). The reinforcing method is used in needling.

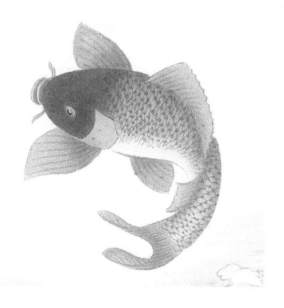

SECTION FOUR • MYOPIA

CASE I: CHENG XINNONG'S MEDICAL RECORD

1. General data

A 31-year-old female, named Ge, visited on August 17, 1984.

2. Chief complaint

Decline of vision for 22 years and aggravated for 4 years.

3. History of present illness

Twenty-two years ago, she suffered from Acute Hepatitis. After it was cured, she noticed that her vision began to decline and it gradually became worse. Tongren Hospital diagnosed her with Myopia. From 4 years ago after delivery of a child, the vision of both eyes declined seriously.

4. Present symptoms

The vision of both eyes was 0.1 and her eyes had a lot of secretion. Appetite and sleep were normal.

5. Tongue and pulse

Pale dark tongue, thin white coating, thready pulse.

6. Differentiation and analysis

The eyes are the organs for seeing. Only with the nourishment of the essential Qi of the five Zang and six Fu organs can the vision be acute. The Liver opens into the eye, and if the Liver Blood is deficient, the vision will decline.

7. Diagnosis

TCM: Myopia (Liver Blood deficiency).

Western medicine: Myopia.

8. Treating principle

Strengthen Spleen and tonify Liver, reinforce deficiency and promote vision.

9. Prescription

Baihui (GV 20), Fengchi (GB 20), Jingming (BL 1), Zanzhu (BL 2), Sibai (ST 2), Zusanli (ST 36), Guangming (GB 37), Sanyinjiao (SP 6), Taichong (LR 3).
　　The reinforcing method.

10. Effect

With 70 treatments, her vision was greatly improved.

11. Essentials

Baihui (GV 20), Zusanli (ST 36), and Sanyinjiao (SP 6) for strengthening the function of Spleen to produce Qi and Blood; Fengchi (GB 20), Guangming (GB 37), and Taichong (LR 3) for clearing the Liver and Gallbladder; Jingming (BL 1), Zanzhu (BL 2), and Sibai (ST 2) for promoting Qi and Blood circulation in the local area of the eyes. In this way, the distal and local points in combination function well to improve the vision.

CASE II: ZHONG MEIQUAN'S MEDICAL RECORD

1. General data

A 9-year-old boy, named Xiao.

2. Chief complaint

He had not been able to see distant objects clearly for 4 years.

3. History of present illness

He couldn't see distant objects clearly, sometimes he had a double vision and his eyes were easily tired. He had been wearing glasses for 1 year already. In the past, he had a bad habit of reading very close up to his eyes.

4. Present symptoms

Failure to see distant objects clearly. Mydri asis examination: the myopia of right eye -1.50 and astigmatism +1.50; the myopia of left eye -1.00 and astigmatism +0.75, and the corrected vision of both eyes 1.2. At both sides of the first cervical vertebra, there were nodules and rope-like objects felt and these were tender. His appetite was good, and urination and defecation normal.

5. Tongue and pulse

Tip of tongue was red, coating thin, and pulse thready and wiry.

6. Differentiation and analysis

The Liver opens into the eyes. The vision depends on the supporting of Liver Blood for nourishment. The patient is deficient in congenital condition and nourished poorly in acquired condition, so the result is myopia.

7. Diagnosis

TCM: Blurred vision (Liver and Kidney deficiency, Heart Blood deficiency).

Western medicine: Myopia.

8. Treating principle

Replenish Heart Blood, tonify Liver and Kidneys.

9. Prescription

Zhengguang (Empirical point), Fengchi (GB 20).

10. Effect

After 1 course of treatment, the eyesight of his right eye was improved from 0.6 to 1.2 and the left eye from 0.6 to 1.5.

In the second course, Neiguan (PC 6) was added in treatment. The eyesight of both his eyes was improved to 1.5. The symptoms disappeared, and he could see clearly with no need to use glasses. The treatment was stopped and he was asked to pay attention to protecting his vision and to do self-massage at Zhengguang point. The follow-up after 7 years found that his vision of both eyes remained at 1.5.

11. Essentials

Myopia is common in teenagers. For treatment, in addition to filiform needle acupuncture, tapping with the plum-blossom needle is also applied. Observation on myopia cases below the age of 20 years old shows that it is possible for the vision to be restored to normal in mild cases, while more than 50% of serious cases may be remarkably improved in vision.

Main points: Zhengguang and Zhengguang$_2$ (Empirical points)

Accompanying points: Fengchi (GB 20), Neiguan (PC 6), Dazhui (GV 14), and Xinshu (BL 15), Ganshu (BL 18), Danshu (BL 19), Shenshu (BL 23).

Tapping: Tap with the plum-blossom needle 20–50 times at the point in the area within 0.5–1.2cm. Once every other day, 15 times as 1 course, half a month for rest, and continue the treatment if necessary. Within half a year to 1 year, the patient should be re-examined and treated once every half a month to 1 month for the purpose to consolidate the therapeutic effect.

Zhengguang (Empirical point) is located at the junction of lateral ¾ and medial ¼ of the supraorbital margin, namely between Zanzhu (BL 2) and Yuyao (EX-HN4), inferior to the supraorbital margin.

Zhengguang$_2$ (Empirical point) is located at the junction of lateral ¼ and medial ¾ of the supraorbital margin, namely between Sizhukong (TE 23) and Yuyao (EX-HN4), inferior to the supraorbital margin.

The selection of above-mentioned points was based on the theory that the Liver opens into the eye and the interrelation between Zang Fu and the body surface. Zhengguang and Zhengguang$_2$ (Empirical points) function to replenish Blood, tonify Liver, and promote vision; Fengchi (GB 20), a point of the Gallbladder Channel which is externally–internally related with the Liver Channel, is effective in soothing the Liver, clearing the Mind and promoting vision; Neiguan (PC 6), a Luo-Connecting point of the Hand Jueyin Pericardium channel, is used to activate Heart Yang and replenish Heart Blood; Dazhui (GV 14), a point of the Governor Vessel which is the meeting of three Yang of hand and foot, is used to regulate Qi and Blood and strengthen the body to tonify Yang; Xinshu (BL 15), Ganshu (BL 18), Danshu (BL 19), Shenshu (BL 23) can remove the obstructed channel Qi; Xinshu (BL 15) unobstructs Heart Qi and replenishes Heart Blood; Ganshu (BL 18) and Danshu (BL 19) are used to soothe the Liver and Gallbladder, replenish Blood and reinforce the Liver. Shenshu (BL 23) is to reinforce the Kidneys to promote Kidney Yang.

SUMMARY

Myopia is an eye disease of ametropia, caused by improper usage of the eyes in reading in a dim light and for a long time, or due to family heredity.

Main points: Chengqi (ST 1), Jingming (BL 1), Fengchi (GB 20), Yiming (EX-HN14), Guangming (GB 37).

Shenshu (BL 23) and Zusanli (ST 36) are added for those who have a prolonged history and weak constitution.

Yiming (EX-HN14) is located 1 cun posterior to Yifeng (TE 17), indicated in eye diseases, such as myopia, hyperopia, early stage of cataract, etc., and headache, dizziness, tinnitus, and psychosis.

SECTION FIVE • VISUAL TIREDNESS

CASE I: RECORD IN *ACUPUNCTURE-MOXIBUSTION FOR DIFFICULT DISEASES*

1. General data

A 28-year-old female, named Fan, visited on November 13, 1999.

2. Chief complaint

Mild blurred vision for 4 months.

3. History of present illness

She was engaged in mental work over a long period and very often worked overtime. She used her eyes too much, causing blurred vision and visual tiredness.

4. Present symptoms

Blurred vision and visual tiredness, listlessness, poor appetite, poor sleep.

5. Tongue and pulse

Pale tongue, white coating, thready weak pulse.

6. Differentiation and analysis

Her visual tiredness is the result of using eyes which have a poor Blood supply over a long time.

7. Diagnosis

TCM: Visual tiredness (Liver Blood deficiency).

Western medicine: Visual tiredness.

8. Treating principle

Regulate Qi and Blood, calm the Mind, promote vision.

9. Prescription

Jingming (BL 1), Chengqi (ST 1), Taichong (LR 3), Zusanli (ST 36), Sanyinjiao (SP 6), Neiguan (PC 6).

   Once a day.

10. Effect

After 5 treatments, she was improved. Another 5 times of treatment, she felt cured.

11. Essentials

TCM holds that the eyes can see clearly only with enough Blood nourishment. Zusanli (ST 36), Sanyinjiao (SP 6) and Taichong (LR 3) reinforce Liver, Spleen and Kidneys and regulate Qi and Blood. Jingming (BL 1) and Chengqi (ST 1) regulate the Qi of channels in the local region. Neiguan (PC 6) relaxes the chest to regulate Qi, and rests the Heart to calm the Mind.

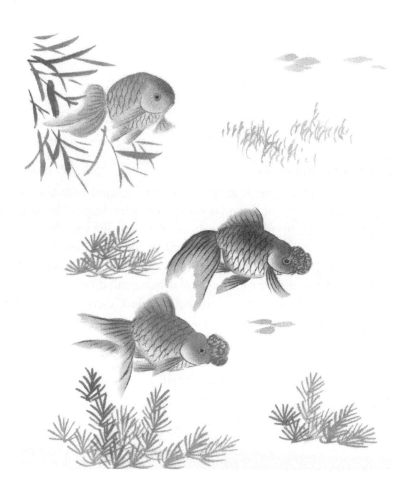

SECTION SIX • BI YUAN (THICK AND STICKY NASAL DISCHARGE)

CASE I: CHENG XINNONG'S MEDICAL RECORD

1. General data

A 25-year-old male, named Wu, visited on January 19, 1982.

2. Chief complaint

Yellow nasal discharge for more than 10 years.

3. History of present illness

He was diagnosed with nasosinusitis, and the therapeutic effect of his treatment was not satisfactory.

4. Present symptoms

Considerable yellow nasal discharge.

5. Tongue and pulse

Thin tongue-coating, a rather slow pulse.

6. Differentiation and analysis

The Lungs dominate Qi and respiration, connecting upward with the trachea and throat and opening into the nose, and outward corresponding to the skin and skin hair. The appearance of Bi Yuan is closely related with the invasion of the Lung Channel by pathogenic factors. Wind Cold attacks the Lungs and later transforms into Fire, the Lungs lose their function in dispersing, thus the nose is obstructed. Although Wind Cold is driven off, the Heat is not cleared out, and this dries the fluid into the turbid and blocks the nose, and therefore there is a lot of thick and sticky nasal discharge.

7. Diagnosis

TCM: Bi Yuan (stagnant Heat in Lung Channel).

Western medicine: Nasosinusitis.

8. Treating principle

Dispel Wind, clear Heat, promote the Lungs in dispersing, remove obstruction of the nose.

9. Prescription

Tongtian (BL 7), Shangxing (GV 23), Shangyingxiang (EX-HN8), Yingxiang (LI 20), Hegu (LI 4), Lieque (LU 7).

The reducing method.

10. Effect

Twenty treatments greatly relieved the symptoms.

11. Essentials

Tongtian (BL 7) acts to dispel Wind, clear Heat and open the nose. Shangxing (GV 23) and Yingxiang (LI 20) are the local points to unobstruct the nose. Shangyingxiang (EX-HN8) is an important point for nose diseases, having an immediate effect on sneezing to open the nose. Hegu (LI 4) and Lieque (LU 7) are the combination of Yuan-Source and Luo-Connecting points, promoting the Lungs in dispersing to open the nose.

SHANGYINGXIANG

Shangyingxiang (EX-HN8) is located on the face, at the junction of the nasal alar cartilage and the nasal conchae, close to the upper portion of the nasolabial groove. It clears Heat to unobstruct the nose, indicated in headache, nasal obstruction and lacrimation, etc.

CASE II: CHENG XINNONG'S MEDICAL RECORD

1. General data

A 55-year-old female, named Li, visited on November 16, 1991.

2. Chief complaint

Nasal obstruction with thick and sticky discharge for 7 years.

3. History of present illness

She had nasal obstruction with thick and sticky discharge for 7 years and the treatment of Chinese and Western medicine had not been very effective for her.

4. Present symptoms

Her complexion was dark, her nose obstructed with thick and sticky discharge which repeatedly occurred when exposed to cold or without obvious reasons. She was coughing, with aversion to cold, lacrimation, and asthmatic breathing when the attack was serious.

5. Tongue and pulse

Tongue tip was red, coating thick sticky and yellow in the middle, pulse wiry, Chi weak.

6. Differentiation and analysis

Damp Heat retention is the cause of this disease.

7. Diagnosis

TCM: Bi Yuan (stagnated Heat in Lung and Gallbladder).

Western medicine: Nasosinusitis.

8. Treating principle

Clear Heat, dissolve Phlegm, unobstruct nose.

9. Prescription

Dazhui (GV 14), Fengchi (GB 20), Yingxiang (LI 20), Tongtian (BL 7), Shangxing (GV 23), Hegu (LI 4), Lieque (LU 7), Taixi (KI 3), Taichong (LR 3).
   The reducing method.

10. Effect

With 6 treatments, the aversion to cold, lacrimation, nasal obstruction with thick and sticky discharge were better, and after 12 treatments, all the symptoms were much relieved, so she stopped coming.

11. Essentials

Plain Questions (*Qi Jue Lun*) says: 'Heat from Gallbladder moving to the brain, there will be tingling in the nose and with thick and sticky discharge.' It points out that the stagnated Heat in the Gallbladde Channel is also one of the causative factors of Bi Yuan.

CASE III: RECORD IN *ACUPUNCTURE-MOXIBUSTION FOR DIFFICULT DISEASES*

1. General data

A 28-year-old male, named Xia, visited on November 8, 1999.

2. Chief complaint

Running nose in the morning and evening for 1 year.

3. History of present illness

He had a running nose in the morning and evening. Diagnosed with Allergic Rhinitis, he was treated in the department of ENT with an antiallergic agent but it was not effective.

4. Present symptoms

Running nose in the morning and evening, itching in the nose, aversion to cold, and catching cold very often.

5. Tongue and pulse

Pale tongue, white coating, thready pulse.

6. Differentiation and analysis

Lung and Spleen Qi deficiency is the causative factor in the production of Phlegm. The disorder of the Lungs in dispersing produces the symptoms of running nose, itching in the nose, aversion to cold, and catching cold very often. Pale tongue, white coating, and thready pulse come from the Qi deficiency.

7. Diagnosis

TCM: Bi Yuan (Wind Cold attacking the Lungs).

Western medicine: Allergic rhinitis.

8. Treating principle

Promote the Lungs in dispersing, remove obstruction of nose.

9. Prescription

Hegu (LI 4), Yingxiang (LI 20), Shenting (GV 24), Feishu (BL 13), Pishu (BL 20), Suliao (GV 25).

Moxibustion was applied to Feishu (BL 13) and Pishu (BL 20). Suliao (GV 25) was inserted 1 cun, penetrating to Yintang (EX-HN3).

10. Effect

With 5 treatments, the symptoms were relieved, and another 5 treatments, all symptoms disappeared, and his common colds were reduced in frequency. The follow-up after 4 months found no recurrence of Bi Yuan.

11. Essentials

Hegu (LI 4), Yingxiang (LI 20), Suliao (GV 25) and Shenting (GV 24) are the first choice points for nose diseases. Feishu (BL 13) and Pishu (BL 20) are the Back-Shu points from where the Qi of the Lungs and Spleen is infused. Moxibustion can clear Heat from the Lungs and dissolve Phlegm, and strengthen the Spleen to dissolve Damp.

CASE IV: HAN BIN'S MEDICAL RECORD

1. General data

Xu, female, 40 years old.

2. Chief complaint

Repeated attacks of nasal itching and obstruction with running nose, and paroxysmal sneezes for 8 years.

3. History of present illness

She was constitutionally weak. Eight years ago, she had nasal obstruction with running nose due to common cold. It was prolonged and intermittently attacked. The symptoms were sometimes better sometimes worse. Her smelling sense was gradually declined. In recent 3 years, the attacks became more frequent. In the attacks, she had itching nose, obstructive nose, running nose, and paroxysmal sneezes. The doctor of the eye, ear, nose and throat department diagnosed her allergic rhinitis.

4. Present symptoms

Itching nose, obstructive nose, running nose, paroxysmal sneezes, especially when exposed to cold and smelled something irritant, accompanied with soreness and weakness of lumbus and knees, being afraid of cold, shortness of breath, tiredness, fullness in epigastric region, poor appetite, and loose stools.

5. Tongue and pulse

Swollen pale tongue, thin white coating; deep weak retarded pulse.

6. Differentiation and analysis

Lung Qi insufficiency, Spleen and Kidney Yang deficiency.

The patient was weak in constitution, insufficient in Lung Qi, not strong in body defence, thus the pathogenic factors invaded her Lungs, causing her obstructed nose, running nose, and frequent sneezes. Kidney Yang deficiency is the cause of cold extremities, and soreness and weakness of the lumbus and knees. Spleen Yang deficiency fails to produce enough Qi and Blood, so she had shortness of breath, tiredness, fullness in the epigastric region, poor appetite, and loose stools.

7. Diagnosis

TCM: Biqiu-allergic rhinitis.

Western medicine: Allergic rhinitis.

8. Treating principle

Dispel Wind, open the nasal orifices, warm and reinforce the Spleen and Kidneys.

Even method for those points of Hand-Yangming. Acupuncture with warming-needle moxibustion for those Back-Shu points of Foot-Taiyang Bladder Meridian.

9. Prescription

Yingxiang (LI 20), Shangxing (GV 23), Yintang (EX-HN3), Hegu (LI 4), Shenshu (BL 23), Pishu (BL 20).

Yintang (EX-HN3) was inserted about 1 cun and the needle manipulated with rotating, letting the needling sensation go to the nose and into the nasal cavity to produce an obvious soreness and distention. Retention of the needles was 30 minutes. Three times a week, 10 times as 1 course, 1 week as the interval for rest before the next course. The effect was observed after 3 courses of treatment.

10. Effect

Clinical symptoms disappeared. After 3 courses, the patient was cured. Followed up after 6 months, she was found to have had no relapse.

11. Essentials

The allergic rhinitis of this patient was caused by the weakness of the Lungs and invasion of Wind Cold. The Lungs, Spleen, and Kidneys were involved in the process of the disease. Those Back-Shu points are the site where the Qi of the Zang Fu organs and meridians infuse to the body surface of the back. Acupuncture and moxibustion at Shenshu (BL 23) and Pishu (BL 20) function to warm the Kidneys and dispel Cold, reinforce Qi and strengthen the Spleen, and to regulate Qi, Blood, and the Zang Fu organs, and promote the immune system to resist diseases to restore the nose and Lungs to their normal functions. Yintang (EX-HN3), an extra point on the running course of the Governor Vessel, is in accordance with the principle of selecting points, 'where the meridian passes, where the disease is cured by using its points'.

SUMMARY

Bi Yuan (thick and sticky nasal discharge) is caused by Wind Cold invading the Lungs and transforming into Heat and obstructing the nose, or the Damp Heat of the Gallbladder Channel forcing upward and blocking the nose. For the treatment, the points are mainly selected from Hand-Taiyin and Hand-Yangming channels to promote the Lungs in dispersing and clearing Heat. Acupuncture is applied with the reducing method.

Main points: Shangxing (GV 23), Yingxiang (LI 20), Hegu (LI 4), Lieque (LU 7).

Fengchi (GB 20) and Dazhu (BL 11) are added for nasal obstruction, Feishu (BL 13) and Taiyuan (LU 9) added for white thin nasal discharge, Dazhui (GV 14), Chize (LU 5) and Shaoshang (LU 11) added for yellow bloody discharge and fever, Taiyang (EX-HN5) and Yintang (EX-HN3) added for headache.

SECTION SEVEN • SORE THROAT

CASE I: YANG YONGXUAN'S MEDICAL RECORD

1. General data

A 21-year-old female, named Chen.

2. Chief complaint

Sore throat for 3 days.

3. History of present illness

Her acute pharyngolaryngitis for 3 days was treated with Western drugs and it was a little better. From yesterday, she had a hoarse voice, and serious sore throat.

4. Present symptoms

Serious sore throat, yellow thick Phlegm, and suffocated breathing.

5. Tongue and pulse

The tongue-coating was thin and dry, pulse thready and rapid.

6. Differentiation and analysis

The acute pharyngolaryngitis, known as sore throat, is mostly caused by invasion of Wind Heat burning the throat, or overwork with the deficiency Fire flaring up to the throat. In a mild case, the patient feels dry and pain in the throat, in serious cases, there will be a difficulty in swallowing, even chills and fever. The patient in this case is a mild case, her sore throat is due to exogenous pathogenic Heat flaring upward and the Body Fluid of the Lungs exhausted by Phlegm Heat.

7. Diagnosis

TCM: Sore throat (invasion of Wind Heat).

Western medicine: Acute pharyngolaryngitis.

8. Treating principle

Clear Heat, dissolve Phlegm, promote the Lung in dispersing.

9. Prescription

Tiantu (CV 22), Neiguan (PC 6), Hegu (LI 4), Taixi (KI 3).

Reinforcing and reducing achieved by rotating of needle was adopted. Tiantu (CV 22) was treated without retaining the needle. For the other points, the needles were retained for 10 minutes.

10. Effect

On the fifth treatment, she was already much relieved of the pain and had a clear voice, but an itching throat. Since the Phlegm was not yet dissolved, Lianquan (CV 23) was added to regulate Qi and remove obstruction of the nose. Lianquan (CV 23) was reduced without retaining the needle. All the symptoms were stopped, she was cured.

11. Essentials

Tiantu (CV 22) is selected to promote the Lungs in dispersing and dissolve Phlegm; Neiguan (PC 6) to circulate Qi in chest; Hegu (LI 4) to treat the Lungs to reduce Heat; Taixi (KI 3) is reinforced to clear the voice and relieve the sore throat. In addition, an empirical point, Liyan (relieve sore throat), even method, is indicated in sore throat. Most of the patient's condition could be relieved of pain 1 hour after needling and cured 5–6 hours later.

LIYAN

Liyan (relieving sore throat), located 0.8 cun lateral to Tianding (LI 17), is inserted 0.5-1 cun, indicated in acute pharyngolaryngitis, acute tonsillitis, and hoarse voice, etc.

CASE II: CHENG XINNONG'S MEDICAL RECORD

1. General data

A 21-year-old female, named Zhang, visited on September 27, 1984.

2. Chief complaint

Dry throat for 5 years.

3. History of present illness

Five years ago, she began to have a dry throat without obvious inducing factors. Diagnosed with pharyngitis in Youdian Hospital, she was administered Western drugs, but they were not effective.

4. Present symptoms

From the morning when she got up, she had a dry and sore throat and hoarse voice, made worse by intake of even a little peppery food.

5. Tongue and pulse

Pale dark tongue with cracks, thready pulse.

6. Differentiation and analysis

Yan Hou means pharynx and larynx. Yan connects with the oesophagus, leading to the Stomach, while Hou connects with the trachea, leading to the Lungs. The exhaustion of essential Qi of the Lungs and Kidneys causing the deficiency Fire flaring up gives rise to dry throat.

7. Diagnosis

TCM: Dry throat (Yin deficiency of Lung and Kidney).

Western medicine: Pharyngitis.

8. Treating principle

Replenish Yin, moisten throat.

9. Prescription

Lieque (LU 7), Taixi (KI 3), Zhaohai (KI 6), Hegu (LI 4), Sanyinjiao (SP 6), Tianding (LI 17).

10. Effect

11. Essentials

Taixi (KI 3) is the Yuan-Source point of Foot-Shaoyin Channel, Zhaohai (KI 6) leads to Yinqiao, these two can replenish Yin to subdue the Fire, bringing down the deficiency Fire, which is important for treating dry throat; Sanyinjiao (SP 6) strengthens Taixi (KI 3) and Zhaohai (KI 6) in replenishing Yin to subdue the Fire; Lieque (LU 7), Luo-Connecting of Hand-Taiyin, Hegu (LI 4), Yuan-Source of Hand-Yangming, and Tianding (LI 17), a point of Hand-Yangming, clear the stagnated Heat of Taiyin and Yangming.

SUMMARY

Sore throat, known as Hou Bi in TCM, is divided into deficiency and excess syndromes. The excess case is from the invasion of exogenous pathogenic Wind Heat burning the Lung system, or the stagnated Heat the of Lung and Stomach channels disturbing upward; and the deficiency case is from the Yin deficiency of the Kidneys causing the deficiency Fire flaring up.

For excess syndrome, the points are mainly selected from Hand and Foot-Yangming channels to dispel Wind Heat, punctured with the reducing method.

Main points: Shaoshang (LU 11), Hegu (LI 4), Neiting (ST 44), Tianrong (SI 17).

For deficiency syndrome, the points are mainly selected from Foot-Shaoyin Channel to replenish Yin and subdue Fire, punctured with the reinforcing method.

Main points: Taixi (KI 3), Yuji (LU 10), Sanyinjiao (SP 6), Zhaohai (KI 6), Lieque (LU 7).

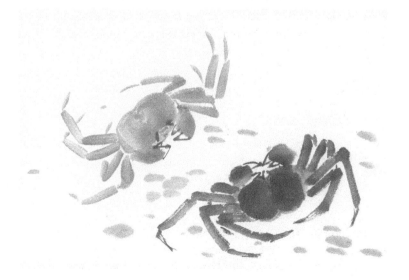

SECTION EIGHT • TOOTHACHE

CASE I: YANG JIEBIN'S MEDICAL RECORD

1. General data

A 23-year-old male, named Duo, visited on December 28, 1996.

2. Chief complaint

Toothache for 7 days.

3. History of present illness

Seven days ago, he began to have toothache and it became worse recently. Taking *tub aspirini composite* was no use.

4. Present symptoms

His toothache which was in a state of being better-and-worse made him unable to eat and unable to sleep, and he had dizziness and chills and fever. His urine was yellow and stools dry.

Examination: Swollen gums and cheeks, foul breath, dental caries on the second cheek tooth of the right lower teeth.

5. Tongue and pulse

Red tongue, no moisture, thin yellow coating, superficial rapid pulse.

6. Differentiation and analysis

The excessive Stomach Fire is manifested in this patient as swollen gums and cheeks, foul breath, yellow urine and dry stools. The internal Heat is evidenced by his red tongue, no moisture, thin yellow coating, superficial rapid pulse.

7. Diagnosis

TCM: Toothache (Stomach Fire excess).

Western medicine: Dental caries.

8. Treating principle

Clear Heat, reduce Fire, dispel Wind, stop pain.

9. Prescription

Jiache (ST 6), Daying (ST 5), Hegu (LI 4), Neiting (ST 44), Ashi points.

The three-edged needle was used to prick Ashi points for bleeding; for other points, the reducing method, with strong stimulation. The needling sensation of soreness, numbness, distention and heaviness was a must. The needles were removed after the pain was stopped. For the duration of retaining, lifting-thrusting and rotating the needles was done once every 3 minutes.

10. Effect

Ten minutes after insertion, the pain was relieved and 30 minutes later the pain stopped. On the following day, the toothache came again and was treated as before for 2 more times, and the swelling of the gums and pain disappeared.

11. Essentials

Hand and Foot-Yangming channels are distributed in teeth. Jiache (ST 6) and Daying (ST 5) are the local points to remove obstruction of channels and collaterals; Hegu (LI 4) is a distal point to dispel Wind to stop pain; Neiting (ST 44) is a Ying-Spring point to send the Qi of the Fu organs downward to clear the Stomach Heat.

CASE II: SHENG XIESUN AND LING XUZHI'S MEDICAL RECORD

1. General data

A 31-year-old male, named Jiang, visited on June 20, 1960.

2. Chief complaint

Swelling and painful gums for 5 days.

3. History of present illness

He was overindulgent in spicy food. Five days ago, his caries began to give a cutting pain and the gums swelled. The analgesic was useless, and the local blocking therapy was effective for a while only.

4. Present symptoms

Swelling and cutting-like pain of gums. Constipation.

5. Tongue and pulse

Tongue-coating was yellow sticky and thick, Chi pulse surging.

6. Differentiation and analysis

The pain shows a nature of excess Heat syndrome caused by Yangming Stomach Fire flaring up. Tongue-coating was yellow sticky and thick, resulting from the accumulation of excess Heat. And the surging pulse points to the excess Heat of Yangming Qi system.

7. Diagnosis

TCM: Toothache (Stomach Fire).

Western medicine: Acute periodontitis.

8. Treating principle

Clear Heat of Stomach to stop pain.

9. Prescription

Erjian (LI 2) (left), Daying (ST 5) (right).
  The reducing method. Retaining needles for 20 minutes.

10. Effect

The pain was relieved. In the afternoon, the pain was sharp again and he came for treatment. Hegu (LI 4) and Jiache (ST 6) were used, the reducing method. But the pain could not be controlled.

  On the following day, Hegu (LI 4), Pianli (LI 6), Fenglong (ST 40) and Lidui (ST 45) (left) were selected, the reducing method, with the needles retained for 40 minutes and manipulated once every 5 minutes. The pain stopped. Later, the same treatment was given twice in succession, his tongue-coating changed to normal and the pain was cured.

11. Essentials

At the first and second time of treatment, the two groups of empirical points, Erjian (LI 2) and Daying (ST 5), Hegu (LI 4) and Jiache (ST 6) were used, but were not effective. On the third treatment, Hegu (LI 4), Pianli (LI 6), Fenglong (ST 40) and Lidui (ST 45) were effective to relieve pain. This is because for the excess Heat syndrome due to Yangming Stomach Fire flaming up, the principle 'for the channel Qi excess, reduce the collateral fullness' should be followed, therefore Pianli (LI 6) and Fenglong (ST 40), the Luo-Connecting points of Hand and Foot-Yangming are used to dredge the obstructed channels to subdue the Stomach Fire. This is also a proven experience of what is said in *Biao You Fu* (*Lyrics of Standard Profoundities*): 'Reduce the collateral with distal points, puncture the foot for the disease on head.'

CASE III: ZHANG ZUOLIN'S MEDICAL RECORD

1. General data

A 68-year-old female, named Huang, visited on October 26, 1987.

2. Chief complaint

Gum pain for half a month.

3. History of present illness

She had had the gum pain for half a month already and it was worse after noon and when tired.

4. Present symptoms

Gum pain, worse after noon and when tired, without a decayed tooth, without swelling and redness of gums.

5. Tongue and pulse

Red tongue tip, without coating, thready rapid pulse.

6. Differentiation and analysis

Her pain is due to Yin deficiency with xu-deficient Fire flaring up, so it is worse in the afternoon and when tired. Red tip of tongue, without coating, thready rapid pulse also come from the Yin deficiency.

7. Diagnosis

TCM: Toothache (Yin deficiency, Fire flaring up).

Western medicine: Periodontitis.

8. Treating principle

Reinforce Yin, tonify the Kidneys, subdue Fire, stop pain.

9. Prescription

Taixi (KI 3).

10. Effect

Three times of acupuncture made her pain stop.

11. Essentials

Taixi (KI 3) is selected to replenish Yin and tonify the Kidneys to check the Fire from flaring up, thus the pain is stopped.

SUMMARY

Toothache, a common disease, is of excess Fire and deficiency Fire in differentiation. The excess toothache is caused by Stomach Heat and invasion of Wind Heat, called Wind Fire toothache; the deficiency toothache results from Kidney Yin deficiency with xu-deficient Fire flaring up.

Main points: Hegu (LI 4), Jiache (ST 6), Xiaguan (ST 7).

Fengchi (GB 20) and Neiting (ST 44) are added for Wind Fire syndrome; and Taixi (KI 3) is added for xu-deficient Fire syndrome.

CHAPTER 4

SKIN DISEASES, EXTERNAL DISEASES

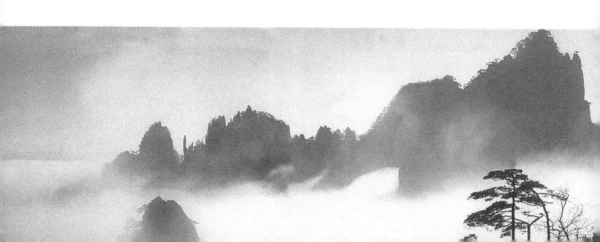

SECTION ONE • ERYSIPELAS

CASE I: LU SHOUYAN'S MEDICAL RECORD

1. General data

Xu, a 45-year-old female, paid her first visit in July 1948.

2. Chief complaint

Her left leg and foot had redness and swelling pain for 3 days.

3. History of present illness

Her left leg and foot was red and swollen with a hot sensation and serious pain without clear reasons.

4. Present symptoms

She couldn't walk because her left leg and foot were swollen, red, with a hot sensation, and seriously painful.

5. Tongue and pulse

The tongue-coating was normal, the pulse soft and rapid.

6. Differentiation and analysis

This condition is caused by the accumulated Heat transformed into Fire flowing to the shank. The swelling and pain is due to obstruction of Qi circulation of the channels. The soft pulse stands for Damp in the interior and rapid pulse is the sign of Heat.

7. Diagnosis

TCM: Liu Huo (flowing Fire) (accumulated Heat transformed into Fire).

Western medicine: Erysipelas.

8. Treating principle

Clear Heat, remove toxins.

9. Prescription

Weizhong (BL 40), Yanglingquan (GB 34), Chengshan (BL 57), Zusanli (ST 36), Fenglong (ST 40).

The reducing method of lifting-thrusting. Weizhong (BL 40) was pricked for bleeding.

10. Effect

The pain was relieved after the first time of acupuncture. Seven times of treatment cured her.

11. Essentials

Erysipelas should be treated by removing the toxic Heat from the affected area and distal points of affected channels. Weizhong (BL 40) pricked for bleeding can remove the toxic Heat of Blood system of lower extremities, and pricking with three-edged needle to cause bleeding is to clear Heat and remove toxins.

SUMMARY

Erysipelas is due to Wind with accumulated Damp Heat infecting the Blood and then the skin and muscles. Arising on shank, it is called Liu Huo or Huo Dan; arising in face, it is called Bao Tou Huo Dan; that moving to the hypochondriac, lumbar and hip regions, called Chi You Dan. It is an acute contagious infectious skin disease characterized by sudden onset of chills, fever, local redness and swelling which may take place on any site of the body and rapid extend. In prolonged cases with repeated attacks the legs become thick swollen, called Da Jiao Feng.

In the local area, the surrounding method with several needles and sallow insertion is applied. Bloodletting and cupping are used to remove the toxic Heat.

Main points: Add Dazhui (GV 14), Quchi (LI 11) and Hegu (LI 4) for chills and fever; add Weizhong (BL 40) and Shixuan (EX-UE11) for pricking for bleeding for high fever with thirst; add Taiyang (EX-HN5) and Fengchi (GB 20) for headache.

SECTION TWO • DING CHUANG (FURUNCLE, BOIL)

CASE I: PENG JINGSHAN'S MEDICAL RECORD

1. General data

Tian, a 22-year-old female, paid her first visit on January 20, 1961.

2. Chief complaint

The tip of the right middle finger had become red and swollen for 1 day.

3. History of present illness

Yesterday in the evening she noticed that her right middle finger had become red and swollen in the region close to the nail.

4. Present symptoms

Her right middle finger was red and swollen at the region close to the nail, and it was getting worse today in the morning, and the colour changed from fresh red to blue purple, with a whitish top, radiating to the medial side of forearm and the ulnar side of cubital region. The pain was unendurable. She had chills and nausea. She was clear in consciousness, with sallow complexion, normal voice and respiration.

5. Tongue and pulse

Thin white tongue-coating, thready rapid pulse.

6. Differentiation and analysis

The boil at the tip of middle finger is the involvement of the Pericardium Channel with pathogenic Damp Heat.

7. Diagnosis

TCM: Ding Chuang (furuncle, boil).

Western medicine: Paronychia.

8. Treating principle

Clear Heat, dissolve Damp.

9. Prescription

Right side: Tianchi (PC 1).
   The reinforcing method of rotating.

10. Effect

The pain was stopped immediately. The sharp-round needle was used to prick along the red thread-like boil from the middle finger up and the pain was relieved, and the nausea and chills stopped as well.

On January 26, she came again. She was cured.

11. Essentials

In this case, the Pericardium channel is involved because the boil is at the tip of middle finger. The Head-Tail method of selecting the point, Tianchi (PC 1) of the affected side, is adopted. Her pulse was thready rapid, belonging to deficiency Heat, so the reinforcing method of needling is employed.

CASE II: PENG JINGSHAN'S MEDICAL RECORD

1. General data

Li, a 40-year-old female, paid her first visit on October 9, 1972.

2. Chief complaint

Numbness of the left palm for half a day.

3. History of present illness

Today in the morning, she felt numbness and pain of her left hand, cold in the body, irritability and nausea.

4. Present symptoms

The pain of her left hand was at the place of Shaofu (HT 8), with a flat swelling without top, without changes of skin colour. Her hand was numb in sensation. She was slim in body figure, with white complexion, feeling cold in the body, irritability and nausea.

5. Tongue and pulse

Red tongue, yellow coating, thready rapid pulse.

6. Differentiation and analysis

The boil in the region of Shaofu (HT 8), and the pulse and symptoms are the signs of deficiency Heat of Heart Channel.

7. Diagnosis

TCM: Ding Du (boil).

Western medicine: Paronychia.

8. Treating principle

Reinforcing Yin to clear the deficiency Heat.

9. Prescription

Jiquan (HT 1).

    The reinforcing method. The needle was retained for 2 minutes.

10. Effect

Her pain, cold feeling in the body and nausea disappeared. She said she felt very comfortable after needling.

11. Essentials

The Head-Tail method of selecting point, Jiquan (HT 1) of the affected channel, is adopted. Based on the treating principle, the reinforcing method of needling is employed.

SUMMARY

Ding Du (boil) is characterized by locating at points. The face, lips, fingers and toes are the starting-ending places of channels. For example, the ending point of the Large Intestine Channel, Yingxiang (LI 20). If the boil is here, the starting point, Shangyang (LI 1), is punctured, and the symptoms such as fever, chills, nausea, pain and irritability, etc., can disappear immediately after needling. The nearby Yuan-Source or Shu-Stream points, and so on, of the affected channels may be selected instead of the Head-Tail points, if necessary.

In cases where lymphatitis (called red thread) exists, the sharp-round needle can be used to prick once every 1 cun in distance to cause bleeding. Squeeze the black Blood out, prick to the end of the red thread. Or place a slice of ginger at the starting or ending point of the red thread, and do moxibustion with cones, until the red thread is finished.

SECTION THREE • PSORIASIS

CASE I: CHENG XINNONG'S MEDICAL RECORD

1. General data

Yi, 60 years old, came on August 23, 1984.

2. Chief complaint

Tinea with itching at the neck and palms for 2 years.

3. History of present illness

Two years ago the patient began to have tinea with itching on the palms and dorsum of the hands without obvious reasons, then with the nape and elbows involved. Diagnosed with Neurodermatitis and treated by various therapies, his itching was not relieved. He couldn't sleep at night because of the itching.

4. Present symptoms

Tinea with itching at palms and dorsum of hands and in the nape and elbows regions, skin as rough as cowskin, serious itching, poor sleep.

5. Tongue and pulse

Red tongue, white coating, wiry pulse.

6. Differentiation and analysis

Based on congenital deficiency, the invasion of Wind Damp Heat makes the channels blocked, causing itching and rough skin.

7. Diagnosis

TCM: Psoriasis (Wind Heat Damp retention, disharmony between Qi and Blood).

Western medicine: Neurodermatitis.

8. Treating principle

Dispel Wind, dissolve Damp, clear Heat, moisten Dryness.

9. Prescription

Fengchi (GB 20), Quchi (LI 11), Waiguan (TE 5), Hegu (LI 4), Baxie (EX-UE9), Xuehai (SP 10), Sanyinjiao (SP 6), Ximen (PC 4), Laogong (PC 8), Yinlingquan (SP 9). Plum-blossom needle was used to tap the nape, elbow and dorsum of hands.
    The reducing method.

10. Effect

11. Essentials

Fengchi (GB 20) is to dispel the Wind; Quchi (LI 11) and Hegu (LI 4), He-Sea and Yuan-Source of Hand-Yangming Large Intestine Channel, clear the Damp Heat on the skin to stop itching and dissolve the Damp Heat of Stomach and intestines; Baxie (EX-UE9) dispels Wind, activates channels to stop itching; Waiguan (TE 5) clears Heat to remove obstruction of the channels; Xuehai (SP 10) replenishes Blood to moisten the Dryness; Sanyinjiao (SP 6) and Yinlingquan (SP 9) remove Dampness and promote diuresis. 'All the pain and itching boils and diseases are related with the Heart.' Reduce Ximen (PC 4) and Laogong (PC 8) to rest the Heart to calm the Mind, to clear the Ying system to stop itching. Tapping the nape, elbow and dorsum of hands with plum-blossom needle is to remove the Wind toxins of the skin and muscles.

CASE II: YANG JIEBIN'S MEDICAL RECORD

1. General data

Qiu, a 30-year-old female, paid her first visit on September 3, 1993.

2. Chief complaint

Her nape and the left elbow had thickened skin with serious itching for 3 months.

3. History of present illness

With no reasons, she began to have thickened skin with serious itching at the nape and elbow for 3 months. She tried many ways of treatment but none helped.

4. Present symptoms

The skin of the nape in an area of 4×8cm and the left cubital fossa in an area of 3 × 5cm became thick, dry and chapped with serious itching, made worse by warmth, and a pink granule-like fluid came out after scratching.

5. Tongue and pulse

6. Differentiation and analysis

According to Professor Yang Jiebin, in prolonged stubborn tinea diseases, the Phlegm Damp and Blood stasis are retained in the channels and collaterals, and the weak constitution caused by prolonged disease causes disharmony between

Ying-nutrient and Wei-defence systems, with the manifestations of Blood deficiency and Wind Dryness.

7. Diagnosis

TCM: Psoriasis (Blood deficiency, Wind Dryness).

Western medicine: Neurodermatitis.

8. Treating principle

Nourish Blood, activate Blood, dispel Wind, moisten Dryness.

9. Prescription

The affected areas were tapped with the cutaneous needle until there was a little bleeding. Cotton moxibustion was done in this way: a thin layer of cotton was placed on the affected area and ignited. This moxibustion was repeated 5 times. Once every 3 days.

10.Effect

After 1 treatment, the itching was greatly relieved. After 2 treatments, the itching was nearly completely over and the skin thickness began to improve. Ten times later, the skin became smooth, nearly normal.

11.Essentials

Following the treating principle, the treatment with pricking to cause bleeding is important to remove the stasis for new Blood production. Cotton moxibustion is combined with this for a better effect. At the beginning of the disease, the Wind Damp Heat stays in the skin, but later, if it is prolonged, there will be Blood deficiency and Wind Dryness, and when the skin is deprived of nourishment, it becomes thick and itchy. Tap with cutaneous needle to regulate and activate Blood, then use cotton moxibustion to dispel Wind and harmonize Ying and Wei. In this way, the Blood circulation is activated and the Wind is eliminated, so the itching is stopped.

CASE III: LIU ZHAOHUI'S MEDICAL RECORD

1. General data

Wang, male, 59 years old, came on November 15, 2002.

2. Chief complaint

Itching of the shank on the medial side and tibial region, accompanied with dark red rashes for a year and a half, aggravated for 2 weeks.

3. History of present illness

Because of scratching, the red miliarias were gradually produced and increased, and later merged to patches, and got bigger and thicker. He took Western and Chinese medicines and had acupuncture treatment as well but without improvement. In the recent 2 weeks, the skin lesions and itching were getting worse owing to milk and meat food.

4. Present symptoms

Itching of the shank on the medial side and tibial region, accompanied with dark red rashes.

Examination: The skin lesion was 12cm × 5cm in size, dark red in colour, thick, 0.2cm higher than the normal skin, dry, scaling, with a few Blood scabs and scratch marks. The patient was emaciated with flushed cheeks. He had poor sleep.

5. Tongue and pulse

Red tongue with little dry coating, wiry, thready and rapid pulse.

6. Differentiation and analysis

This patient has a typical Yin-deficiency body constitution, such as a thin body, emaciated with the flushed cheeks, and poor sleep. Yin and Blood deficiency will cause internal Heat which lead to neurodermatitis.

7. Diagnosis

TCM: Neurodermatitis (Yin-Blood deficiency with internal Heat, Wind and Dryness syndrome).

Western medicine: Neurodermatitis.

8. Treating principle

Expel internal Wind through promoting Blood circulation, eliminate internal Heat by opening the pores of the local lesion.

9. Prescription

Moxibustion was selected for his treatment since the medicine and acupuncture were not helpful for him before. Method: The four moxa-sticks were bundled up and ignited and blown to make the Fire stronger. The moxibustion was done once every other day with the Heat according to the endurance of the patient at the affected area and around it.

10. Effect

During the treatment, the patient felt that the itching was worse, but it gradually relieved with the Heat penetrating and moving. After 2 treatments, the itching was remarkably reduced. The colour turned to light red and the lesions became thinner and basically not higher than normal skin. After 5 treatments, the itching disappeared, the skin became normal in height and in colour with only a little bit of pigmentation left. Another 5 treatments were done to support the good result. He was told not to eat much oily, fishy and milky food. The 6-month follow-up found no recurrence of neurodermatitis.

11. Essentials

Yin deficiency and Blood Heat are always contraindicated in moxibustion. But for the patient in this case, the author got a good result. The reason is that the reducing method is used and only done on the affected area, not to the points. The purpose is to clear the local Heat and Dryness from the Blood. When the Blood is circulating well, the Wind will be automatically stopped.

The Elementary Medicine: 'For Heat syndrome, moxibustion is to lead the stagnated Heat out and the Fire to approach the Dryness.' This tells us that moxibustion is applicable for Heat cases. Dr. Zhu Danxi thought that moxibustion for Heat syndromes is to follow the principle that treating Yang makes Yin increase. The important thing in treating Heat syndrome with moxibustion is to perform the reducing properly, otherwise, an unexpected result may present.

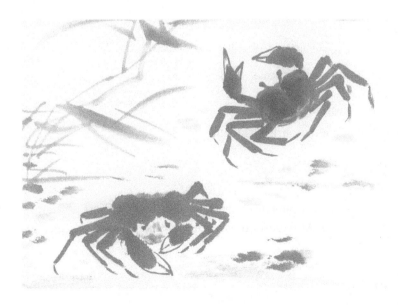

SECTION FOUR • LEUCODERMA

CASE I: HE PUREN'S MEDICAL RECORD

1. General data
Liu, an 18-year-old girl.

2. Chief complaint
Many white patches all over the body for 7 years.

3. History of present illness
Seven years ago, she noticed a white patch sized about 1cm on the lateral side of her left lower limb. One year ago, her wrist regions, ankle regions and the right hypochondrium began to have white patches too.

4. Present symptoms
Many white patches on the body with the biggest one 5 × 7cm in size.

5. Tongue and pulse
Red tongue with toothmarks on borders, thin white coating, thready pulse.

6. Differentiation and analysis
Based on the comprehensive condition of the patient, including her tongue and pulse, her skin problem is thought to be caused by Qi and Blood deficiency, leading to poor nourishment of the skin and muscles.

7. Diagnosis
TCM: Leucoderma (disharmony between Qi and Blood, skin lack of nourishment).

Western medicine: Leucoderma.

8. Treating principle
Regulate Qi and Blood, nourish skin and muscles.

9. Prescription
Ashi points, Xiabai (LU 4).

The white patch was punctured densely with several short filiform needles retained for 30 minutes. Moxibustion was done at Xiabai (LU 4) for 30 minutes.

10. Effect

In total, 10 treatments were given and the white patches became considerably smaller, and the one on the left wrist almost disappeared.

11. Essentials

The micro-removing method, Wei Tong Fa, in which a filiform needle is used, and the warm-removing method, Wen Tong Fa, in which moxibustion is adopted, are applied to reinforce Qi and Blood to strengthen the anti-pathogenic Qi and dispel pathogenic Qi, and moxibustion is done at Xiabai (LU 4) to regulate the Qi of the Lungs. The Lungs dominate skin and skin hair, being white in colour, so the appearance of leucoderma is classified as one of the diseases of the Lungs. *Plain Questions* says: 'All kinds of Qi relate to the Lungs.' and 'Convergence of vessels is in the Lungs.' Therefore, moxibustion done at Xiabai (LU 4) functions to regulate the Qi and Blood of the whole body to nourish skin and muscles.

CASE II: HE PUREN'S MEDICAL RECORD

1. General data

Fu, a 27-year-old lady.

2. Chief complaint

White patch on the right shoulder for several months.

3. History of present illness

Several months ago, she noticed a white patch on her right shoulder, without any discomfort in the local area. Application of medicine was not effective.

4. Present symptoms

A white patch on her right shoulder, 3 × 2cm in size.

5. Tongue and pulse

Pale tongue, white sticky coating, rolling pulse.

6. Differentiation and analysis

According to her tongue and pulse, this is differentiated as the syndrome of Damp retention, as a result of which, Qi and Blood are not harmonized with each other, failing to nourish skin and muscles well.

7. Diagnosis

TCM: Leucoderma (Damp retention).

Western medicine: Leucoderma.

8. Treating principle

Regulate Qi and Blood, nourish skin and muscles.

9. Prescription

Ashi points in the patch area.
    The patch was pricked with a thin Fire-needle. Twice a week.

10. Effect

With 5 treatments, the patch disappeared.

11. Essentials

As the Damp is a Yin pathogenic factor, the Fire needling is to promote Yang, thus, the Fire-needle therapy of the Warm-removing method is employed to warm and remove obstruction of channels, circulate Qi and activate Blood. By doing this, the Damp retained in the channels is driven out by the anti-pathogenic Qi.

CASE III: HE PUREN'S MEDICAL RECORD

1. General data

Sun, a 30-year-old male.

2. Chief complaint

White patch on the dorsum of left hand for half a month.

3. History of present illness

Half a month ago, he noticed a white patch on the dorsum of his left hand after a quarrel with somebody.

4. Present symptoms

A white patch on the dorsum of his left hand, 3×6cm in size.

5. Tongue and pulse

Red tongue, thin white coating, rolling pulse.

6. Differentiation and analysis

His patch is thought to be related with anger which damages the Liver, causing Liver Qi stagnation. 'Qi is the commander of Blood, Blood is the mother of Qi.' The Qi stagnation leads to Blood stasis, thus skin and muscles lack nourishment, resulting in leucoderma.

7. Diagnosis

TCM: Leucoderma (Qi stagnation, Blood stasis).

Western medicine: Leucoderma.

8. Treating principle

Regulate Qi and Blood, nourish skin and muscles.

9. Prescription

Ashi points.

The white patch was pricked with an ensiform needle and cupped to cause bleeding. Once a week.

10. Effect

A total of 4 treatments made his patch disappear.

11. Essentials

Bleeding with the ensiform needle, which is the strong-removing method, Qiang Tong Fa, can remove Blood stasis directly. The channels are cleared of obstruction, so the Qi and Blood circulate well to nourish skin and muscles.

SUMMARY

Leucoderma, called Bai Bo Feng, is a localized disease of pigment metabolism, due to hereditary, autoimmune and nervous factors. In TCM, the cause is emotional disturbance, Qi stagnation, invasion of exogenous pathogenic factors, the failure of Lung defence, Qi and Blood disharmony, thus giving poor nourishment to the skin. Professor He Puren says that the skin patches are only the outward manifestation of disease, the pathogenesis, and the root of disease is the disharmonious Qi and Blood. For treatment, the principle to replenish Blood, dispel Wind, regulate Qi and Blood to nourish the skin should be followed. The three-removing method (San Tong Fa), with different needles used is adopted according to the individual conditions of patients.

For those with Qi and Blood deficiency, the micro-removing method (Wei Tong Fa), with the filiform needle to puncture is used together with the warm-removing method (Wen Tong Fa), moxibustion, to replenish Qi and Blood to strengthen Zheng Qi (anti-pathogenic Qi) to eliminate Xie Qi (pathogenic Qi).

For those with Damp retention, the warm-removing method with the Fire needling to reinforce Yang to dissolve Damp is selected to warm the channels and collaterals to circulate Qi to activate Blood.

For those with Qi stagnation and Blood stasis, the strong-removing method (Qiang Tong Fa), with the ensiform needle to prick to cause bleeding for dredging the channels and collaterals is applied to remove stasis directly.

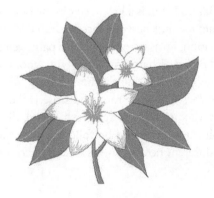

SECTION FIVE • YIN ZHEN (URTICARIA)

CASE I: RECORD IN *ACUPUNCTURE-MOXIBUSTION FOR DIFFICULT DISEASES*

1. General data

Zhou, a 34-year-old female, paid her first visit on June 10, 1999.

2. Chief complaint

Skin itching for 1 year.

3. History of present illness

She had scattered skin rashes with itching without inducing factors. An antiallergic agent didn't help.

4. Present symptoms

Scattered skin rashes, red in colour, a little higher than the skin, in patches, with itching. Accompanied by irritability, thirst, and yellow urine.

5. Tongue and pulse

Red tongue, slightly yellow coating, superficial and wiry pulse.

6. Differentiation and analysis

Pathogenic Wind Heat attacking the superficial areas of the body is the cause of skin rashes of red colour, higher than the skin, in patches, with itching. Irritability, thirst, and the manifestations of tongue and pulse evidence the invasion of Wind Heat as well.

7. Diagnosis

TCM: Yin Zhen (Wind Heat attacking body surface).

Western medicine: Urticaria.

8. Treating principle

Dispel Wind, harmonize Ying system.

9. Prescription

Xuehai (SP 10), Quchi (LI 11), Fengshi (GB 31), Sanyinjiao (SP 6), Dazhui (GV 14).

Once a day, 12 times as 1 course.

10. Effect

After 2 courses, she was cured.

11. Essentials

Xuehai (SP 10) is to clear the Blood Heat; Quchi (LI 11) to clear Wind Heat, remove rashes and stop itching; Fengshi (GB 31), the door from where the Wind invades, to dispel Wind; Sanyinjiao (SP 6) to reinforce Qi and Blood; Dazhui (GV 14), a meeting point of Yang channels, to drive Wind Heat out.

CASE II: LIU TAOXIN'S MEDICAL RECORD

1. General data

Alf, male, 65 yeas old, first visited on February 13, 2001.

2. Chief complaint

Severe urticaria over the whole body for 8–9 years.

3. History of present illness

Skin itching started 8–9 years ago and the rash appeared immediately after scratching the skin. The rash felt slightly hard and looked reddish or white in colour. The itching became more and more severe over time and could appear anywhere in the body, and later the rash was all over the body. More frequent attacks caused him considerable suffering. Attacks did not have much to do with the change of cold or hot climate and he could take baths normally. He did not notice what caused this but felt concern about his work because of frequent contact with chemicals. His skin has been allergic to sunlight.

Chronic urticaria was the diagnosis of Western medicine and he was treated with antiallergic tablets. He became reliant on the tablets to control it and the effect was not so good.

Everything such as his emotions and sleep has been bothered by the trouble. His stools were sometimes dry.

His appetite was good. His urination was normal. His blood pressure was normal.

He denied pain in the body, thirst and heart disease. No other complaints.

History of cigarette smoking.

4. Present symptoms

Rash all over the body and limbs, above normal skin, more reddish in colour, with slightly itching sensation. Skin is dry and lustreless. Rash did not feel warm but a bit hard. Xuehai (SP 10), and Sanyinjiao (SP 6) painful upon pressure.

5. Tongue and pulse

Red tongue with a little coating. Cun and Guan pulse feels wiry and slightly rapid and Chi position weak.

6. Differentiation and analysis

External evil Qi attacking the body and staying in the skin and muscles; deficiency of Yin-Blood producing Wind Heat affecting body surface.

The patient worked in the laboratory of an aluminium-making factory for many years and came into contact with a lot of chemicals which could be harmful to the body. His skin and muscles were poorly nourished and troubled by internal Wind Heat both because of deficiency of Yin-Blood. Skin allergic to sunlight, dry stool, dry skin, red tongue and rather rapid pulse all indicate internal Heat due to Yin deficiency.

7. Diagnosis

TCM: Chronic urticaria.

Western medicine: Chronic urticaria.

8. Treating principle

To dispel Wind and clear away Heat; to stop itching and rash by nourishing Yin and replenishing Blood.

9. Prescription

Methods of treatment: Acupuncture and cupping.

Prescription of points: Three Sima points (Middle Sima – 3 cun anterior to G 31, Upper Sima – 2 cun above Middle Sima and Lower Sima – 2 cun below Middle Sima) and Fengshi (GB 31) to stop Wind and itching; Xuehai (SP 10) and Sanyinjiao (SP 6) to nourish Yin, replenish and regulate Blood. Cupping on Shenque (Ren 8) to stop itching.

10. Effect

Second treatment on 15 Feb: No change. Adding bleeding method. Pricked a small blood vessel in the back of the ear on both sides to clear away Heat.

Third treatment on 17 Feb: No change. Pricked Weizhong (B 40) in order to clear more Heat.

Fourth treatment on 23 Feb: Patient's conditions became worse after last treatment. Stopped bleeding method. Punctured Quchi (LI 11), Xuehai (SP 10) and Taixi (KI 3). Cupping on Shenque (Ren 8).

Fifth treatment on 27 Feb: No change. Careful study was done. The patient had deficiency when he started to have this problem and his age and the disease lasting 8 years made his condition much more deficient. His deficiency was worsened by the wrong treatment of over-doing bleeding so that there was no effect. The treatment principle should be changed and reinforcing the Spleen and Stomach to build up body resistance to get rid of evil Qi was adopted as a new treatment. Punctured Zhongwan (Ren 12), Jianli (Ren 11), Zusanli (ST 36) and Sanyinjiao (SP 6) to strengthen the postnatal foundation of the body and punctured Baihui (Du 20) and Taichong (LR 3) to move Qi and Blood and harmonize the Liver and Spleen.

This prescription worked very well and then became the basic prescription until all rash and itching disappeared and tablets stopped.

Sixth treatment on 2 Mar: He felt better. The same treatment.

Seventh treatment on 6 Mar: Much better. The same prescription plus Shangwan (Ren 13) and Xiawan (Ren 10 in order to get more improvement.

Eighth treatment on 9 Mar: Started to reduce the amount of tablet from 25mg to 20mg per day.

Ninth treatment on 13 Mar: Dosage reduced to 15mg.

Tenth treatment on 16 Mar: Dosage reduced to 10mg.

Eleventh treatment on 20 Mar: He felt very good and wanted a treatment to stop smoking. The same prescription plus Tianmeixue (tender point in between LI 5 and LU7) and Shenmen (HT 7).

Twelfth treatment on 23 Mar: Dosage reduced to 7.5mg. Told the patient to slow down dosage reduction.

Fourteenth treatment on 29 Mar: Dosage reduced to 5mg.

Eighteenth treatment on 20 Apr: Dosage reduced to 2.5mg.

Twenty-fourth treatment on 6 May: Stopped Western medicine.

Altogether 25 treatments were given and the rash disappeared, the itching stopped and the tablets stopped. The doctor had to leave so he advised the patient to have more spaced-out treatment to keep the effect and not to eat seafood and to eat less food of a hot nature. He also asked the patient to maintain a regular bowel movement.

11. Essentials

It was a case of long-lasting disease and the patient thought that it was hopeless to cure it. Effective treatment of this stubborn case was actually enlightened by our ancient Medical Sage Zhang Zhongjing's principle of treatment in relieving exterior syndrome 'To treat exterior syndrome, apply sweating method to the strong and reinforcing the Middle (Burner) method to the weak'. Urticaria is not an exterior syndrome but the diseased area is on the body surface. A saying which goes 'Protracted disease results in deficiency and deficiency makes pathogenic factors stay' explains the transformation of a disease from an acute to a chronic condition. Reinforcing Spleen and Stomach (strengthening the middle) method is an essential and important method to treat deficiency because when the postnatal foundation becomes strong, Qi can be strengthened and its ascending and descending movement can be regulated, Blood can be replenished, and Phlegm and Dampness can be resolved. Hence reinforcing the Spleen and Stomach method should not be ignored in treating any sort of chronic disease.

SUMMARY

Yin Zhen (hidden rash), also called Feng Zhen, is known as urticaria in Western medicine. It is an allergic skin disease induced by multiple pathogenic factors, symptomized by itching, skin rashes as large as broad beans, in wheals, coming and going, and without any marks left after disappearance.

Main points: Quchi (LI 11), Hegu (LI 4), Xuehai (SP 10), Fengchi (GB 20).

Add Geshu (BL 17) and Quze (PC 3) (pricked to cause bleeding) for those with rashes red in colour; add Zusanli (ST 36) for those with the rashes white in colour; add Neiguan (PC 6) and Zhongwan (CV 12) for those with epigastric pain.

SECTION SIX • ACNE

CASE I: FENG LI'S MEDICAL RECORD

1. General data

Gao, a 30-year-old female.

2. Chief complaint

Acne on face with repeated attacks for 6 months.

3. History of present illness

The acne on her face appeared densely whenever she ate deep-oil-fried or seafood and drank wine, so she came for acupuncture.

4. Present symptoms

The acne on her face was yellow-bean or millet size, with a white granule-like substance in it, accompanied by dry mouth and foul breath, and constipation.

5. Tongue and pulse

Red tongue, yellow sticky coating, rolling rapid pulse.

6. Differentiation and analysis

The patient preferred sweet deep-oil-fried rich food, which produces Heat of the Lungs and Stomach. Accumulated Heat, prolonged, changes into Fire, and attacks up to the facial region. This is the causative factor of her acne. Red tongue, yellow sticky coating, and rolling rapid pulse are the manifestations of Damp Heat and excess Heat.

7. Diagnosis

TCM: Acne (accumulated Heat in the Lungs and Stomach).

Western medicine: Acne.

8. Treating principle

Promote the Lungs in dispersing, clear Heat, dissolve Damp.

9. Prescription

Dazhui (GV 14), Feishu (BL 13), Xinshu (BL 15), Geshu (BL 17), Weishu (BL 21), Dachangshu (BL 25).

  Three-edged needle was used for pricking, each time 3–4 points, then cupping for 5 minutes to draw a little Blood out. Once a day, 10 times as 1 course.

Auricular points: Lung, Large Intestine, Endocrine, Adrenal, Cheek, Forehead.

Herbal seeds were applied to press the ear points. Each ear was used in turn. The points were pressed 3 times a day, 10 days as 1 course.

10. Effect

After the first course of treatment, her acne was reduced, and her stools smooth. After 3 courses, all acne disappeared, she was cured.

11. Essentials

Pricking Dazhui (GV 14) to clear Heat toxins, dispersing the pathogenic factors from the skin and muscles; Feishu (BL 13) and Weishu (BL 21) clear Heat of the Lungs and Stomach; prick Geshu (BL 17), the Influential point of Blood, to activate Blood for removing Heat toxins from Blood; Dachangshu (BL 25) dredges the Large Intestine to restore its transmission to treat constipation. After pricking with a three-edged needle, cupping is done to strengthen the function of removing stasis and driving out the pathogenic Heat, namely, 'Stasis should be driven out.' Acne is always associated with Yangming Fire hyperactivity. The Lungs and Large Intestine are externally–internally related. The auricle point of the Large Intestine is selected to clear the Yangming Fire. 'All kinds of pain, itching and boils are relating to Heart', so Heart is selected to clear Fire, stopping itching. Endocrine and Adrenal are selected to regulate the endocrine system. Cheek and Forehead are corresponding points of acne on the face, improving Blood circulation of the facial region to treat inflammation. Deep fried and peppery food should be avoided, more fruits and vegetables should be taken to prevent constipation, and facial cleaning and physical exercises should be strengthened to cure acne from the root cause.

CASE II: WEI LIXIN'S MEDICAL RECORD

1. General data

Zhao, female, 35 years old.

2. Chief complaint

Acne for 1 month.

3. History of present illness

One month ago, she learnt how to drive in a driving school and was exposed to sunlight too much. She used a lot of sunscreen cream. Acne appeared on her face and she had a red and swollen face. Generally she preferred Western-style fast-food, had a good appetite and was often constipated, with a bowel movement once every 2–3 days.

4. Present symptoms

Acne, especially on the cheeks, big and merged into patches, red in colour, with pus-tops, slightly painful, but without itching. Eating a lot but always feeling hungry, thirst. Constipation. Sleep normal.

5. Tongue and pulse

Red tongue, thin yellow coating, slightly sticky; rolling pulse, a little bit rapid.

6. Differentiation and analysis

Exposed to sunlight and using a lot of sunscreen cream, she got acne. This is the affecting of the Lungs by exogenous pathogenic factor because the Lungs dominate the body surface. She preferred high Heat food, so the Heat accumulated in the Stomach. The Heat goes up along the Stomach Meridian to the face, manifesting as a red and swollen face. The Heat of the Stomach causes her voracious eating while still feeling hungry, and the thirst and constipation. The signs of Heat are also seen in her red tongue, yellow coating and rapid pulse. The sticky tongue-coating and rolling pulse indicate Damp, which is the result of Heat condensing the Body Fluid.

7. Diagnosis

TCM: Acne (accumulation of Heat in the Lung and Stomach).

Western medicine: Acne.

8. Treating principle

Clear the accumulated Heat in the Lungs and Stomach.

9. Prescription

Acne local areas, Quchi (LI 11), Hegu (LI 4), Tianshu (ST 25), Xuehai (SP 10), Fenglong (ST 40), Sanyinjiao (SP 6), Taichong (LR 3), Neiting (ST 44).

Acupuncture. Pricking bleeding cupping at Dazhui (GV 14), Feishu (BL 13), and Geshu (BL 17).

10. Effect

After 10 treatments, her acne was greatly reduced, the pus-top and pain and redness disappeared. Acne disappeared after 20 treatments. Voracious eating but still feeling hungry, thirst, and constipation were all getting better.

11. Essentials

Bloodletting is the quickest and most effective method for all the skin diseases of Heat type, bleeding cupping especially gets an instant result. In addition, a regular bowel movement is very important for eliminating Heat from the intestines, so treating constipation is also urgent.

CASE III: YANG JINHONG'S MEDICAL RECORD

1. General data

Wang, female, 42 years old.

2. Chief complaint

Papulonodules on the face and chest and back for years, worse for 1 month.

3. History of present illness

For some years the patient had papulonodules on the face and chest and back of dark colour and with tenderness, dark yellow complexion, pigment patches on the face, heaviness in the body, difficulty in falling asleep, bitter taste in the mouth, abdominal distention, sticky loose stools, cold feeling in the lower abdomen and ex-tremities, and scanty menstrual flow of dark colour. Herbal treatment helped her at the beginning, but later it was not effective for relapses. Now it had become worse in the recent 1 month.

4. Present symptoms

Papulonodules on the face and chest and back, abdominal distension, sticky loose stools.

5. Tongue and pulse

Swollen dark tongue with toothmarks on the borders, thin white yellow coating; deep thready pulse.

6. Differentiation and analysis

Irregular food intake or overeating cold and raw food damages the Spleen in its function of transportation and transformation, and there will be abdominal dis-tention and heaviness in the body. Water Damp staying in skin causes oedema. Emotional depression, Liver Qi stagnation, dysfunction of Chong and Ren, and Blood stasis explain the pathogenesis of this case in dark yellow complexion, pig-ment patches on the face, and scanty dark menstrual flow.

7. Diagnosis

TCM: Acne (dysfunction of Chong and Ren).

Western medicine: Acne.

8. Treating principle

Soothe the Liver, strengthen the Spleen, regulate Chong and Ren, activate Blood circulation, and remove Blood stasis.

9. Prescription

Ashi, Lingtai (GV 10), Hegu (LI 4), Quchi (LI 11), Zhongting (CV 16), Guanyuan (CV 4), Sanyinjiao (SP 6), Taichong (LR 3), Feishu (BL 13), Pishu (BL 20), Ganshu (BL 18), Geshu (BL 17), Shenshu (BL 23).

The reducing method for Taichong (LR 3), Quchi (LI 11) and Hegu (LI 4). The reinforcing method for Pishu (BL 20). Even method for the rest of points. Retaining of needles was 30 minutes. Once every other day.

TDP lamp radiation was used for the lower abdomen.

Pricking bleeding cupping was used on Feishu (BL 13) and Lingtai (GV 10), once a week.

In total the patient was treated 30 times.

10. Effect

Remarkably effective. The acne disappeared and no new acne appeared. The menstrual flow was increased. The cold feeling in the lower abdomen and extremities was getting better. The stools were improved.

11. Essentials

- The patient is 42 years old, so this is not a case of puberty acne, so regulating Chong and Ren is the key link for treatment.

- This is a complicated case of deficiency and excess, upper Heat with lower Cold. Bleeding cupping to clear Heat and remove stasis and reinforcing the Spleen and Kidneys at the same time are to treat both the root cause and symptoms.

SUMMARY

Acne is a chronic inflammatory skin disease of the hair follicles and sebaceous glands, mostly seen in the facial region of teenagers and middle-aged females, forming papilla, comedo or pustule, affecting the looks seriously. TCM holds that overeating rich food, damaging Spleen and Stomach, then producing Damp Heat that steams upward, or with the basis of accumulated Heat in the Lungs, invasion of Wind, or cold water washing, blocking the Blood Heat in the interior, are the causes of acne.

Syndrome of accumulated Heat in Lungs: Early stage of acne, with redness, swelling, pain, itching, dry mouth, yellow urine, dry stools, red tongue, yellow coating, superficial rapid pulse.

Syndrome of Damp Heat in the Spleen and Stomach: Acne falls and rises, yellowish greasy embolism or pus can be squeezed out, oily face, foul breath, bitter taste in the mouth, sometimes poor appetite, sticky stools not smooth in discharge, red tongue, yellow sticky coating, wiry rapid pulse.

Syndrome of Qi and Blood stagnation: Prolonged, purple dark acnes, in which papilla, pustule, nodule, and cyst are all present, known as 'compound acne'.

Prescription I: Hegu (LI 4), Fengchi (GB 20).

Local points: Quanliao (SI 18), Xiaguan (ST 7), Yingxiang (LI 20), Sibai (ST 2). Add Feishu (BL 13) and Lieque (LU 7) for Wind Heat in the Lungs; add Quchi (LI 11), Fenglong (ST 40), Yinlingquan (SP 9) and Sanyinjiao (SP 6) for Damp Heat of the Spleen and Stomach; add Xuehai (SP 10), Sanyinjiao (SP 6) and Taichong (LR 3) for Qi and Blood stagnation; add Zhigou (TE 6), Daheng (SP 15), Zhaohai (KI 6) and Sanyinjiao (SP 6) for constipation.

Prescription II: Dazhui (GV 14), Pishu (BL 20), Zusanli (ST 36), Hegu (LI 4), Sanyinjiao (SP 6).

Ear points: Lung, Shenmen, Sympathetic nerve, Endocrine, Adrenal, Subcortex.

Manipulation: Stick vaccaria seed (Wang Bu Liu Xing Zi) with adhesive plaster to the ear points. Press the points 3 times a day, 10 minutes each time.

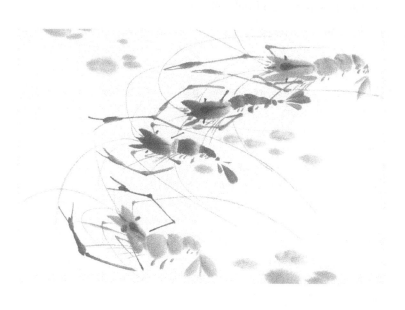

SECTION SEVEN • CHLOASMA

CASE I: FENG LI'S MEDICAL RECORD

1. General data

Zhang, female, 42 years old.

2. Chief complaint

Facial pigmentation for 1 year.

3. History of present illness

One year ago, she began to have facial pigmentation and it gradually became darker.

4. Present symptoms

Facial pigmentation, accompanied by listlessness, insomnia, scanty menstrual flow light in colour.

5. Tongue and pulse

Pale tongue, white coating, thready pulse.

6. Differentiation and analysis

The pigmentation of this case is from the Qi and Blood deficiency, facial skin lacks nourishment.

7. Diagnosis

TCM: Chloasma (Qi and Blood deficiency).

Western medicine: Chloasma.

8. Treating principle

Regulate the Zang Fu organs, replenish Qi and Blood, remove pigmentation, promote the looks.

9. Prescription

Pigmentation area, Hegu (LI 4), Sanyinjiao (SP 6), Zusanli (ST 36), Pishu (BL 20), Shenshu (BL 23), Ganshu (BL 18). Ear points: Cheek, Lung, Liver, Spleen, Kidney, Endocrine, Shenmen, Ovary, Internal Genitalia, Uterus.

The body points were punctured with retention of needles for 30 minutes after the arrival of Qi, once a day, 10 times as 1 course. The ear points were stimulated with vaccaria seeds, each ear used in turn.

10. Effect

After the first course of treatment, the pigmentation became light in colour and the accompanying symptoms were relieved. After 5 courses, the chloasma disappeared. The follow-up after 1 year found no recurrence.

11. Essentials

Puncturing the local area may regulate Qi, activate Blood, improve facial nourishment, strengthen cell regeneration, remove accumulated waste, and promote disappearance of pigmentation.

Hegu (LI 4) is for all diseases of facial region. Sanyinjiao (SP 6) is for regulating Qi of the Liver, Spleen and Kidneys. Zusanli (ST 36) is for strengthening the Spleen and Stomach, and tonifying the acquired foundation of the human body. Ganshu (BL 18), Pishu (BL 20) and Shenshu (BL 23) are for promoting the Spleen, Liver and Kidneys.

Ear points for chloasma follow the theory of ear-Zang Fu-channels relation: 'Ear is the convergence of all channels', and 'Qi and Blood of 12 channels and 365 collaterals go up to the face and ear. Hearing is formed with the Qi of divergent channels going to the ear.' Stimulation to those points relating to chloasma may remove obstruction of channels, regulate Qi and Blood, dissolve stasis, and reinforce the Liver and Kidneys, with the effect of improving the looks.

SUMMARY

Chloasma is the colour change of the facial skin to brown or light brown, mostly seen in the cheek and forehead regions, before and after delivery.

Prescription I: Feishu (BL 13), Ganshu (BL 18), Pishu (BL 20), Danshu (BL 19), Shenshu (BL 23), Sanjiaoshu (BL 22), Xuehai (SP 10), Taixi (KI 3), Taichong (LR 3).

Cupping is adopted at the Back-Shu points after needling.

Prescription II: Dazhui (GV 14), Feishu (BL 13), Geshu (BL 17), Xinshu (BL 15), Ganshu (BL 18).

Use one point each time, disinfect, prick with three-edged needle to cause bleeding, or tap with cutaneous needle until skin becomes reddish, then do cupping. The points are used in turn, once a day for strong patients and once every 2–3 days for weak ones. Five times as 1 course, 3–5 days for rest before the next course.

Ear points: Endocrine, Ovary, Cheek.

Added points: Subcortex, Lung, Liver, Spleen, Heart, Kidney, Adrenal, Internal Genitalia, Eye, Mouth, Forehead, Temple.

Select points according to the affected Zang Fu and channels and the locations of the brown spots. Endocrine, Subcortex and Internal Genitalia will be used in turn.

Manipulation: Stick vaccaria seed (Wang Bu Liu Xing Zi) with adhesive plaster to the ear points. The patient is asked to press 3 times a day, 10 minutes each time. Change seeds once every 3–4 days in summer and 5–6 days in other seasons. The ears are used alternately.

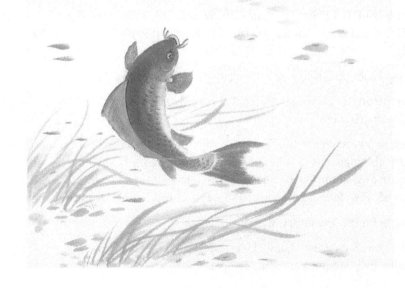

SECTION EIGHT • SPRAIN AND CONTUSION

CASE I: YANG JIEBIN'S MEDICAL RECORD

1. General data

Xu, female, 16 years old.

2. Chief complaint

Swelling and pain of the right ankle joint for 1 day.

3. History of present illness

One day ago, she got her right ankle joint sprained as a result of walking carelessly. Immediately the joint became swollen and blue purple with serious pain. She couldn't walk at all and couldn't sleep either because of the pain.

4. Present symptoms

The right ankle joint was swollen with serious pain, with the inability for the foot to touch the ground without pain. In palpation, there was no fracture and dislocation of bones.

5. Tongue and pulse

Light red tongue, thin white coating, superficial tight pulse.

6. Differentiation and analysis

The swelling and pain of ankle joint is from Blood stasis and Qi stagnation. The obstruction causes the pain and swelling.

7. Diagnosis

TCM: Sprain (Blood stasis, Qi stagnation).

Western medicine: Soft tissue injury.

8. Treating principle

Activate Blood, dissolve stasis, relieve swelling, stop pain.

9. Prescription

Qiuxu (GB 40), Kunlun (BL 60), Jiexi (ST 41), Ashi points.

Affected side only. Three-edged needle was used to prick for bleeding about 1ml, and cupping for drawing all Blood stasis out.

10. Effect

After needling, the pain was relieved. On the following day, the same treatment was given, the swelling basically disappeared. After the third session, her swelling and pain stopped completely and she could walk freely.

11. Essentials

Ankle sprain falls into the category of Shang Jin (injury of tendons) in TCM and soft tissue injury in Western medicine. *Plain Questions* (*Yin Yang Ying Xiang Da Lun*) says: 'Qi is injured, causing pain, tissue is injured, causing swelling.' So the manifestation is swelling and pain. The treating principle is to activate Blood, remove obstruction of the channels, relieve swelling and stop pain. Points of the affected channels in the local area are selected as the main ones to be pricked and cupped to 'remove the Blood stasis from channels to restore the balance of Yinyang', so she is cured.

SUMMARY

Sprain and contusion here refer to the injury of the soft tissues, including skin, muscles and tendons without fracture, dislocation or wound, caused by violent movement, awkward posture of the body, bruising, falling, traction or overtwisting, resulting in local stagnation of Qi and Blood in the channels of the diseased areas, with manifestation of pain and swelling of the injured areas, and motor impairment of the joints. For the treatment, Ashi points are used as principal ones with the combination of distal points of involved channels to ease tendons and activate Blood circulation. Pricking and cupping to cause bleeding in the local area, and moxibustion applied if necessary, are adopted to relieve swelling and pain and speed up the recovery of the injured tissues.

SECTION NINE • GANGLION

CASE I: YANG YONGXUAN'S MEDICAL RECORD

1. General data

Sun, a 56-year-old female.

2. Chief complaint

A cyst on the dorsum of her right wrist for several months.

3. History of present illness

The cyst appeared without a clear reason. She hadn't received any treatment yet.

4. Present symptoms

The cyst was as big as a peach seed, movable, painful when pressed.

5. Tongue and pulse

6. Differentiation and analysis

Ganglion, called Jin Jie (tendon knot) in TCM, is a hard cyst often occurring at the wrist or ankle joint regions, caused by tiredness damaging the tendons.

7. Diagnosis

TCM: Jin Jie (obstruction of channels by Phlegm Damp retention).

Western medicine: Ganglion.

8. Treating principle

Remove stagnation, warm and unobstruct channels.

9. Prescription

In the cyst area, Qi Ci Needling (Triple Puncture) was applied, in which the needles were inserted at three spots simultaneously with one in the centre and two on both sides. Warming-needle moxibustion was used in combination.

10. Effect

The cyst got smaller and soft gradually, and was cured 4 treatments later.

11. Essentials

Qi Ci Needling (Triple Puncture) and warming-needle moxibustion are used in combination to warm channels and collaterals to dissolve the mass and swelling.

SUMMARY

For the treatment of ganglion, the jelly fluid should be drained out with one of the following methods:

- Use a thick acupuncture needle, prick to break the ganglion from its top, squeeze the jelly fluid out. One week later, repeat the procedure if the cyst appears again.

- Warming-needle method. In a mild case, insert one needle into the centre of ganglion deeply to its base, put a piece of moxa-stick on the needle to do warming-needle moxibustion. After several treatments in this way, the ganglion will disappear. For prolonged cases, Qi Ci Needling (Triple Puncture) should be applied, in which the needles are inserted at three spots simultaneously with one in the centre and two on both sides, to strengthen the stimulation.

- Surrounding with filiform needles. Insert two needles at the base of ganglion transversely, making a '+' inside it, and insert one needle on its top. After removing the needles, press to force the jelly fluid out to lie between skin and muscles.

- Fire needling. Push the ganglion away to one side, Heat the needle on the alcohol burner to red, prick the ganglion deeply, avoiding blood vessels, and squeeze the jelly fluid out.

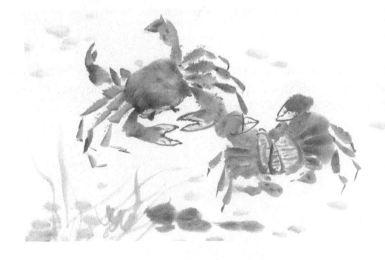

SECTION TEN • HEEL PAIN

CASE I: HU JINSHENG'S MEDICAL RECORD

1. General data

Liang, female, 46 years old.

2. Chief complaint

Heel pain for 3 months.

3. History of present illness

She got heel pain, especially on the left side, without any clear reasons. In the morning when she got up touching the ground the pain started and became worse and worse in walking.

4. Present symptoms

Severe tenderness at the sole and slight tenderness on both sides of the plantae. X-ray film showed a slight hyperosteogeny of heel.

5. Tongue and pulse

Slim tongue, light red, little coating; deep thready pulse.

6. Differentiation and analysis

The Kidneys dominate the bones, including the heel. The Kidney Meridian passes through and winds round and enters the heel. The patient has the symptoms of Kidney deficiency, soreness in the lumbus and tiredness. The heel pain is the manifestation of Kidney deficiency, because the bone is lacking in nourishment from the Kidney Essence.

7. Diagnosis

TCM: Heel pain (due to the Kidney deficiency).

Western medicine: Slight hyperosteogeny of heel.

8. Treating principle

Reinforce the Kidneys, calm the Mind.

9. Prescription

Zusanli (ST 36), Sanyinjiao (SP 6), Taixi (KI 3), Shenmen (HT 7), Neiguan (PC 6), Ashi.

10. Effect

The points were selected according to the syndrome differentiation. Ashi points were used together. After one time of acupuncture, the pain was getting better. Five treatments relieved the heel pain greatly. After 1 course of treatment, the heel pain on the right side stopped. Totally 15 times of treatment cured her.

11. Essentials

For heel pain, the Ashi points are more important. One to four needles can be used according to the severity of the pain. For the mild case, one needle is inserted in the centre of the painful area. For the serious case, the both sides and the back part of the heel were punctured respectively.

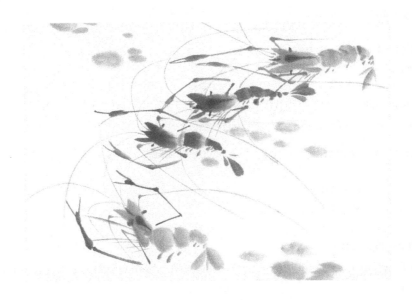

SECTION ELEVEN • LOCKJAW

CASE I: WU ZHONGCHAO'S MEDICAL RECORD

1. General data

Chen, male, 58 years old.

2. Chief complaint

Lockjaw (bird-beak like) for half a year.

3. History of present illness

Three months ago, one day in the morning, the patient felt that his mouth was uncomfortable, and subsequently discovered that it was difficult to open his mouth. He could only open his mouth as big as a bird mouth. He had to use a straw to drink water and ate bit by bit with chopsticks. In hospital, the doctor in oral surgery thought it was a problem of the mandibular joint, but there were no abnormal findings in various examinations; the doctor in the neurology department thought it was a disease of the brain, but there were no abnormal findings in various examinations; while the doctor in orthopedics thought it was a bone tumour, but there were no abnormal findings in various examinations. Treatment with mouth-gag, injection of muscle relaxant, and nerve block therapy was not applied because of the unclear diagnosis and side effects. The medication of oryzanol and herbs plus acupuncture was not helpful in relieving the symptoms.

4. Present symptoms

Lockjaw (bird-beak like), depression, emaciation, sallow complexion.

5. Tongue and pulse

Tongue tip red, Blood spots on the borders; pulse weak and string-taut.

6. Diagnosis

TCM: Lockjaw (Qi deficiency, Liver stagnation).

Western medicine: Unclear.

7. Differentiation and analysis

From the patient's appearance and the pulse as well as the progress of the disease, we knew that at present the main aspect of his condition was 'deficiency', which was caused by the difficulty in opening his mouth. Based on the principle that 'treat the Biao-symptom first when it is acute and treat the Ben-root after the acute symptom is relieved', opening his mouth was the most important thing for treatment. Otherwise, the deficiency will result in stagnation until he could eat and express his emotions.

8. Treating principle

Treat the acute symptom first, open his mouth.

9. Prescription

Hegu (LI 4) and Taichong (LR 3) of both sides.

Four doctors punctured him at the same time. The needles were inserted in the routine way, after arrival of Qi, the four doctors manipulate the needles continuously in a large amplitude with an even method to produce strong stimulation until he could open his mouth. Then the needles were removed without retaining.

Hegu (LI 4) is the point for all diseases of the face and mouth. To open the mouth of this patient, Hegu (LI 4) is used as a first point. The patient had a serious psychological burden, manifested as the Liver stagnation, therefore, his pulse was string-taut. Taichong (LR 3) which is the Yuan-Primary point of the Liver Meridian is also important. Because his lockjaw is of 3 months duration already, repeated treatment had lowered the points' sensitivity, so strong stimulation should be given for the result.

10. Effect

The manipulation of needles was continuous until the patient could open his mouth. One treatment cured him.

11. Essentials

Lockjaw, trismus, means the mouth is closed. To open the mouth means to open the gate. Hegu (LI 4) and Taichong (LR 3) are known as the 'Four Gates' points. Gate and gate are put in communication with each other, when one of them is open the other will be open too.

During these three months, the patient had had acupuncture many times already, including Hegu (LI 4) and Taichong (LR 3), but without an effective result, the reason being that the stimulation was not strong enough. First, his condition was prolonged, so he was not sensitive to the general stimulation any more. Second, his weak constitution with deficiency of meridian Qi needed the external help to move the meridian Qi to the facial region to relax the locked joint.

Postscript: Next day in the morning, I came to the clinic and discovered that this patient was sitting there and was waiting for me. He had continuous hiccups. He said he began to have the hiccups since last night after his meal. After seeing his tongue, I understood that his Stomach Qi had become weakened because of the long period of no eating. Yesterday he had overeaten, and his Spleen and Stomach could not receive such a big burden all of a sudden. I pressed his tongue root with a tongue depressor. After vomiting a lot of vomitus he was cured completely.

SECTION TWELVE • OLD TRAUMATIC INJURY COMPLICATED WITH INFECTION

CASE I: LIU ZHAOHUI'S MEDICAL RECORD

1. General data

Liu, female, 70 years old, came on December 25, 2001.

2. Chief complaint

The right index and middle fingers were red, swollen and painful for 1 month.

3. History of present illness

One month ago, her right index and middle fingers were injured by the window frame falling down. The pain was serious and the two nails became blue with Blood stasis. She herself dressed the wound with the gauze sterilized with Rivanol and had the dressing changed once every 3 days. One month later, the pain and swelling still existed.

4. Present symptoms

The right index and middle fingers were dark red and swelling, the oozing of the yellowish fluid was from around the nails. The pain, especially at night, was serious, making her sleep disturbed. The motor impairment of two fingers was normal. The patient was emaciated, pale, looking tired and thin.

5. Tongue and pulse

Pale tongue with white coating, thready weak pulse.

6. Differentiation and analysis

The old lady of this age was deficient in Qi and Blood, the wound was at the ending of a limb, and the obstructed Qi and Blood had existed for a long time and transformed into Heat causing infection.

7. Diagnosis

TCM: Fingers' traumatic injury with infection (Qi stagnation with Blood stasis transforming into Heat).

Western medicine: Fingers' traumatic injury complicated with infection.

8. Treating principle

Promote Blood circulation to dissolve Blood stasis, clear internal head.

9. Prescription

Moxibustion was selected. Method: The bundle with 3 moxa-sticks in it was ignited and blown to make the Fire strong. The moving moxibustion was done at the affected area with Heat according to the endurance of the patient for 10–15 minutes.

10. Effect

After treatment for 3 days in succession, the redness and swelling and the pain were greatly relieved and the oozing stopped. The moxibustion changed to once every other day. After 5 treatments, the redness and swelling disappeared, the nails fell off. The pain stopped. The joints moved freely. There was only a slight numbness of tips of fingers.

11. Essentials

Western medicine alone was not enough to remove this Blood stasis. But the reducing moxibustion acts to clear the local Heat and to activate Qi and Blood to produce new Blood. Thus the functions of moxibustion in stopping pain and promoting the growth of new muscles for anti-inflammation make the healing of the wound quicker.

OTHER CONDITIONS

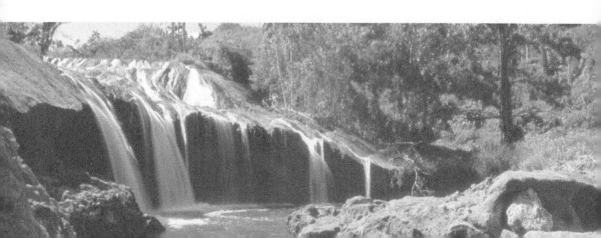

SECTION ONE • SUNSTROKE

CASE I: YANG JIEBIN'S MEDICAL RECORD

1. General data

Xia, female, 29.

2. Chief complaint

Headache and nausea for 2 hours.

3. History of present illness

It was in summer. She felt a splitting headache and had irritability and nausea. She came for acupuncture.

4. Present symptoms

Splitting headache, sickly complexion, rough breathing, congested vessels like red threads in eyes, irritability, strong thirst, profuse sweating, and nausea.

Examination: Temperature: 41°C.

5. Tongue and pulse

Yellow sticky coating, soft rapid pulse.

6. Differentiation and analysis

In the height of summer, invasion of the Damp and summer Heat mists the Heart, the ascending of clean Yang is disturbed, so there is headache and nausea. Summer Heat consumes Qi and Body Fluid, causing strong thirst and profuse sweating. The manifestations of her tongue and pulse are also the signs of summer Heat.

7. Diagnosis

TCM: Sunstroke (Yang Summer-Heat syndrome, Heat damaging the Mind stored in the Heart).

Western medicine: Sunstroke.

8. Treating principle

Promote resuscitation, reduce body temperature, remove Heat caused by Summer Heat.

9. Prescription

Dazhui (GV 14), Taiyang (EX-HN5), Shangyang (LI 1), Zhongchong (PC 9), Shaoze (SI 1), Weizhong (BL 40).

Dazhui (GV 14) was pricked and cupped for bleeding. Other points were pricked with ensiform needle for bleeding. She was given warm light saline to drink.

10. Effect

Two hours later, her fever was reduced and her Mind was clear again. She went home by herself.

11. Essentials

The serious case of sunstroke may manifest as loss of consciousness, profuse sweating, cold extremities, shallow and abrupt respiration, and feeble pulse. For the treatment, Professor Yang Jiebin's Five Centre points, namely, Baihui (GV 20), the brain centre, both Laogong (PC 8), two palm centres, and both Yongquan (KI 1), two sole centres, is suggested. The effect is better and quicker if acupuncture and moxibustion are used together or in combination with Renzhong (GV 26) and Shixuan (EX-UE11).

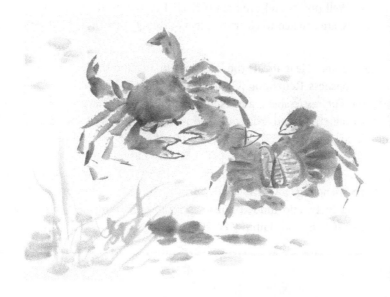

SUMMARY

Sunstroke is an acute disease in which the disordered thermotaxic function or even peripheral circulatory failure is caused by working under the scorching sun or in a place of high temperature. Often seen in summer, it is generally called Fa Sha. With symptoms such as dizziness, headache, and nausea, it is Shang Shu; with sudden loss of consciousness, it is Yun Jue; with convulsions, it is Shu Feng. Professor Yang Jiebin treats it with the pricking-bleeding method, and the result is very good. Over many years clinical practice, he summarized two groups of points named the Clearing Summer-Heat Prescription.

1. Dazhui (GV 14), Taiyang (EX-HN5), Shangyang (LI 1), Zhongchong (PC 9), Shaoze (SI 1), Weizhong (BL 40).

2. Dazhu (BL 11), Zanzhu (BL 2), Shaoshang (LU 11), Guanchong (TE 1), Shixuan (EX-UE11), Quze (PC 3).

Usage: After routine disinfection, prick Dazhui (GV 14) and Dazhu (BL 11) with the ensiform needle and cup to draw 4–5ml of the dark Blood out. Other points are pricked to bleed 0.5–1ml, Quze (PC 3) and Weizhong (BL 40) can bleed 3–4ml.

Explanation: The extreme hot weather in summer can cause sunstroke based on the weak constitution. Dazhui (GV 14) and Dazhu (BL 11) are selected to clear Heat through pricking bleeding. Taiyang (EX-HN5) and Zanzhu (BL 2) can clear the Heat of the Upper Burner. Summer Heat is a Yang pathogenic factor, likely to affect the Pericardium and damage the Qi and Yin of the human body. Quze (PC 3) and Weizhong (BL 40) may reduce the Heat of the Pericardium and Blood system. Jing-Well points and Shixuan (EX-UE11), the meeting places of Yin and Yang channels, are pricked to clear the Heat of the Qi and Yin systems to promote resuscitation.

In case the Summer Heat affects the Pericardium, misting the Heart, manifested as loss of consciousness, Renzhong (GV 26) and Baihui (GV 20) are added to promote resuscitation. For restlessness, add Neiguan (PC 6) and Shenmen (HT 7) to rest the Heart to calm the Mind. For convulsions, add Houxi (SI 3), Yanglingquan (GB 34) and Chengshan (BL 57) to relax the muscles. For vomiting and diarrhoea, add Zhongwan (CV 12), Tianshu (ST 25) and Zusanli (ST 36) to harmonize the Middle Burner and regulate the Fu-intestine Qi. For dizziness and blurred vision, add Sishencong (EX-HN1) and Taichong (LR 3) to remove Wind Yang. For sweating, cold limbs and hidden pulse, apply moxibustion heavily at Guanyuan (CV 4), Qihai (CV 6) and Baihui (GV 20) to restore Yang to treat collapse.

SECTION TWO • OBESITY

CASE I: TAN XIAOHONG'S MEDICAL RECORD

1. General data

Anonymous female, 53, came on January 8, 1995.

2. Chief complaint

Obesity for 12 years.

3. History of present illness

She had a history of obesity for 12 years. She came for acupuncture.

4. Present symptoms

Her body weight was about 300 pounds. She had a voracious appetite and shortness of breath which was worse on exertion.

5. Tongue and pulse

Yellow and slightly sticky coating, rolling pulse.

6. Differentiation and analysis

Obesity, according to TCM, it is due to Phlegm. 'Fat people have Phlegm and slim people have Fire.' Phlegm retained for a long time will be transformed into Heat. The Stomach with Heat in it will digest quickly and feel hungry all the time. So the patient always eats voraciously.

7. Diagnosis

TCM: Obesity (Phlegm Damp retention).

Western medicine: Obesity.

8. Treating principle

Dissolve Phlegm Damp, regulate Qi of Middle Burner.

9. Prescription

Liangqiu (ST 34), Gongsun (SP 4), Neiguan (PC 6), Fenglong (ST 40), Zusanli (ST 36). Ear points: Lung, Endocrine, Triple Burner, Stomach, Intestine, Shenmen (HT 7), Hunger.

The reducing method was used for the body points. Twice a week. Ear points were pressed with herbal vaccaria seeds, which were changed once every 3 days. Each ear were used by turn.

She was asked to press the ear points several times before meals, to be on a diet of more vegetables and less oily food, and do more exercises.

10. Effect

After the first 2 treatments in the first week, she felt very well. She said that by pressing the ear points, her appetite could be reduced. Her body weight was reduced by 4 pounds. She felt confident. With more than 20 treatments, her weight was reduced by 3–4 pounds each week and in total 42 pounds. The symptoms of palpitations and shortness of breath disappeared. She was in a good mood.

11. Essentials

The points selected from Spleen and Stomach channels are the main ones for her treatment. Fenglong (ST 40) and Zusanli (ST 36) to strengthen the Spleen to dissolve Phlegm. Liangqiu (ST 34), Xi-Cleft point, Gongsun (SP 4), Luo-Connecting point, to regulate the Spleen and Stomach, dissolve Phlegm, and reduce Stomach Heat. Neiguan (PC 6) to regulate Stomach Qi. Western medicine reports that puncturing Gongsun (SP 4), Neiguan (PC 6) and Liangqiu (ST 34) functions to inhibit the gastric acid secretion; puncturing Gongsun (SP 4) weakens the gastric peristalsis. The ear points Lung, Triple Burner, Spleen and Stomach have the functions to regulate absorption and excretion, and promote metabolism and induce diuresis; Endocrine to regulate the endocrine system. With the combination of body and ear points, the metabolism of the human body is regulated, the voracious appetite reduced, thus, the body weight decreased.

SUMMARY

When the fat of human body is over accumulated and the body weight is 20% more than normal, it is known as obesity.

Standard body weight: height (cm)−105 = weight (kg). If the weight (kg)/[height (metre)]^2 24 (for Chinese body type) this constitutes obesity. In simple obesity, secondary obesity and other cases, acupuncture is mainly used for the simple cases.

Main points: Zhongwan (CV 12), Shuifen (CV 9), Guanyuan (CV 4), Sanyinjiao (SP 6), Wailing (ST 26), Tianshu (ST 25), Huaroumen (ST 24).

Accompanying points: Add Quchi (LI 11), Hegu (LI 4), Shangjuxu (ST 37), Neiting (ST 44) for excess Heat of Stomach and intestines; add Zusanli (ST 36), Fenglong (ST 40), Yinlingquan (SP 9) for Phlegm Damp retention; add Zusanli (ST 36), Sanyinjiao (SP 6), Pishu (BL 20), Shenshu (BL 23) for Spleen and Kidney Qi deficiency; add Zhigou (TE 6) penetrating to Neiguan (PC 6), Zusanli (ST 36), Shangjuxu (ST 37) for constipation; add Quchi (LI 11) and Taichong (LR 3) for hypertension; add Neiguan (PC 6), Sanyinjiao (SP 6), Shanzhong (CV 17) for coronary heart diseases; add Zusanli (ST 36), Sanyinjiao (SP 6), Yangchi (TE 4) for diabetes.

Shangwan (CV 13), Guanmen (ST 22), Huaroumen (ST 24) are selected to reduce the fat of the abdomen above the umbilicus; Fujie (SP 14), Daju (ST 27), Shuidao (ST 28) for reducing the fat of the abdomen below the umbilicus Daimai (GB 26), Fengshi (GB 31), Zhishi (BL 52) for reducing the fat in the waist region; Zhibian (BL 54), Chengfu (BL 36), Ashi points for reducing the fat in the hip region; Binao (LI 14), Jianyu (LI 15), Quchi (LI 11) for reducing the fat of the upper limbs; Futu (ST 32), Liangqiu (ST 34), Fenglong (ST 40), Ashi points for reducing the fat of the lower limbs.

Generally, 2–3 cun filiform needles are used, puncture with the reducing or even method, once every day or every other day, retain for 30–60 minutes, 15 times as 1 course, 3 days rest before the next course.

Ear points: Endocrine, Brain Point, Stomach, Spleen, Kidney, Liver, Large Intestine, Lung, Heart.

Five or six points are selected each time, once or twice a week. Each ear is used in turn. Press before meals every day.

At the same time, you need to pay attention to the diet and lifestyle and do exercises as well. Especially, when the effect is achieved in weight loss, the patient should be very careful about the diet and good lifestyle and should do exercises to prevent weight gain again.

SECTION THREE • CHRONIC FATIGUE SYNDROME

CASE I: HE PUREN'S MEDICAL RECORD

1. General data

Anonymous male, 41, came on September 6, 2004.

2. Chief complaint

Insomnia for 2 weeks, headache for 1 week.

3. History of present illness

He was a policeman, began to have insomnia 2 weeks ago because of the work pressure.

4. Present symptoms

Insomnia, headache, fatigue, hot temper and irritability.

Examination: BP: 140/80mmHg.

5. Tongue and pulse

Tip and borders of tongue red, coating yellow sticky and slightly dry, pulse wiry and rolling.

6. Differentiation and analysis

Hard work is the cause of dysfunctions of the Liver in keeping the free flow of Qi. Later the stagnated Liver Qi is transformed into Fire. The Mind stored in the Heart gets disturbed for the Liver Fire flares up. That's why he has insomnia. The Liver Fire flaring affects the head, resulting in headache, hot temper, and irritability. His red tongue and yellow sticky coating and wiry rolling pulse are also the manifestations of Liver Fire excess.

7. Diagnosis

TCM: Insomnia (Liver Yang hyperactivity).

Western medicine: Chronic fatigue syndrome.

8. Treating principle

Soothe the Liver, clear Heat.

9. Prescription

Gaohuang (BL 43), Geshu (BL 17), Danshu (BL 19).

Strong-removing method (Qiang Tong Fa) was adopted. Manipulation: Pinch the punctured area with the left hand, hold the three-edged needle with the right hand and prick the points quickly, squeeze to bleed. Then, do cupping at the punctured points to bleed again with the cups retained for 5–10 minutes until 10–15m1 Blood was drawn out. Less bleeding, less effect. Once a week. Generally, with 1–3 times of treatment, a satisfactory result would be achieved.

10. Effect

After 1 treatment, the patient felt relieved and his sleep improved. After 3 treatments, his sleep symptoms stopped. He was cured later with herbal medication.

11. Essentials

Gaohuang (BL 43), located below the spinous process of the fourth thoracic vertebra and 3 cun lateral to the midline, Geshu (BL 17), located below the spinous process of the seventh thoracic vertebra and 1.5 cun lateral to the midline, and Danshu (BL 19), located below the spinous process of the tenth thoracic vertebra and 1.5 cun lateral to the midline. The latter two are known as the Four-Flower points. The ancient acupuncture literature reported that these points were used to treat chronic deficiency diseases which are similar to the subhealthy state of many nowadays. Massive clinical reports and lab experiments have also proved the good effect of these points for deficiency diseases.

STRONG-REMOVING METHOD (QIANG TONG FA)
One of the He's three-removing methods (San Tong Fa), namely, prick with the three-edged needle the superficial veins at certain areas of the body to bleed so as to regulate the Blood, by doing which, to regulate Qi, to restore the functions of Qi and Blood of the Zang Fu organs.

SUMMARY

Chronic fatigue syndrome (CFS), known as the subhealthy state or the third state, referring to a low quality state between diseased and healthy state of health, with the manifestations of somatic and psychological symptoms. The somatic symptoms are chronic fatigue of the body, lasting and difficult to recover from tiredness, accompanied by sleep disturbance, headache, lowered resistance and disordered metabolism, while the psychological symptoms are anxiety, depression, irritability, restlessness, hot temper, and always feeling scared.

Prescription I: Gaohuang (BL 43), Four-Flower points. He's strong-removing method (Qiang Tong Fa).

Prescription II: Xinshu (BL 15), Ganshu (BL 18), Pishu (BL 20), Shenshu (BL 23), Feishu (BL 13).

Added points: Zusanli (ST 36) and Baihui (GV 20) for Qi deficiency, Guanyuan (CV 4) and Qihai (CV 6) for Qi and Blood deficiency; Sanyinjiao (SP 6) and Qihai (CV 6) for Qi and Yin deficiency; Taichong (LR 3) and Zusanli (ST 36) for Qi deficiency and Liver Qi stagnation; Zusanli (ST 36) and Sanyinjiao (SP 6) for Qi deficiency with Blood stasis; Taichong (LR 3) and Yinlingquan (SP 9) for disharmony between Liver and Spleen; Mingmen (GV 4) and Dachangshu (BL 25) for Spleen and Kidney Yang deficiency; Taixi (KI 3) and Taichong (LR 3) for Liver and Kidney Yin deficiency.

The Back-Shu points are the sites where the Qi of the Zang Fu organs is infused. Puncturing the Back-Shu points can regulate the Qi of the Zang Fu organs. With normal circulation of Qi and Blood, all the tissues and organs of human body are well nourished and the patient does not feel tired.

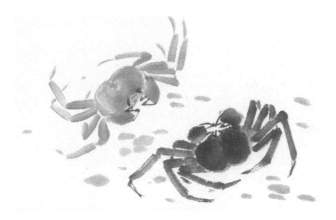

SECTION FOUR • ABSTINENCE SYNDROME

CASE I: TAN XIAOHONG'S MEDICAL RECORD

1. General data

Anonymous female, 63, paid her first visit on February 18, 1995.

2. Chief complaint

Smoking cigarettes for 35 years.

3. History of present illness

Every day she smoked more than 35 cigarettes. She tried many times to stop smoking but failed. She heard that acupuncture could help stop smoking, so she came to try.

4. Present symptoms

She smoked like a chimney, every day more than 35 cigarettes.

5. Tongue and pulse

6. Differentiation and analysis

Smoking produces Heat, consuming the Heart Yin Blood. The Mind stored in the Heart gets disturbed, so she is addicted to smoking.

7. Diagnosis

TCM: Smoking withdrawal syndrome.

Western medicine: Smoking withdrawal syndrome.

8. Treating principle

Replenish Yin and Blood, ease the Heart, calm the Mind.

9. Prescription

Tianmei (a new point for stopping smoking).

She was asked to inhale and hold the breath when the needle was inserted and after insertion to exhale. The needle was rotated. Ten minutes later, she tried to smoke and the cigarette felt tasteless and she had no desire to finish this cigarette. The needle was removed after 20 minutes of retaining.

Ear points: Mouth, Lung, Triple Burner, Endocrine.

Herbal vaccaria seeds were stuck at ear points and the patient pressed them several times a day.

10. Effect

On the fouth day, she came and said that she stopped smoking completely, the only problem was that she felt like something was lost and she didn't know what to do with both hands. The same treatment was given and she was told not to worry. One week later, she felt everything was normal and she was in a good mood. The follow-up after 1 month found she had not begun smoking again.

11. Essentials

Tianmei is a specific point for stopping smoking discovered by accident by the American doctor James. S. Olms. Tianmei means that after stopping smoking the patient can taste the deliciousness of food. Its location is generally described at the midpoint between Yangxi (LI 5) and Lieque (LU 7). But treatment given on these points is not very effective. According to Dr. James S. Olms, it is at about one finger-breadth from the border of styloid process of radius, in the small soft depression near Lieque (LU 7). Olms thinks that most patients have difficulty reaching this depression by touching by hand, but if you use a pair of curved nose pliers to press around Lieque (LU 7), it is easy to get it. The needle can be inserted into the depression 3–4mm without falling down, like a key into a lock. In case it is not exactly located, with the error only 1–2mm from it, the needle cannot stand, and the result will not be as good as it should be. Tianmei is a good point to stop smoking, the important thing is whether it is exactly located or not.

CASE II: FAN HONG'S MEDICAL RECORD

1. General data

Wang, female, 25.

2. Chief complaint

Addiction to heroin for 7 years.

3. History of present illness

Seven years ago, she began to smoke heroin because she was curious about it. Gradually she smoked as much as 3g, 5–6 times in a day, and fell asleep; 3 hours later, she woke up and smoked again, so all day long she was in a half anaesthesia state. When she stopped smoking she had abstinence symptoms and when she started smoking again the symptoms disappeared. She tried 7 times to stop smoking but failed. When she came to drug-relief reformatory, it was 30 hours after her last time of smoking.

4. Present symptoms

Clear consciousness, listlessness, pupils 0. 25cm, symmetrical, sensitive light reflex, heart rate 96/min, regular rhythm, body weight 47kg, skin looking like chicken skin, yawning all the time and with tears, nausea, vomiting, irritability with a sensation like a cat scratching her Heart and ants walking in her bones.

5. Tongue and pulse

6. Differentiation and analysis

Drug smoking can exhaust the Qi, Blood, Yin and Yang of human body, leading to the decline of functions of the Zang Fu organs, there occurs various symptoms.

7. Diagnosis

TCM: Heroin withdrawal syndrome.

Western medicine: Heroin withdrawal syndrome.

8. Treating principle

Reinforce the functions of the Zang Fu organs.

9. Prescription

Dazhui (GV 14), Shenmen (HT 7), Neiguan (PC 6), Shixuan (EX-UE11).

The needle was rotated continuously for 5 minutes with strong stimulation. Bleeding was at Shixuan (EX-UE11). Dazhui (GV 14) and Neiguan (PC 6) were used alternatively each time. The added points were selected accordingly.

10. Effect

On the following day, her nausea, vomiting, running nose and tears were obviously less, and sleep was better. Now she felt soreness and tiredness in the lower back, and her chicken skin was much relieved. Shangyang (LI 1) and Zulinqi (GB 41) were added for treatment.

On the third day, the withdrawal symptoms were basically stopped. Now she was easily woken up and it was difficult to fall asleep again. There was no more chicken skin. Yongquan (KI 1) and Baihui (GV 20) were added.

On the fourth day, her sleep was not good. She had soreness in the lower back. The pupils, heart rate, blood pressure and skin were normal.

On the seventh day, the urine test showed a heroin negative. Her addiction disappeared. The body weight increased to 49kg. The treatment for heroin withdrawal syndrome was successful.

11. Essentials

The main points are Neiguan (PC 6) and Dazhui (GV 14). Each time use one of them. On the first day, Shaochong (HT 9) and Shenmen (HT 7) are added; on the second day, Shangyang (LI 1) and Zulinqi (GB 41) added; on the third day, Hegu (LI 4) and Zusanli (ST 36) or Gongsun (SP 4) and Zhigou (TE 6) added for dysfunctions of gastrointestinal tract; Shenmen (HT 7) and Sanyinjiao (SP 6) or Baihui (GV 20) and Yongquan (KI 1) added for insomnia; Shuigou (GV 26) and Yongquan (KI 1) added for unconsciousness; Zhongchong (PC 9) and Laogong (PC 8) or Shixuan (EX-UE11) and Dazhui (GV 14) added for serious irritability.

Neiguan (PC 6) rests the Heart to calm the Mind, regulates Qi in chest, harmonizes Stomach to stop vomiting; Dazhui (GV 14) ascends Yang and reinforces Qi, removes Heat and tonifies deficiency; Shaochong (HT 9) promotes resuscitation, clears the Mind and reduces toxic Heat; Shenmen (HT 7) calms the Mind, removes Fire from the Ying system; Shangyang (LI 1) promotes resuscitation, clears Heat and stops spasm; Zulinqi (GB 41) dispels Wind, reduces Fire and clears the Mind; Hegu (LI 4) harmonizes the Stomach and removes obstruction of intestines; Zusanli (ST 36) regulates intestines and Stomach to reinforce anti-pathogenic Qi; Gongsun (SP 4), Luo-Connecting point, connecting with Chong Vessel, regulates Spleen and Stomach and Chong Vessel; Zhigou (TE 6) clears Heat and promotes bowel movements; Sanyinjiao (SP 6), a meeting point of three Yin channels of the foot, especially strengthens the Spleen and calms the Mind; Baihui (GV 20), known as Three-Yang Five-Hui, especially calms the Mind and soothes the Liver; Shuigou (GV 26), Yongquan (KI 1), Zhongchong (PC 9), Laogong (PC 8) and Shixuan (EX-UE11) promote resuscitation and clear Heart Fire.

The above-mentioned points activate channel Qi, reinforce anti-pathogenic Qi, remove pathogenic Qi, regulate Yinyang, treating Biao-symptom and Ben-root at the same time to stop drug-addiction.

This case report comes from Shanghai Rehabilitation Centre of Police Bureau. In the report, Neiguan (PC 6) and Dazhui (GV 14) are used as the main points for the treatment of 20 cases of Heroin Abstinence syndrome. During the treatment, all morphine receptor excitants are not allowed and they are without any sedatives for help either. The result is that 19 of them steadily pass through the withdrawal fastigium, indicating that acupuncture can relieve the abstinence symptoms of heroin reliers, and is helpful for abstinence from drugs.

CASE III: CI SHUIXIN AND SHANG YINJIA'S MEDICAL RECORD

1. General data

Anonymous male, 27, paid his first visit on November 14, 1993.

2. Chief complaint

Heroin smoking for 6 years.

3. History of present illness

He smoked heroin 6 years ago, and later became addicted to it. Every day he smoked about 1g, 2–3 times. In the recent 2 years, being aware of its harmfulness, he tried to withdraw but failed twice. Now he came for acupuncture treatment. He felt dizziness with blurred vision and weakness in the whole body. He had nasal obstruction, poor appetite, insomnia, forgetfulness, and at night he could only fall asleep by taking 30 diazepam tablets.

4. Present symptoms

Emaciation, listlessness, dull eyes, dark complexion, running tears and nose.

5. Tongue and pulse

Light red tongue, thin white coating, deep weak pulse.

6. Differentiation and analysis

Drug addiction consumes the anti-pathogenic Qi, making Yin Yang Qi Blood consumed, then the functions of the Zang Fu organs decline. The pathogenic condition of this patient is Yang deficiency with drug toxin deposited in the interior. His Qi and Blood both became deficient.

7. Diagnosis

TCM: Heroin withdrawal syndrome (Yang deficiency with toxin deposited in the interior).

Western medicine: Heroin withdrawal syndrome.

8. Treating principle

Restore Yang, conduct toxin out.

9. Prescription

Zhigou (TE 6), Baihui (GV 20).

Even method, with the needles retained for 50 minutes. With the gentle and comfortable needling sensation, the patient felt the nasal obstruction removed

5 minutes later and was clear minded. His tears and running nose stopped. The needles were manipulated every 10 minutes by scratching the handle 9 times, which is a Yang figure, with the meaning to lead to Yang.

10. Effect

The patient felt comfortable similar to being relaxed by smoking heroin during the acupuncture treatment which lasted 50 minutes. That night he didn't take any medicine and fell asleep. At midnight he was woken up by the drug addiction with pain in all joints, irritability, and running tears and nose. With the help of massage and 4 diazepam tablets he slept again with difficulty.

The second visit: Baihui (GV 20), Zhigou (TE 6), Quchi (LI 11), Hegu (LI 4), Taichong (LR 3), Sanyinjiao (SP 6).

The same technique was adopted. About 10 minutes later, the patient felt irritable and aching all over the body. The adjustment of needling sensation and spiritual comfort calmed him again. The needles were retained for 2 hours, during which he twice slept briefly. Two hours later, his dizziness and pain stopped, he felt hungry and clear minded.

In total he was treated 10 times. He became energetic again and went back to work.

11. Essentials

Following the treating principle, the treatment should aim at restoring Yang and driving the toxin out.

Zhigou (TE 6) is to regulate Sanjiao, Triple Burner and promote Yang Qi to drive the toxin out; Baihui (GV 20) is to restore Yang and reinforce Qi.

Acupuncture-moxibustion is an effective and simple way to stop heroin addiction and eliminate heroin poisoning, worth becoming more widely known.

SUMMARY

Abstinence syndrome refers to the group of symptoms that appear in smoking-withdrawal, alcohol-withdrawal and drug-withdrawal. Acupuncture is an ideal therapy in treating addiction to various substances. Its advantage is not only to change the addiction behaviour temporarily but also to make this a lasting change, thus worth spreading information about it. Although massive clinical and experimental studies have already been carried out, the selection of points and their functional mechanism need to be studied further, and what is more, some animal experiments have not yet provided convincing achievements. Here are some successful cases described for reference.

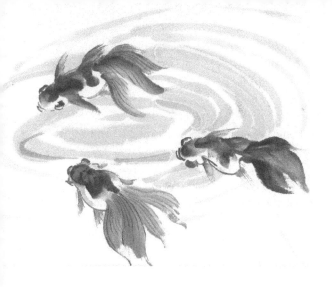

GLOSSARY

Angioneurotic   Relating to angioneuroses (conditions attributed to the dysfunction of the vasomotor system).

Antral gastritis   A digestive condition characterized by the inflammation of the antrum (the lower portion of the stomach).

Aphasia   Partial or total loss of the ability to articulate ideas or comprehend spoken or written language, resulting from damage to the brain caused by injury or disease.

Ascariasis   A genus of parasitic nematode worms.

Atrophic gastritis   A digestive condition characterized by the chronic inflammation of the mucous lining of the stomach.

Cholecystitis   The inflammation of the gall bladder.

Colitis   Inflammation of the colon.

Diaphoresis   The process of sweating, usually referring to excessive sweating.

Duodenal bulbar ulcer   An ulcer in the duodenum, caused by the action of acid and pepsin on the duodenal lining.

Dyscrasia   An abnormal state of the body or part of the body, especially one due to abnormal development or metabolism.

Dysphonia   Difficulty in voice production.

Dyspnoea   Difficulty breathing.

Dysuria   Difficult or painful urination.

Ecchymosis   A bruise.

Ensiform   Sword-shaped.

Enteritis   Inflammation of the small intestine.

Epigastric   Pertaining to the upper central region of the abdomen.

Erysipelas   A bacterial infection of the skin, especially the face, characterized by redness and swelling.

Formication   A prickling sensation in the skin.

Galea aponeurotica   A flat sheet of fibrous tissue that caps the skull and links the two parts of the muscle of the scalp.

Glandular hyperplasia   The increased production and growth of normal glandular cells in a tissue or organ without an increase in the size of the cells.

Gonitis   Inflammation of the knee joint.

Haemostatics   Agents that stop or prevent bleeding.

Haematemesis   The vomiting of blood.

Haematochezia   The passing of bright red, bloody stools.

Haematuria   The passing of blood in the urine.

Haemoptysis   The coughing up of blood from the trachea, larynx, bronchi or lungs.

Hyperaemia   The presence of excess blood in the vessels supplying a part of the body.

Hyperosteogeny   Excessive bone development.

Hypochondrium   The upper lateral part of the abdomen, beneath the lower ribs.

Hypogeusia   A condition in which the sense of taste is abnormally weak.

Intestinal tuberculosis   An infectious bacterial disease characterized by the formation of nodular legions in the tissues of the intestine.

Leucoderma   Loss of pigment in areas of the skin, resulting in the appearance of white patches.

Lymphatitis   Inflammation of the lymphatic vessels of lymph nodes.

Mastoideum   The bone that covers the mastoid cells in the ear.

Menophania   First sign of the menses at puberty.

Miliaria   Small and itchy rashes that appear when a patient suffers from 'prickly heat' or a sweat rash.

Myasthenia gravis   A chronic disease characterized by abnormal fatigability and weakness of selected muscles.

Myatrophy   Muscular atrophy; a decrease of mass in the muscle.

Myelitis   An inflammatory disease of the spinal cord.

Myodynamia   Muscular strength.

Neuritis   A disease of the peripheral nerves showing the pathological changes of inflammation.

Palpebral   Relating to the eyelid.

Petechiae   Small round flat dark-red spot caused by bleeding into the skin or beneath the mucous membrane.

Pleurisy   Inflammation of the pleura (covering of the lungs and inner surface of the chest wall), often due to pneumonia.

Precordial   Related to the region of the thorax immediately over the heart.

Prolactin   A hormone that stimulates milk production after childbirth and also stimulated progesterone production in the ovary.

Prostatic hypertrophy   Abnormal growth of the prostate.

Ptosis   The drooping of a body part.

Pyelitis   Inflammation of the pelvis of the kidney (the part of the kidney from which urine drains into the ureter).

Rales   The clicking, rattling, or crackling noises that may be made by one or both lungs of a human with a respiratory disease during inhalation.

Tarsus   The seven bones of the ankle and proximal part of the foot.

Tenesmus   Straining, especially ineffective and painful straining, during a bowel movement or urination.

Tetany   A type of cramping which activates all of the nerve endings in the body.

Tinea   A fungus infection of the skin, scalp or nails. Also known as ringworm.

Torticollis   An irresistible turning movement of the neck that becomes persistent, so that eventually the head is held continually to one side.

Trigeminal neuralgia   A severe burning or stabbing pain following the course of the trigeminal nerve in the face.

Tympanitis   Inflammation of the inner ear.

Xiphoid process   The lowermost section of the breastbone.

GLOSSARY OF CHINESE TERMS

Bai Bo Feng   Leucoderma.

Beng Lou   Uterine bleeding.

Bi Yuan   Thick and sticky nasal discharge.

Bu Mei   Insomnia.

Chan syndrome   Tremor syndrome.

Ding Chuang   Furuncle, boil.

Ding Du   Boil.

Fa Sha   Sunstroke.

Feng Zhen   Urticaria (hidden rash), also called Yin Zhen.

Ha Ma Wen   Mumps.

Hou Bi   Sore throat.

Lin Zheng   Urination disturbance.

Long Bi   Urination disturbance.

Lou Ru   Abnormal lactation; milk flowing from the breast when not breast feeding.

Luo Zhen   Torticollis.

Qi Ci needling   Triple puncture.

Qiang Tong Fa   The strong-removing method.

Re Bi   Febrile Bi.

Ru Pi   Nodules in the breast.

Ru Nü   Nipple bleeding.

San Tong Fa   The three-removing method.

Shang Jin   Injury of tendons.

Shang Shu   Sunstroke with dizziness, headache and nausea.

Shu Feng   Sunstroke with convulsions.

Tong Bi   Painful Bi.

Wei Tong Fa   The micro-removing method.

Wen Tong Fa   The warm-removing method.

Xiao Ke   Diabetes.

Xie Qi   Pathogenic Qi.

Xing Bi   Wandering Bi.

Xuan Yun   Dizziness.

Yin Ting   Prolapse of the uterus.

Yin Zhen   Urticaria (hidden rash), also called Feng Zhen.

Yun Jue   Sunstroke with sudden loss of consciousness.

Zha Sai   Mumps.

Zheng Qi   Anti-pathogenic Qi.

Zhuo Bi   Fixed Bi.

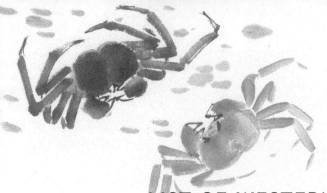

LIST OF WESTERN CONDITIONS

Acne
    Chapter 4, Section six, Case 1,
    2, 3.
Amenorrhoea
    Chapter 2, Section two, Case 1, 2.
Anxiety
    Chapter 1, Section fifteen, Case 4.
Arthritis
    Chapter 1, Section twenty-four,
    Case 1.
    Chapter 1, Section twenty-five,
    Case 1.
    Chapter 1, Section twenty-six,
    Case 1.
    Chapter 1, Section twenty-seven,
    Case 2.
Ascariasis of biliary tract
    Chapter 1, Section seven, Case 2.
Asthma
    Chapter 1, Section three, Case
    1, 2, 3.

Blepharoconjunctivitis
    Chapter 3, Section two, Case 1.
Bronchitis
    Chapter 1, Section two, Case 1,
    2, 3.

Cerebral arteriosclerosis
    Chapter 1, Section seventeen,
    Case 1.
Cerebral infarction
    Chapter 1, Section twenty, Case
    4, 5.
Cervical spondylosis
    Chapter 1, Section twenty-three,
    Case 1, 2, 3.
Chloasma
    Chapter 4, Section seven, Case 1.
Cholecystitis
    Chapter 1, Section five, Case 2.

Chronic fatigue syndrome
    Chapter 5, Section three, Case 1.
Common cold
    Chapter 1, Section one, Case 1,
    2, 3, 4.
Constipation
    Chapter 1, Section nine, Case
    1, 2.
Coronary heart disease
    Chapter 1, Section fourteen,
    Case 3.

Degeneration of lumbar spine
    Chapter 1, Section twenty-one,
    Case 2.
Dentalcaries
    Chapter 3, Section eight, Case 1.
Depression
    Chapter 1, Section thirty-six,
    Case 3.
Diabetes II
    Chapter 1, Section thirteen,
    Case 1.
Diarrhoea
    Chapter 1, Section eight, Case
    1, 2,3.
Duodenal ulcer
    Chapter 1, Section five, Case 1, 3.
Dysfunctional uterine bleeding
    Chapter 2, Section three, Case
    1, 2.
Dysmenorrhoea
    Chapter 2, Section one, Case 1.
Dysuria
    Chapter 1, Section ten, Case 1.

Enuresis
    Chapter 2, Section ten, Case 1,
    2, 3.
Epilepsy
    Chapter 1, Section thirty-four,
    Case 1, 2.

Erysipelas
    Chapter 4, Section one, Case 1.

Facial spasm
    Chapter 1, Section thirty-one,
    Case 1, 2.

Ganglion
    Chapter 4, Section nine, Case 1.
Gastroptosis
    Chapter 1, Section five, Case 4.
Generalized stress ulcer
    Chapter 1, Section forty-one,
    Case 1.
Gonitis
    Chapter 1, Section twenty-five,
    Case 2.

Headache
    Chapter 1, Section sixteen, Case
    1, 2, 3, 4, 5.
Hernia
    Chapter 1, Section thirty-eight,
    Case 1, 2.
Heroin withdrawal syndrome
    Chapter 5, Section four, Case
    2, 3.
    Chapter 1, Section thirty-five,
    Case 2.
Hyperosteogeny of heel
    Chapter 4, Section ten, Case 1.
Hyperplasia of mammary glands
    Chapter 2, Section four, Case 1,
    2, 3.
Hysteria
    Chapter 1, Section thirty-five,
    Case 1, 3.
    Chapter 1, Section thirty-five,
    Case 2.
Hysteric aphasia
    Chapter 1, Section thirty-five,
    Case 2.

Impotence
Chapter 1, Section thirty-seven, Case 1, 2.
Insomnia
Chapter 1, Section fifteen, Case 1, 2, 3.
Intellectual disturbance
Chapter 1, Section thirty-three, Case 1.

Leucoderma
Chapter 4, Section four, Case 1, 2, 3.
Lumbago
Chapter 4, Section twenty-one, Case 3, 4.
Lumbar sprain
Chapter 1, Section twenty-one, Case 1.

Macromastia
Chapter 2, Section seven, Case 1.
Maldevelopment of breasts
Chapter 1, Section twenty-nine, Case 1.
Mammary development problem of males
Chapter 2, Section four, Case 5.
Mammary development problem of young girls
Chapter 2, Section four, Case 4.
Meniere's disease
Chapter 1, Section seventeen, Case 3, 4.
Muscular atrophy
Chapter 1, Section twenty-nine, Case 2.
Myasthenia gravis
Chapter 1, Section thirty, Case 2.
Myopia
Chapter 3, Section four, Case 1, 2.

Nasosinusitis
Chapter 3, Section six, Case 1, 2.
Neck pain
Chapter 1, Section twenty-two, Case 1.
Neurodermatitis
Chapter 4, Section three, Case 1, 2, 3.
Numbness of extremities
Chapter 1, Section twenty-eight, Case 1, 2.

Obesity
Chapter 5, Section two, Case 1.

Oedema
Chapter 1, Section twelve, Case 1, 2.
Old traumatic injury complicated with infection
Chapter 4, Section twelve, Case 1.
Optic atrophy
Chapter 3, Section three, Case 1.
Osteoarthritis
Chapter 1, Section twenty-five, Case 3.

Palpitations
Chapter 1, Section fourteen, Case 1, 2.
Paronychia
Chapter 4, Section two, Case 1, 2.
Parotitis
Chapter 2, Section eleven, Case 1.
Periodontitis
Chapter 3, Section eight, Case 2, 3.
Peripheral facial paralysis
Chapter 1, Section nineteen, Case 1, 2, 3, 4, 5, 6.
Pharyngeal neurosis
Chapter 1, Section thirty-six, Case 1.
Pharyngitis
Chapter 3, Section seven, Case 2.
Pharyngolaryngitis
Chapter 3, Section seven, Case 1.
Phrenospasm
Chapter 1, Section six, Case 1.
Precordial pain
Chapter 1, Section four, Case 1.
Prolapse of rectum
Chapter 1, Section thirty-nine, Case 1, 2.
Prolapse of uterus
Chapter 2, Section eight, Case 1.
Prostatic hypertrophy
Chapter 1, Section eleven, Case 1.
Protrusion of lumbar intervertebral disc
Chapter 1, Section twenty-one, Case 5.
Ptosis
Chapter 1, Section thirty, Case 1.
Pulmonary tuberculosis
Chapter 1, Section two, Case 4.

Retention of urine
Chapter 1, Section ten, Case 2, 3.
Rhinitis
Chapter 3, Section six, Case 3, 4.

Scapulohumeral periarthritis
Chapter 1, Section twenty-four, Case 2.
Chapter 1, Section twenty-seven, Case 1.
Sciatic neuritis
Chapter 1, Section twenty-six, Case 2.
Sciatica
Chapter 1, Section twenty-one, Case 5.
Sequelae of cerebral paralysis
Chapter 1, Section twenty-nine, Case 4.
Sequelae of poliomyelitis
Chapter 1, Section twenty-nine, Case 3.
Smoking withdrawal syndrome
Chapter 5, Section four, Case 1.
Soft tissue injury
Chapter 4, Section eight, Case 1.
Sterility
Chapter 2, Section nine, Case 1.
Stroke
Chapter 1, Section twenty, Case 1, 2, 3, 6.
Sudden deafness
Chapter 3, Section one, Case 1, 2, 3.
Sunstroke
Chapter 5, Section one, Case 1.

Torticollis
Chapter 1, Section twenty-two, Case 2.
Trigeminal neuralgia
Chapter 1, Section eighteen, Case 1, 2, 3.
Tumour in the mammary duct
Chapter 2, Section six, Case 1.

Urticaria
Chapter 4, Section five, Case 1, 2.

Vestibular neuritis
Chapter 1, Section seventeen, Case 2.
Visual tiredness
Chapter 3, Section five, Case 1.

Xerophthalmia
Chapter 3, Section two, Case 2.